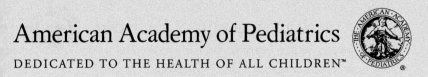

American Academy of Pediatrics
DEDICATED TO THE HEALTH OF ALL CHILDREN™

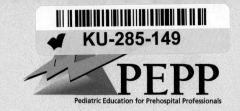

PEPP
Pediatric Education for Prehospital Professionals

Paediatric Education
for Prehospital Professionals

REVISED THIRD EDITION

Editors

Susan Fuchs, MD, FAAP, FACEP
Bruce L. Klein, MD, FAAP

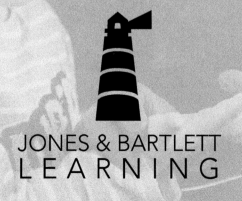

JONES & BARTLETT
LEARNING

American Academy of Pediatrics
DEDICATED TO THE HEALTH OF ALL CHILDREN™

World Headquarters
Jones & Bartlett Learning
5 Wall Street
Burlington, MA 01803
978-443-5000
info@jblearning.com
www.jblearning.com

Melissa Marx, Manager, AAP Life Support Programs
Michael Greenier, MPH, Life Support Simulation and Course Specialist
Karen Kostakis, AAP Life Support Programs Assistant
Wendy Simon, MA, CAE, Senior Director, AAP Global Life Support Initiatives
American Academy of Pediatrics
345 Park Boulevard
Itasca, IL 60143
www.PEPPSite.com
www.aap.org

Production Credits
Cover Image: © Class Publishing/Nigel Wilson

To order this product, use ISBN: 978-1-284-05072-1

6048

Brief Contents

Contents

UK Foreword

The College of Paramedics is delighted to be working with the American Academy of Pediatrics, Public Safety Group, and Class Publishing, who deliver the Paediatric Education for Prehospital Professionals (PEPP) products and texts in the UK and Europe. With the support of Class Publishing, the College has been involved in developing quality educational products for paramedics and other prehospital personnel for many years and has welcomed the opportunity to review the PEPP product to ensure its relevance to the UK market.

The PEPP course has been developed in the USA over the last 25 years through several iterations, is led by the American Academy of Pediatrics (AAP) in partnership with the Jones & Bartlett Learning Public Safety Group. In 2015, the National Association of Emergency Medical Technicians (NAEMT) adopted the PEPP textbook for use in its paediatric courses. There has been significant expert input over this lengthy period of development and refinement, resulting in a high quality course that will substantially enhance the knowledge and skills of current practitioners.

Almost all practitioners who work in the out-of-hospital setting and whose primary role is to respond to a wide range of unscheduled care cases will acknowledge that paediatrics can present extreme challenges. The PEPP course builds on pre-registration skills and knowledge and provides students with systematic assessment and continuity of care processes when managing paediatrics.

The College of Paramedics is delighted to have had the opportunity to review the course to ensure its relevance in the UK setting and to improve the clinical skills and knowledge of practitioners who manage these complex paediatric conditions.

This is a really exciting development for the College of Paramedics and for the paramedic profession in general in the UK and we hope it will lead to a long and successful relationship with AAP and NAEMT. Along with the strong relationship between the College and Class Publishing, I firmly believe that the localised UK PEPP course represents another important step in delivering high quality training here in the UK.

Gerry Egan
Chief Executive
College of Paramedics

Acknowledgments

UK Editors-in-Chief

Lewis Andrews
  Head of Quality Improvement
  East of England Ambulance Service NHS Trust

Tracy Nicholls
  Director of Clinical Quality and Improvement
  East of England Ambulance Service NHS Trust

UK Editor

Will Broughton, BSc (Hons) PGCert MSc FHEA MCPara
  Trustee Official for Professional Practice
  College of Paramedics, UK
  Senior Lecturer, University of Hertfordshire

UK Contributors

David Brown
  Clinical Skills Tutor
  Anglia Ruskin University

Vince Clarke
  Senior Lecturer
  University of Hertfordshire

Dr. Ed England
  Pharmacist
  South Central Ambulance Service NHS Foundation Trust

Tim Hayes
  Deputy Head of the Department of Allied Health
  Anglia Ruskin University

Erica Ley
  Critical Care Paramedic
  East of England Ambulance Service

Steven Moore
  Senior Specialist Operations Manager
  East of England Ambulance Service NHS Trust

Richard Nicholson
  Lecturer in Paramedic Science
  Anglia Ruskin University

Ursula Rolfe
  Senior Lecturer in Emergency Care
  Bournemouth University

Clare Sutton
  Discipline Leader in Paramedicine
  Charles Sturt University

Alan Taylor
  Head of Safeguarding and Prevent
  London Ambulance Service NHS Trust

Aidan Ward
  Senior Lecturer
  University of Northampton

Aimee Yarrington BSc (Hons) MCPara
  Paramedic, West Midlands Ambulance Service NHS
    Foundation Trust
  Midwife, Shrewsbury and Telford NHS Trust

Acknowledgments

The American Academy of Pediatrics wishes to acknowledge the following PEPP Steering Committee members for their contributions as reviewers in the development of this resource.

Stanford Heath Ackley, MD, MPH, FAAP
Representative — AAP General Member
Seattle Children's Hospital
Seattle, WA

Kathleen M. Brown, MD, FAAP, FACEP
Representative — American College of
    Emergency Physicians
The George Washington University School of Medicine
Children's National Medical Center
Washington, DC

Joelle Donofrio, DO, FAAP
Representative — National Association of
    EMS Physicians
UC San Diego School of Medicine
Rady Children's Hospital of San Diego
San Diego, CA

Susan Fuchs, MD, FAAP, FACEP
Co-Editor, *PEPP Revised Third Edition*
Representative — American Heart Association
Feinberg School of Medicine
Northwestern University
Ann and Robert H. Lurie Children's Hospital of Chicago
Chicago, IL

Bruce L. Klein, MD, FAAP
Chair, PEPP Steering Committee
Co-Editor, *PEPP Revised Third Edition*
Representative — AAP Section on Transport Medicine
Johns Hopkins Children's Center
Baltimore, MD

Toni Petrillo, MD, FAAP
Representative — AAP General Member
Emory University School of Medicine
Children's Healthcare of Atlanta
Atlanta, GA

Michael Stoner, MD, FAAP
Representative — AAP General Member
Nationwide Children's Hospital
Columbus, OH

Michael H. Stroud, MD, FAAP
Representative — AAP Section of Transport Medicine
University of Arkansas for Medical Sciences
Arkansas Children's Hospital
Little Rock, AR

PEPP Steering Committee

American Academy of Pediatrics
DEDICATED TO THE HEALTH OF ALL CHILDREN™

Stanford Heath Ackley, MD, MPH, FAAP
Representative – AAP General Member
Seattle Children's Hospital
Seattle, WA

Thomas Breyer, FF/NRP
Representative – International Association of Fire
Fighters
Washington, DC

Kathleen M. Brown, MD, FAAP, FACEP
Representative – American College of
Emergency Physicians
The George Washington University School
of Medicine
Children's National Medical Center
Washington, DC

Ann Dietrich, MD, FAAP
Representative – National Association of Emergency
Medical Technicians
Nationwide Children's Hospital
Columbus, OH

Joelle Donofrio, DO, FAAP
Representative – National Association of
EMS Physicians
UC San Diego School of Medicine
Rady Children's Hospital of San Diego
San Diego, CA

**Joyce Foresman-Capuzzi, MSN, APRN, CCNS, CEN,
CPEN, CTRN, TCRN, CPN, EMT-P, FAEN**
Representative – Emergency Nurses Association
Prospect Park, PA

Susan Fuchs, MD, FAAP, FACEP
Co-Editor, *PEPP Revised Third Edition*
Representative – American Heart Association
Feinberg School of Medicine
Northwestern University
Ann and Robert H. Lurie Children's Hospital of Chicago
Chicago, IL

Brandon Kelley
Representative – National Association of State
EMS Officials
Cheyenne, WY

Bruce L. Klein, MD, FAAP
Chair, PEPP Steering Committee
Co-Editor, *PEPP Revised Third Edition*
Representative – AAP Section on Transport Medicine
Johns Hopkins Children's Center
Baltimore, MD

Corolla Lauck
Representative – National Association of State
EMS Officials
Sioux Falls, SD

Rich Martin
Representative – International Association of
Fire Chiefs
Castle Rock, CO

Toni Petrillo, MD, FAAP
Representative – AAP General Member
Emory University School of Medicine
Children's Healthcare of Atlanta
Atlanta, GA

Michael Stoner, MD, FAAP
Representative – AAP General Member
Nationwide Children's Hospital
Columbus, OH

Michael H. Stroud, MD, FAAP
Representative – AAP Section of Transport Medicine
University of Arkansas for Medical Sciences
Arkansas Children's Hospital
Little Rock, AR

Keith Widmeier, BA, NRP, CCEMT-P, EMSI
Representative – National Association of
EMS Educators
Cincinnati, OH

Acknowledgments

Editors: Susan Fuchs, MD, FAAP, FACEP, and Bruce L. Klein, MD, FAAP

Authors

The American Academy of Pediatrics and Editors acknowledge with appreciation the contributions of the following individuals in the development of this resource.

Andrew Bartkus, RN, MSN, JD, CEN, CCRN, CFRN, NREMT-P, FP-C
Albuquerque, NM

Angela M. Bowen, RN, BSN, CPEN, NREMT-P
East Tennessee Children's Hospital
Knoxville, TN

Kelly Buddenhagen, NREMT-P
ElliJay, GA

Glen W. Clegg
Zephyrhills, FL

Twink Dalton, RN, MS, CNS, NREMT-P
Longmont, CO

Fidel O. Garcia, Paramedic
Grand Junction, CO

Carol Gupton, BS, NREMT-P
Omaha, NE

Bryan Hess, NREMT-P
Gunnison, CO

Gail Larkin, BS, NREMT-P
Long Island City, NY

Jennifer McCarthy, MAS, MICP
Crawford, NJ

Shannon Watson, NREMT-P
St. Louis, MO

Elizabeth M. Wertz Evans, RN, BSN, MPM, FACMPE, CPHQ, CPHIMS, FHIMSS
Cranberry Township, PA

Keith Widmeier, NREMT-P, BA
Somerset, KY

Contributors

The American Academy of Pediatrics and Editors acknowledge with appreciation the contributions of the following individuals in the development of the Procedures.

Bruce L. Klein, MD, FAAP
Johns Hopkins Children's Center
Baltimore, MD

Kristen Nelson McMillan, MD, FAAP
Johns Hopkins University School of Medicine
Baltimore, MD

Karen Schneider, MD, MPH, FAAP
Johns Hopkins University
Baltimore, MD

Physician Reviewers

The American Academy of Pediatrics and Editors acknowledge with appreciation the contributions of the following individuals in the development of this resource.

Terry Adirim, MD, MPH, FAAP
Director, Office of Special Health Affairs
Health Resources and Services Administration

Jeffrey R. Avner, MD, FAAP
Children's Hospital of Montefiore

Carol D. Berkowitz, MD, FAAP, FACEP
Harbor-UCLA Medical Center

Deena Brecher, MSN, RN, APN, ACNS-BC, CEN, CPEN
Representative – Emergency Nurses Association
Cincinnati, OH

Thomas Breyer, FF/NRP
Representative – International Association of Fire Fighters

Kathleen M. Brown, MD, FAAP, FACEP
Representative – American College of
Emergency Physicians

Casey Buitenhuys, MD
Stanford University Hospital and Clinics

Marilyn J. Bull, MD, FAAP
Riley Hospital for Children at IU Health

James M. Callahan, MD, FAAP, FACEP
The Children's Hospital of Philadelphia

William A. Carey, MD, FAAP
Mayo Clinic

Meta L. Carroll, MD, FAAP
Northwestern University Feinberg School of Medicine

Christopher E. Colby, MD, FAAP
Mayo Clinic

Ronald Dieckmann, MD, MPH, FAAP, FACEP
University of California, San Francisco

Timothy Erickson, MD, FACEP, FAACT, FACMT
University of Illinois College of Medicine

George L. Foltin, MD, FAAP, FACEP
NYU School of Medicine

Susan Fuchs, MD, FAAP, FACEP
Co-Editor, *PEPP Revised Third Edition*

Marianne Gausche-Hill, MD, FAAP, FACEP
Harbor-UCLA Medical Center

Phyllis L. Hendry, MD, FAAP, FACEP
University of Florida Health Science Center, Jacksonville

Stephen R. Karl, MD, FAAP, FACS
Avera McKenna Hospital and University Health Center

Brandon Kelley
Representative – National Association of State
EMS Officials

Bruce L. Klein, MD, FAAP
Chair, PEPP Steering Committee
Co-Editor, *PEPP Revised Third Edition*

Katherine Remick, MD, FAAP
Austin/Travis County EMS System

Peter Di Rocco, MD
John A. Burns School of Medicine

Steven M. Selbst, MD, FAAP
Jefferson Medical College

Ghazala Q. Sharieff, MD, FACEP, FAAEM
University of California, San Diego

Stephen G. Simon, MS, EMT-P, EFO
Roanoke County Fire & Rescue

Paul E. Sirbaugh, DO, FAAP
Baylor College of Medicine/TCH

Michael G. Tunik, MD, FAAP
NYU School of Medicine

Keith Widmeier, BA, NRP, CCEMT-P, EMSI
Representative – National Association of
EMS Educators

Cynthia Wright-Johnson, MSN, RNC
Maryland Institute for Emergency Medical
Services Systems

Board Reviewers

The editors would like to acknowledge the work of the American Academy of Pediatrics Board-appointed reviewer.

Carden Johnston, MD, FAAP, FRCP
University of Alabama at Birmingham School
of Medicine

EMS Reviewers

Jason Ambrose, EMT-P, NCEE
Virginia Beach, VA

Gary R. Anderson, AEMT
Layton, UT

Steven K. Frye, BS, NREMT-P
College Park, MD

Kevin M. Gurney, BS, CCEMT-P, I/C
Waterville, ME

Peter D. Johnson, EMSI/NREMT-P
Oxford, CT

Deb Kaye, BS, NREMT
Willmar, MN

Greg LaMay, BS, NREMT-P, NCEE
Tyler, TX

Judith Lynch, AA
Oakville, CT

Shannon McDaniel, EMS-I
Seymour, CT

Charlene Phelps, EMT-I
Starksboro, VT

Katharine P. Rickey, BS, NRParamedic
Barnstead, NH

Superintendent Roland Webb, PCP
Delta, BC, Canada

Susan Siorek, RN, BSN, TNS
Maywood, IL

Pamela N. Taylor, EMT-P, PI
Westfield, IN

Photoshoot Acknowledgments

We would like to thank the following people and institutions for their collaboration on the photoshoots for this project. Their assistance was greatly appreciated.

Erica D'Errico
Schenectady, NY

Glen E. Ellman
Fort Worth Fire Department
Fort Worth, TX

Medical Advisor: Anthony Caliguire, Lieutenant REMT-P
Scotia Fire Department
Scotia, NY

Paul Felts
Ballston Lake, NY

PEPP History

The Pediatric Education for Prehospital Professionals (PEPP) Course is a tapestry of 25 years of collaboration, brainstorming, review, revision, and refinement by hundreds of physicians, nurses, paramedics, EMTs, and EMS educators dedicated to improving prehospital care of children. It is the most widely used and most extensively referenced course in pediatric prehospital care. The PEPP learning system is an honored cornerstone of EMS and pediatric life support education in the United States and worldwide.

The earliest history of the course dates back to 1990, to a period in American EMS when very little evidence-based information was available about safe and effective practices in prehospital care of infants and children. The original course was officially born in Dr. Ron Dieckmann's back office at San Francisco General Hospital, as a project of the California Pediatric Emergency and Critical Care Coalition, to address widening alarm over dangers and deficiencies in prehospital care of children being documented in medical journals and the lay media. The California EMS Authority funded the initial project through a federal block grant to a new committee formed by the Coalition named the California "PEP (Pediatric Education for Paramedics) Task Force."

After two years of fact-finding, deliberation and collaboration with representatives from the AAP, American College of Emergency Physicians (ACEP) and National Association of EMS Physicians (NAEMSP), the original California PEP Task Force published *Pediatric Education Guidelines for Paramedics* in 1993. The manuscript outlined desired educational goals, learning objectives, and components for a pediatric-specific curriculum for paramedics. The *Guidelines* were formally approved for all California paramedic training programs by the California EMS Commission and concurrently adopted and published by ACEP as the first national consensus document on prehospital pediatric care.

That same year, ACEP established a national committee on pediatric prehospital care, which became the "National PEP Task Force." Chaired by Dr. Dieckmann, the committee translated the California *Guidelines* into a practical "curriculum" for primary paramedic education in pediatrics. Then, in 1996, the Task Force released the first complete "PEP Course" with coordinated state-of-the art learning materials customized for prehospital providers. The course reflected the inspirational work of multiple state EMSC projects—especially the Washington Pediatric Prehospital Care Project, headed by Dena Brownstein in Seattle, and the California Pediatric Airway Project, directed by Dr. Marianne Gausche-Hill in Los Angeles. The new course was an interactive, highly visual, assessment-based "learning system" that included multiple linked components: a student manual, instructor manual, PowerPoint slide set, and an instructional video. Moreover, the learning system was developed and archived electronically and disseminated on a CD to allow rapid and inexpensive national distribution to site instructors, as well as easy modification with anticipated ongoing enhancements in prehospital clinical care.

1998 was a watershed moment in the course's history. That year, the AAP, the country's largest professional pediatric organization, identified prehospital care of children as a critical element of community pediatric services, and invested its vast clinical expertise and administrative and educational resources in the systematic dissemination of the course nationally and internationally. The AAP assumed financial and administrative ownership of the broadening PEP initiative, under the dedicated and visionary leadership of Linda Lipinsky, AAP Director of Life Support Programs. To oversee ongoing course development, improvements in teaching materials, and establishment of a sustainable national training network and fiscal infrastructure, the AAP appointed a permanent oversight group, the "National PEPP Steering Committee," with representatives from all organizations countrywide involved in pediatric prehospital care. The original committee included Bob Bailey, Pam Baker, Dr. Dena Brownstein, Dr. David Burchfield, Dr. Art Cooper, Dr. Susan Fuchs, Dr. Marianne Gausche-Hill, Tricia Kunz-Howard, Dr. Deborah Mulligan-Smith, Michael Pante, Gary Rainey, Steve Strawderman, Dr. Robert Wiebe, and Dr. George Woodward. Dr. Dieckmann served as first PEPP chairperson.

In the transition of the course to the AAP, a significant modification occurred in the scope and overall vision of the initiative: the earlier moniker "PEP" was changed to "PEPP" or "Pediatric Education for Prehospital Professionals." Every letter and word in the course's new name reflected strongly-held tenets of the Steering Committee: "Pediatric" to embody the full emphasis of the course on care of children; "Education" to reflect the goal for a broader cognitive and affective context for learning beyond conventional training; "Prehospital" to convey a special focus on the unique aspects of care delivery in the out-of-hospital environment; "Professionals" to promote commitment of both BLS *and* ALS personnel to effective pediatric care delivery.

At the beginning of the national rollout, the AAP entered into a key business partnership with Jones & Bartlett Learning, who had long experience in the arena of EMS educational publications. A major proponent in the production and dissemination of PEPP as a state-of-the art learning system was Jones & Bartlett's executive publisher, Kimberly Brophy, who became an invaluable ex-officio member of the PEPP Committee and vigorous advocate in the PEPP national effort.

A significant development in the early proceedings of the committee was the adoption of the Pediatric Assessment Triangle (PAT) as the centerpiece of the PEPP learning system. This paradigm was created by Drs. Dieckmann, Brownstein, and Gausche-Hill to introduce an integrative, visual, easily-remembered approach to assessment of infants and children.* Soon after introduction of the course, the PAT became the PEPP "brand" and the ongoing course logo. Then, in 2005, following the enthusiastic adoption of the PAT by PEPP learners, the PAT was established as the approved assessment model for all American pediatric life support courses in a national consensus meeting sponsored by the Federal EMSC Program. Since then, the PAT has become the recommended approach to assessment of children not only in PEPP, but also in APLS: The Pediatric Emergency Medicine Resource, the Emergency Nurse Pediatric Course (ENPC) for nurses, and in all pediatric

life support programs countrywide. Studies in Los Angeles and elsewhere have confirmed that the PAT is a valuable tool when applied by nurses at triage and when used accurately by paramedics to drive prehospital pediatric care.

The inaugural fully-packaged PEPP course enjoyed meteoric success. The first edition of the 2000 "PEPP Manual" sold 91,233 copies—an astounding volume for a medical reference in any field. A year later, PEPP received its first major national accolade: the "EMSC National Heroes Award" from the Emergency Medical Services for Children Program, Maternal and Child Health Bureau, and National Highway Traffic Safety Administration, to recognize outstanding achievements in improving care of infants and children.

After the release of the first edition, the National PEPP Steering Committee pushed to extend its reach further into the prehospital provider communities. The second edition of the highly popular PEPP student manual was published in 2006 by Jones and Bartlett and sold 100,795 copies! The concepts and teaching methods outlined in the second edition were further embellished by the addition of the first online, interactive PEPP refresher course. This electronic program represented a further evolution of the learning system to accommodate providers who had previously completed the primary PEPP course and needed continuing refresher education. The online course offered a new option—learners could study pediatric concepts and perform self-assessment remotely, any time, at their convenience, with only a computer and web access.

After the release of the second edition, Dr. Brownstein who had helped usher the course through its first 15 years of history became the national chairperson. Thereafter, Dr. Susan Fuchs, a national leader in EMSC and original PEPP Committee member assumed the co-chairpersonship of the committee along with Michael Pante, a New Jersey paramedic, representative from the National Association of EMS Educators and also original PEPP Steering Committee member.

In 2008, a final piece of the original vision of the Steering Committee for an inclusive educational product for all prehospital provider levels was implemented when the AAP published the first PEPP student manual specifically for BLS providers. Since the course's introduction, the AAP has awarded 57,742 PEPP certificates of completion to BLS students.

In 2013, the AAP announced a partnership with the National Association of Emergency Medical Technicians (NAEMT). The AAP and NAEMTs agreement recognizes the value of collaborating with all providers in the continuum of pediatric emergency care.

The third edition of the student manual was released in 2014, amid a widening scope of influence of the course in multiple other countries in the Western world, who have adopted PEPP as the international standard of pediatric prehospital education. Following the release of the third edition manual, NAEMT adopted the third edition of the PEPP textbook for use within their Emergency Pediatric Care (EPC) course.

Historical summary prepared by Ron Dieckmann, MD, MPH University of California, San Francisco

*Dieckmann RA, Brownstein D, Gausche-Hill M. The Pediatric Assessment Triangle: A Novel Approach to Pediatric Assessment. *Pediatric Emergency Care*, Vol 26, No 4, 2010: 312–315.

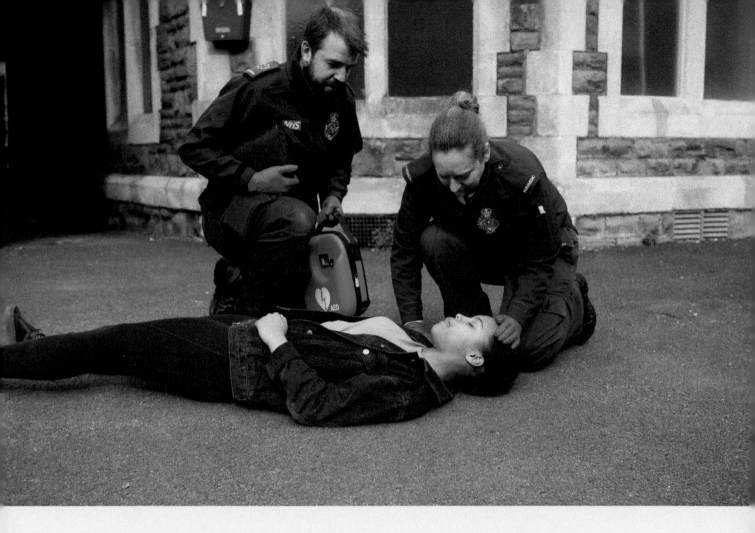

Learning Objectives

1. Discuss the special challenges for the prehospital professional in paediatric assessment.

2. Recognise the key features of prearrival preparation and the scene assessment.

3. Differentiate the three elements of the Paediatric Assessment Triangle (PAT) in the primary (initial) assessment.

4. Describe the important paediatric considerations for each step in the hands-on <C>ABCDE sequence of the primary assessment.

5. Recognise clinical situations requiring pain assessment and management.

6. Discuss guidelines for when to stay on scene and treat, and when to immediately transport an ill or injured child, including appropriate mode of transport.

7. Outline the unique considerations in the additional assessment of a child, including history taking, secondary assessment, monitoring devices, and reassessment.

Paediatric Assessment

Introduction

Caring for a critically ill or injured infant or child can be one of the most stressful duties of the prehospital professional. Key history may be unreliable or unknown because the patient may be too young to have descriptive language, or the child may be afraid and unable to accurately recount the key events. The caregiver may be sobbing, frightened, and anxious for reassurance. Examination may be difficult because of the child's small size and resistance to hands-on evaluation, but this should not be a barrier to effective care. Observations and vital signs require careful attention due to normal age-based variations, and therefore they must be accurately obtained. It is the job of the prehospital professional to bring comfort to the child, caregiver, or family, and to bring calm to an incident. The prehospital professional must conduct an accurate assessment and deliver effective emergency treatment to the child.

The *Paediatric Education for Prehospital Professionals* (PEPP) course, developed by the American Academy of Paediatrics (AAP), started out as an American course that provides the core cognitive knowledge and skills to prepare prehospital professionals for comprehensive assessment and management of critically ill and injured infants and children. It has now been rewritten in a UK context.

Effective emergency care of children involves many professionals inside and outside of the hospital setting. Two of the most important concepts for comprehensive and high-quality out-of-hospital paediatric emergency care are teamwork and prevention. Teamwork involves professionals working together to develop and implement comprehensive clinical services, professional education, and appropriate administrative oversight specifically for children. Prevention involves professionals recognising the limitations of an emergency care system oriented toward treatment after an illness or injury occurs, and working to change potentially dangerous conditions before an event of this type occurs. Of all community activities that can improve children's overall health and well-being, prevention of acute injury and illness is by far the most cost-effective. "Making a difference", involves new roles for prehospital professionals in injury and illness prevention, in their professional day-to-day duties, and as part of their activities as community leaders and health advocates.

Accurate assessment of a child with a serious illness or injury requires special knowledge and skills. For patients of all ages, the prehospital professional's evaluation includes five steps:

1. Scene assessment
2. Primary (initial) assessment <C>ABCDE using the Paediatric Assessment Triangle (PAT)
3. History taking
4. Secondary assessment including physical examination and monitoring devices
5. Reassessment

Case Study 1

A 7-year-old boy, not wearing a helmet, rode his bicycle out of his driveway into the path of an oncoming car. According to witnesses, the car was travelling at about 30 mph (50 kph), the victim was struck and thrown approximately 4.5 m, and he was unconscious for 1–2 minutes. On your arrival, he is crying and anxious but responds appropriately to questions. He is complaining that his stomach hurts. He has no abnormal airway sounds, grunting, flaring, or retracting. His skin is pale. The respiratory rate is 30 breaths/min, there are equal breath sounds with good air exchange, and the pulse oximetry reading is 98% on room air. His heart rate is 150 beats/min, and his blood pressure is 80/40 mm Hg. The radial pulse is absent, and the femoral pulse is weak. Capillary refill time is 4 seconds.

1. How badly injured is this child, and which physiological process requires your immediate attention?

2. Should this child's pain be treated?

The primary and secondary assessments have well-defined components that follow the same sequence used for adult patients. However, all five steps in assessment have important paediatric modifications. In the emergency department (ED), doctors and nurses may continue the assessment with an additional step, diagnostic testing, often with the benefit of ancillary tests.

Summary of Assessment Flowchart

This chapter introduces a flowchart that reflects the sequence of paediatric assessment taught by the PEPP course. The flowchart reinforces the interconnecting relationships of the different assessment components. Sometimes the assessment sequence must be stopped after the primary assessment to allow the prehospital professional to treat potentially life-threatening problems and initiate transport. For example, when a child has a critical injury, the secondary assessment must be deferred until after the child has been resuscitated and stabilised. Reassessment, however, is required in every case to monitor response to treatment, guide further interventions, and assist with transport and triage decisions. While monitoring devices such as a pulse oximeter or a blood glucose meter do provide diagnostic testing, if further diagnostic testing is required then hospital-based evaluation may include laboratory tests and radiologic procedures.

Scene Assessment

On the way to the scene, prepare mentally to approach and treat an infant or child, and to interact with a distressed family. This means planning for a paediatric scene assessment, paediatric equipment and medication requirements, and age-appropriate assessment. All paediatric equipment and medications should be routinely checked, because they are rarely used by most prehospital professionals and it is easy to become unfamiliar with their application. The information from dispatch on age and gender of the child, location of the scene, and chief complaint or mechanism of injury (or both) is the basis for pre-arrival preparation.

At the scene, begin the assessment by looking for possible safety threats to the child, caregiver, bystanders, or prehospital professionals. Examples of safety threats include spilled toxins, open containers of alcohol, drug paraphernalia, weapons, or fire. The child actually may be a safety threat if he or she has an infectious disease, such as chickenpox or meningitis.

Evaluating the setting includes an inspection of the physical environment and watching family-child or caregiver-child interactions (**Figure 1-1**). For example, documenting observations of dangerous scene conditions and inappropriate

Scene Assessment
↓
Primary Assessment
Using the PAT
Hands-on <C>ABCDE
Transport Decision: Stay or Go
↓
History Taking
↓
Secondary Assessment
Physical Examination
Monitoring Devices
↓
Reassessment

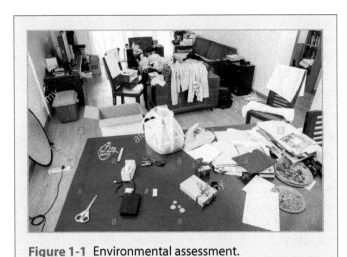

Figure 1-1 Environmental assessment.
© Jones & Bartlett Learning

statements from caregivers greatly assists child protective services if the child is later determined to be a victim of inflicted injury. On the scene, be like a sponge; soak up as much useful information as possible to ensure scene safety. These two aspects all make up your global overview of the scene.

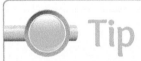

On the way to the scene, mentally rehearse your approach to the assessment and treatment of an infant or child, and the expected interaction with a caregiver or family. Dispatch information, when available, about the child's age can be helpful to mentally prepare for age-appropriate developmental considerations and for anticipating equipment and medication requirements for assessment and treatment.

Primary Assessment: The Paediatric Assessment Triangle

After the scene assessment and global overview, begin a primary assessment of the child. The primary assessment must have a developmentally appropriate approach. This assessment includes a visual and auditory "general impression" of the child, and uses the PAT as a standardised method to gather this information.

Rapid assessment is essential to determine level of acuity and urgency for treatment and transport. Ask yourself, "is the patient sick or not sick?" In the case of a child who is a victim of trauma with a known mechanism of injury, or of a child with a clear-cut complaint of pain in a specific anatomical location, the assessment may be straightforward.

Still, careful evaluation is needed to identify less obvious, but potentially serious injuries or physiological instability. For a child with an illness, the assessment may be much trickier. The prehospital professional must elicit information on the onset, duration, severity, and progression of symptoms, often from a child who cannot accurately provide such history. Moreover, illness complaints may be vague and less specific to an anatomical region. Whether the child has an injury or an illness, the PAT helps to identify physiological instability, direct resuscitation priorities, and determine the timing of transport.

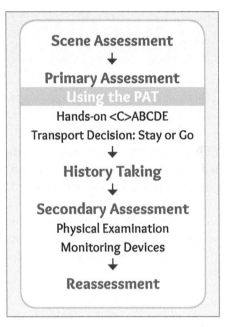

Scene Assessment
↓
Primary Assessment
Using the PAT
Hands-on <C>ABCDE
Transport Decision: Stay or Go
↓
History Taking
↓
Secondary Assessment
Physical Examination
Monitoring Devices
↓
Reassessment

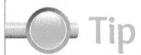

Use the PAT at the point of initial contact with every child, regardless of age or presenting complaint.

Developing a General Impression: The PAT

The PAT is an easy tool to use during the rapid, primary assessment of any child (**Figure 1-2**). It allows the prehospital professional to develop a first general impression of the patient's status with only visual and auditory clues. By using the PAT at the point of first contact with the patient, the prehospital professional can immediately establish a level of severity, determine urgency for life support, and identify the general type of physiological problem. Continued use of the PAT gives the prehospital professional a way to track response to therapy and determine timing of transport. It also allows for communication among medical professionals about the child's physiological status.

There are three components of the PAT that together reflect the child's overall physiological status: (1) appearance,

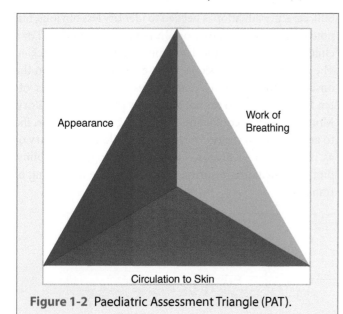

Figure 1-2 Paediatric Assessment Triangle (PAT).

(2) work of breathing, and (3) circulation to the skin. The PAT is based on listening and seeing, and does not require a stethoscope, blood pressure cuff, cardiac monitor, or pulse oximeter. The PAT does not require numbers. The PAT should be completed in less than 30 seconds and is designed to organise a time-honoured process of "across the room assessment", an intuitive process that experienced clinicians do instinctively.

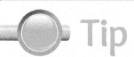

The elements of the PAT incorporate auditory and visual clues that should be obtained from "across the room", without appearing threatening to an already anxious child.

The PAT

Together, the physical characteristics of the PAT provide an accurate initial picture of the child's underlying cardiopulmonary status and level of consciousness. Although the PAT does not necessarily lead to a diagnosis, it identifies the general category of the physiological problem and establishes urgency for treatment or transport. The PAT does not replace traditional observations and the <C>ABCDE assessment, which are part of the primary assessment in the next phase of the physical evaluation.

The patient characteristics emphasised by the three arms of the PAT did not originate with PEPP. Experienced health care professionals have always intuitively used these characteristics to obtain a rapid first "general impression" of ill or injured children. What is unique about the PAT is its systematic approach to making, integrating, and communicating

these observations. The PAT is the cornerstone of the PEPP course. Use the PAT in every encounter with every child. Over time, it will become an indispensable and spontaneous method for making a rapid initial "sick or not sick" assessment of ill or injured children of all ages.

Appearance

Characteristics of Appearance. The child's general appearance is the most important factor in determining the severity of the illness or injury, the need for treatment, and the response to therapy. Appearance reflects the adequacy of ventilation, oxygenation, brain **perfusion**, body **homeostasis**, and **central nervous system (CNS)** function. There are many characteristics of appearance; the most important are summarised in the "tickles" (TICLS) mnemonic: tone, interactiveness, consolability, look/gaze, and speech/cry (**Table 1-1**).

Identifying abnormal appearance is a better way to detect subtle abnormalities in behaviour than the conventional **"alert, verbal, pain, unresponsive" (AVPU) scale** or the Paediatric Glasgow Coma Scale (GCS) for neurological evaluation. Most children with mild to moderate illness or injury are "alert" on the AVPU or "15" on the Paediatric GCS, although some may have an abnormal appearance and a potentially serious underlying problem. Therefore, assessing a child's appearance is the most useful first thing to do in evaluating every paediatric patient.

Table 1-1 Characteristics of Appearance: The "Tickles" (TICLS) Mnemonic

Characteristic features to look for
• Tone Is she moving or vigorously resisting examination? Does she have good muscle tone? Or is she limp, listless, or flaccid?
• Interactiveness How alert is she? How readily does a person, object, or sound distract her or draw her attention? Will she reach for, grasp, and play with a toy or examination instrument, such as a penlight? Or is she uninterested in playing or interacting with the caregiver?
• Consolability Can she be consoled or comforted by the caregiver? Or is her crying or agitation unrelieved by gentle reassurance?
• Look/Gaze Does she fix her gaze on a face? Or is there a vacant, glassy-eyed stare?
• Speech/Cry Is her speech or cry strong and spontaneous? Or is it weak, muffled, or hoarse?

Adapted from Dieckmann RA, Brownstein D, Gausche-Hill M. The Pediatric Assessment Triangle: A novel approach to pediatric assessment. *Pediatr. Emerg Care.* 2010:26;312–315.

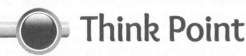

Think Point

In assessing patients with mild to moderate illness or injury, numerical "scoring" methodologies and severity scales for levels of consciousness are rarely useful. These classical neurological evaluation systems work best in patients with severe injury or illness and serious brain dysfunction.

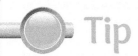

Tip

Never ignore the pale infant, the "vacant stare", or the infant who does not respond appropriately to stimulation.

Techniques to Assess Appearance. Assess the child's appearance from the doorway. This is Step 1 in the PAT. Techniques for assessment of a conscious child's appearance include observing from a distance; allowing the child to remain in the caregiver's lap or arms; using distraction tools, such as bright lights or toys, to measure the child's ability to interact; and kneeling down to be at eye level with the child. An immediate "hands-on" approach may cause agitation and crying, and may complicate the assessment. Unless a child is unconscious or obviously critically ill, get as much information as possible by observing the child before touching the child or taking observations.

One example of a child with a normal appearance is an infant who holds himself or herself upright in the caregiver's arms, makes good eye contact, and has good colour (**Figure 1-3**). An example of an infant with a worrisome appearance is a

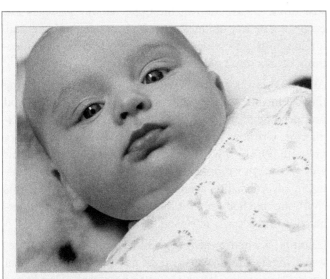

Figure 1-3 A child making good eye contact is normal and a sign of a good appearance.
© Photos.com

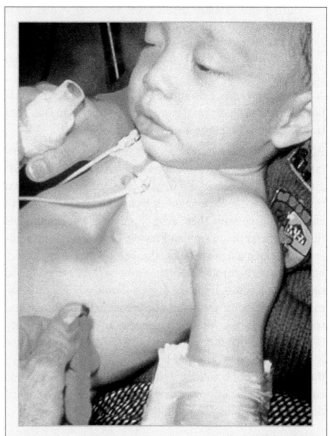

Figure 1-4 A limp, pale child unable to make eye contact or a child with retractions may be critically ill or injured.
Courtesy of the Health Resources and Services Administration (HRSA), Maternal and Child Health Bureau (MCHB), Emergency Medical Services for Children (EMSC Program.

toddler who makes poor eye contact with the caregiver or prehospital professional and is pale and listless (**Figure 1-4**).

An abnormal appearance may have many causes: inadequate oxygenation, ventilation, or brain perfusion; systemic abnormalities, such as poisoning, infection, or hypoglycaemia; or acute or chronic brain injury. Regardless of the cause, a child with a grossly abnormal appearance is seriously ill or injured and needs immediate life support efforts to increase oxygenation, ventilation, and perfusion.

Although an alert, interactive child is usually not critically ill, there are some cases where a child may have life-threatening problems despite an initially normal appearance. Toxicological or traumatic emergencies are good examples:

1. A child with paracetamol, iron, or a tricyclic antidepressant overdose may not show symptoms immediately after ingestion. Despite the child's normal appearance, he or she may develop deadly complications in the coming minutes or hours.

2. A child with blunt trauma and solid organ injury may be able to maintain adequate core perfusion, despite internal bleeding, by increasing cardiac output and systemic vascular resistance; therefore, he or she may appear normal

during the primary assessment. However, when these compensatory mechanisms fail, the child may acutely "crash", with rapid progression to decompensated shock. Pallor may be the only finding on the PAT that suggests impending disaster.

A benign appearance should never justify a denial of transport. However, a normal appearance usually means that transport with "lights and siren" is not necessary.

Age differences are associated with important developmental differences in psychomotor and social skills. "Normal" appearance and behaviour vary by age group, as discussed in the *Using a Developmental Approach* chapter. Children of all ages engage with their environment: newborns do this through energetic sucking and crying; older infants, by smiling or tracking a light; toddlers through physical exploration; and adolescents through speech. Knowledge of normal child development through the age groups should guide the assessment of appearance and result in more accurate treatment and transport decisions. Although appearance reflects the severity of illness or injury, it does not identify the cause. Appearance is the "screening" portion of the PAT. The other elements of the PAT (work of breathing and circulation to the skin) provide more specific information about the type of physiological derangement, while giving additional clues about severity.

Work of Breathing

Characteristics of Work of Breathing. In children, work of breathing is a more accurate indicator of oxygenation and ventilation than respiratory rate or breath sounds on auscultation, the standard measures of breathing effectiveness in adults. Work of breathing reflects the child's attempt to compensate for abnormalities in oxygenation and ventilation, and it is an indication of the effectiveness of gas exchange. This component of the PAT requires listening carefully for abnormal airway sounds and looking for signs of increased breathing effort. It is another "hands-off" evaluation method that does not require a stethoscope or pulse oximeter. **Table 1-2** summarises the key characteristics of work of breathing.

Table 1-2 Characteristics of Work of Breathing

Characteristic	Features to Look for
Abnormal airway sounds	Snoring, muffled or hoarse speech, stridor, grunting, wheezing
Abnormal positioning	Sniffing position, tripoding, refusing to lie down
Retractions	Supraclavicular, intercostal, or substernal retractions of the chest wall; head bobbing in infants
Flaring	Flaring of the nares on inspiration

Abnormal Airway Sounds. Examples of abnormal airway sounds that can be heard without a stethoscope are snoring, muffled or hoarse speech, stridor, grunting, and wheezing. Abnormal airway sounds provide information about the physiology and anatomical location of the breathing problem.

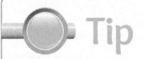

Tip

The child's general appearance is the single most important feature when assessing severity of illness or injury, need for treatment, and response to therapy.

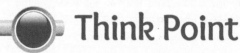

Think Point

Although an alert, interactive child is usually not critically ill, there are some exceptions to the reliability of general appearance as an indicator of stable cardiopulmonary and neurological function. The most common exceptions are ingestions with delayed physiological effects and blunt injury with slow internal bleeding.

Snoring, muffled or hoarse speech, and stridor suggest an upper airway obstruction. Snoring or gurgling occurs when the oropharynx is partially obstructed by the tongue and soft tissues. Muffled or hoarse speech reflects inflammation of the glottis or supraglottic structures. Stridor is a high-pitched sound heard on inspiration, or during inspiration and expiration, reflecting an obstruction at the level of the glottis or subglottic trachea. All of these sounds reflect abnormal airflow through partially obstructed upper airway structures. Obstruction of the upper airway passages can occur in a variety of illnesses and injuries, including croup, foreign body aspiration, and bacterial upper airway infections, or as a result of bleeding or oedema.

Abnormal lower airway sounds that may be heard during the PAT include grunting and wheezing. Grunting is a sound produced by partial closure of the glottis on the end of expiration. Grunting is a form of auto positive end-expiratory pressure (PEEP), a way to distend lower respiratory tract air sacs (alveoli) to promote maximum gas exchange. Grunting involves exhaling against a partially closed glottis. This short, low-pitched sound is best heard at the end of the exhalation and is easily mistaken for whimpering.

Grunting is often present in children with moderate to severe hypoxia, and it reflects poor gas exchange because of obstruction in the lower airways and alveoli. Conditions that cause hypoxia and grunting are pneumonia, pulmonary contusion (bruising of the lungs), pulmonary oedema (fluid in air sacs).

Wheezing is the result of movement of air across partially blocked small airways. At first, wheezing usually occurs during exhalation and can be heard only by auscultation of the chest with a stethoscope. As the airway obstruction increases and breathing requires more work, wheezing is often present during inhalation and exhalation. With more obstruction, wheezing may be audible without a stethoscope. Finally, if respiratory failure develops, work of breathing may diminish and the wheezing may not be heard at all. The most common cause of wheezing in childhood is asthma, although wheezing may also be associated with bronchiolitis (a viral respiratory infection in infants) and lower airway foreign body aspiration.

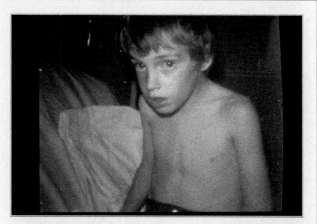

Figure 1-5 The sniffing position opens up the airways to improve patency.

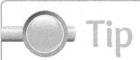 **Tip**

Abnormal airway sounds can provide excellent information about breathing effort, type of breathing problem, location of the breathing problem, and potential degree of hypoxia.

Visual Signs of Increased Work of Breathing. There are several useful visual signs of increased work of breathing. These signs reflect an increased breathing effort by the child to improve oxygenation and ventilation. The presence of certain physical features, such as abnormal positioning, retractions, and nasal flaring, reflect overall illness or injury severity. Abnormal positioning is usually evident from the doorway. There are several types of abnormal postures that can indicate the child is struggling to improve airflow. A child who is in the sniffing position is trying to align the axes of the airways to improve patency and increase airflow (**Figure 1-5**). This position is usually the result of severe upper airway obstruction. The child who refuses to lie down, or who leans forward on outstretched arms (tripoding), is creating optimal mechanical positioning to use accessory muscles of respiration (**Figure 1-6**). The sniffing position and tripoding are abnormal and indicate airway obstruction, increased work of breathing, and severe respiratory distress.

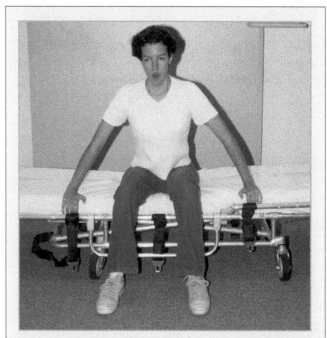

Figure 1-6 The abnormal tripod position indicates the patient's attempts to maximise accessory muscle use.
© Jones & Bartlett Learning

Retractions are physical signs of increased work of breathing. Retractions represent the recruitment of accessory muscles of respiration to provide more "muscle power" to move air into the lungs in the face of airway or lung disease or injury. To optimally observe retractions, expose the child's chest. Retractions are a more useful measure of work of breathing in children than in adults because a child's chest wall is less muscular, and the inward excursion of skin and soft-tissue between the ribs is more apparent. Retractions may be in the supraclavicular area (above the clavicle), the intercostal area (between the ribs), or the substernal area

(under the sternum), as illustrated in **Figure 1-7**. Another form of accessory muscle use seen only in infants is "head bobbing", which is the use of neck muscles to assist breathing during times of severe hypoxia. The infant extends the neck as he or she inhales, and then allows the head to fall forward as he or she exhales.

Nasal flaring is another sign of accessory muscle use that reflects significant increased work of breathing (**Figure 1-8**). Nasal flaring is the exaggerated opening of the nostrils during laboured inspiration and indicates moderate to severe hypoxia. It reflects the child's extra effort to breathe during hypoxic stress, usually caused by such conditions as croup, pneumonia, asthma, bronchiolitis, or pulmonary contusion.

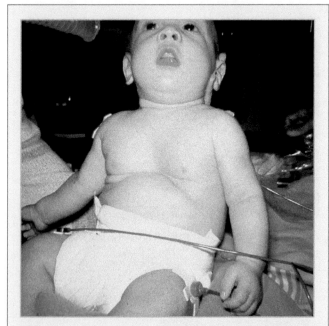

Figure 1-7 Retractions indicate increased work of breathing and may occur in the supraclavicular, intercostal, and substernal areas.

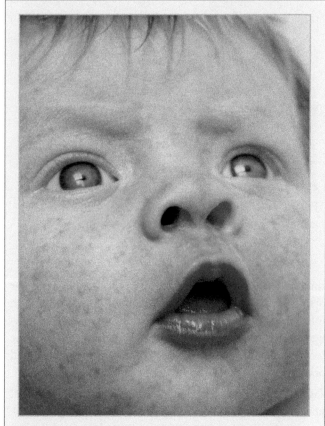

Figure 1-8 Nasal flaring indicates increased work of breathing and moderate to severe hypoxia.
© Hemera/Thinkstock

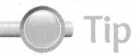

Tip

Head bobbing is a form of accessory muscle use specific to infants and is indicative of increased work of breathing.

Techniques to Assess Work of Breathing. Step 2 in the PAT is assessing work of breathing. Begin by listening carefully from a distance for abnormal airway sounds. Next, look for key physical signs. Note if the child has an abnormal posture, most notably the sniffing position or tripoding. Next, have the caregiver uncover the chest of the child for direct inspection, or have the child undress on the caregiver's lap. Look for intercostal, supraclavicular, and substernal retractions, and note if there is head bobbing in infants. After examining for retractions, inspect for nasal flaring. This stepwise process is critical for gathering accurate information. After an infant or child begins to cry, assessment of work of breathing becomes more difficult.

Children may have increased work of breathing because of abnormalities anywhere in their upper or lower airways, alveoli (air sacs), **pleura** (membrane surrounding the lungs and lining the walls of the pleural cavity), or chest wall. The type of abnormal airway sounds gives an important clue to the anatomical location of the illness or injury process, whereas the number and type of physical signs of increased work of breathing helps in determining the degree of physiological stress.

Combining assessment of appearance and work of breathing can also help establish the severity of the child's illness or injury. A child with a normal appearance and increased work of breathing is in respiratory distress. An abnormal appearance and increased work of breathing suggests respiratory failure. An abnormal appearance and abnormally decreased work of breathing implies impending respiratory arrest.

Circulation to Skin

Characteristics of Circulation to Skin. The goal of rapid circulatory assessment is to determine the adequacy of cardiac output and core perfusion, or perfusion of the vital organs. The child's appearance is one indicator of brain perfusion, but abnormal appearance may be caused by other conditions unrelated to circulation, such as hypoxia, hypoglycaemia, brain injury, or intoxication. For this reason, other signs of adequacy of perfusion must be added to the evaluation of appearance to assess the child's true circulatory status.

An important sign of core perfusion is circulation to the skin. When cardiac output is inadequate, the body shuts down circulation to non-essential anatomical areas, such as

Table 1-3 Characteristics of Circulation to Skin

Characteristic	Features to Look for
Pallor	White or pale or mucous membrane colouration from inadequate blood flow
Mottling	Patchy skin discolouration caused by vasoconstriction or vasodilation
Cyanosis	Bluish discolouration of skin and mucous membranes

the skin and mucous membranes, to preserve blood supply to the most vital organs (brain, heart, and kidneys). Therefore, circulation to the skin reflects the overall status of core circulation. Pallor, mottling, and cyanosis are key visual indicators of reduced circulation to the skin and mucous membranes. **Table 1-3** summarises these characteristics.

Pallor may be the first sign of poor skin or mucous membrane perfusion. Pallor may be the only visual sign apparent in a child with compensated shock, and indicates reflex peripheral vasoconstriction to shunt blood away from the skin to the core. Pallor may also be a sign of anaemia or hypoxia. Mottling is another sign of inadequate skin perfusion, reflecting vasomotor instability (abnormal blood vessel tone) in the capillary beds of the skin. Mottled skin has patchy areas of vasoconstriction (pallor) mixed with areas of vasodilation (cyanosis or erythema). Mottling may also be a normal physiological response in a child exposed to cold environmental temperatures.

Cyanosis is blue discolouration of the skin and mucous membranes. It is the most extreme visual indicator of poor perfusion or poor oxygenation. Do not confuse acrocyanosis (blue hands and feet in a newborn or infant less than 2 months of age) with true cyanosis. Acrocyanosis is a normal finding when a young infant is cold, and it reflects vasomotor instability rather than hypoxia or shock. True cyanosis is a late finding of respiratory failure or shock. A hypoxic child is likely to show other physical abnormalities long before turning blue. These abnormalities may include abnormal appearance with agitation or lethargy, and increased work of breathing. A child in shock may also have pallor or mottling. Never wait for cyanosis to begin treatment with supplemental oxygen. However, the presence of cyanosis is always a critical sign that requires immediate intervention with breathing support.

Abnormal circulation to the skin, in combination with an abnormal appearance, suggests shock. However, the abnormalities in appearance in early phases of compensated shock may be subtle, and some children may remain alert. As perfusion worsens and compensatory mechanisms fail, appearance becomes abnormal, reflecting inadequate delivery

of oxygen and glucose to the brain. Another clue to the presence of shock is effortless tachypnoea, or tachypnoea without signs of increased work of breathing. Effortless tachypnoea is a reflex mechanism that allows the body to blow off carbon dioxide to compensate for the metabolic acidosis caused by poor peripheral perfusion (lactic acidosis). Hypocarbia (low blood CO_2 levels) generates a respiratory alkalosis and helps to restore normal pH (blood acid-base balance). Effortless tachypnoea is different from the rapid and laboured respirations that are present with illnesses and injuries associated with airway or lung pathology.

Techniques to Assess Circulation to Skin. Step 3 in the PAT is evaluating circulation to the skin. Be sure the child is exposed long enough for visual inspection, but not long enough to become cold. A cold child may have normal core perfusion, but abnormal circulation to the skin. Cold circulating air temperature is the most common reason for misinterpretation of skin signs, and an exposed young infant may become hypothermic quickly, even at normal ambient temperatures.

Inspect the skin and mucous membranes for pallor, mottling, and cyanosis. Look at the face, chest, abdomen, and extremities, and then inspect the lips for cyanosis. In black and minority ethnic (BME) children, circulation to the skin is sometimes more difficult to assess, and the lips, mucous membranes, and nail beds are the best places to look for pallor or cyanosis (**Figure 1-9**). Combining assessment of appearance and circulation to the skin can also help establish the severity of the child's illness or injury. A child with a normal appearance and poor circulation to the skin is possibly cold. An abnormal appearance and circulation to the skin suggests the child is in shock.

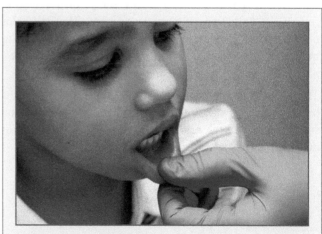

Figure 1-9 In BME children, circulation to the skin is sometimes more difficult to assess, and the lips, mucous membranes, and nail beds may be the best places to look for pallor or cyanosis.
© Jones & Bartlett Learning

Using the PAT to Evaluate Severity and Illness or Injury. The PAT provides a general impression of the paediatric patient. The intent is to provide a standardised approach to the "general impression" and an immediate picture of the child's physiological status. By combining the three components of the PAT, the prehospital professional should be able to answer three critical questions:

1. How severe is the child's illness or injury?

2. What is the most likely physiological abnormality?

3. What is the urgency for treatment?

This information helps the prehospital professional select the most important actions: how fast to intervene, what type of general and specific treatment to give, and how rapidly to transport.

The three elements of the PAT work together and allow a rapid assessment of the child's overall physiological stability. For example, if a child is interactive and pink, but has mild intercostal retractions, the prehospital professional can take time to approach the child in a developmentally appropriate manner to complete the primary assessment. However, if the child is limp, with unlaboured rapid breathing and pale or mottled skin, shock is likely. In this case, the prehospital professional must move rapidly through the primary assessment and begin resuscitation. A child who has an abnormal appearance, but normal work of breathing and normal circulation to skin, probably has a primary brain dysfunction or a major metabolic or systemic problem, such as postictal state, subdural haemorrhage, concussion, intoxication, hypoglycaemia, or sepsis.

The PAT has two important advantages. First, it allows the clinician to quickly obtain critical information about the child's physiological status before touching or agitating the child. Second, the PAT helps set priorities for the rest of the hands-on primary assessment. The PAT takes only seconds, it helps to identify the need for life-saving interventions, and it assists in the transition into the next phase of hands-on physical assessment.

The three components of the PAT (appearance, work of breathing, and circulation to the skin) can be assessed in any sequence, unlike the ordered <C>ABCDE of resuscitation discussed next.

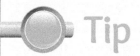

Tip

By combining the three components of the PAT, the prehospital professional can answer three critical questions: (1) How sick or injured is the child? (2) What is the most likely physiological abnormality? (3) What is the urgency for treatment?

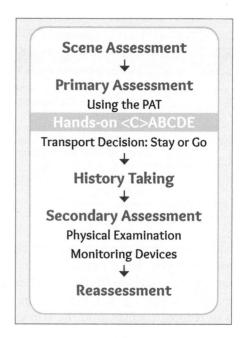

Scene Assessment
↓
Primary Assessment
Using the PAT
Hands-on <C>ABCDE
Transport Decision: Stay or Go
↓
History Taking
↓
Secondary Assessment
Physical Examination
Monitoring Devices
↓
Reassessment

Primary Assessment: <C>ABCDE
Hands-on <C>ABCDE

The primary assessment continues to try to identify life-threatening conditions using an ordered hands-on physical evaluation of the <C>ABCDE. It provides a prioritised sequence of life-support interventions to reverse critical physiological abnormalities. As in adults, there is a specific order for treating life-threatening problems as they are identified, before moving to the next step. The steps are also the same as with adults, but there are important paediatric differences in anatomy, physiology, and signs of distress. <C>ABCDE assessment involves the following components:

1. Catastrophic Bleeding

2. Airway

3. Breathing

4. Circulation

5. Disability

6. Exposure

Catastrophic Bleeding

The immediate control of catastrophic bleeding is a core component of the primary survey and is considered essential for survival. Control of external catastrophic bleeding can be performed with the use of direct and indirect pressure, elevation, tourniquets and haemostatic dressings. Suspected internal catastrophic bleeding may be managed with traction, splinting and with the administration of medicine like tranexamic acid.

Airway

The PAT may identify the presence of an airway obstruction based on the presence of abnormal airway sounds. However, the loudness of the stridor or wheezing is not necessarily related to the amount of airway obstruction. For example, children with asthma in severe distress may have little or no wheezing. Similarly, children with an upper airway foreign body below the <u>vocal cords</u> may have minimal stridor. Abnormal positioning and retractions provide further information about the degree of obstruction, as does the quality of air entry on auscultation during the hands-on assessment.

If the airway is open, ensure that the chest rises with each breath. If a child has assumed a position that maximises his or her ability to maintain a spontaneously open airway, allow the child to remain in that position of comfort. If gurgling is present, there may be mucus, blood, or a foreign body in the mouth or upper airway. Oropharyngeal suctioning of mucus or blood, or removal of a visible foreign body, very often restores patency. If the airway is totally obstructed, then advanced airway management is required.

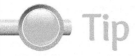

"Red flag" respiratory rates are less than 20 breaths/min for children younger than 5 years of age and less than 12 breaths/min for children younger than 18 years of age.

Breathing

Respiratory Rate. Verify the respiratory rate per minute by counting the number of chest rises in 60 seconds, then doubling that number. Interpret the respiratory rate carefully. Normal infants may show "periodic breathing" or variable respiratory rate with short (<20 second) periods of apnoea. Therefore, counting for only 10–15 seconds may give a falsely low respiratory rate.

Respiratory rates are highly sensitive for serious illness and injury in children and the significance of respiratory rates must not be overlooked. Record an accurate respiratory rate for all children, regardless of presenting complaint. Rapid respiratory rates may reflect high fever, anxiety, pain, or excitement. Normal rates, however, may occur in a child who has been breathing rapidly with increased work of breathing for some time and is now becoming fatigued. In the child who is distressed and crying, you can gauge an approximate respiratory rate by counting the 'pauses' in between cries over 1 minute. Finally, interpretation requires knowledge of normal values for age (**Table 1-4**).

Serial assessment of respiratory rates may be especially useful, and the trend is sometimes more accurate than any single value. A sustained increase or decrease in respiratory rate is usually significant.

Pay close attention to extremes of respiratory rate. A very rapid respiratory rate (>60 breaths/min for any age), especially with abnormal appearance or marked retractions, indicates respiratory distress and possibly respiratory failure. An abnormally

Table 1-4 Normal Child Respiratory Rate for Age

Age	Respiratory Rate (breaths/min)
Birth–11 mos	30–40
12–24 mos	25–35
2–4 yr	25–30
5–11 yr	20–25
12 years plus	15–20

Source: JRCALC, 2016.

slow respiratory rate is always worrisome because it might mean respiratory failure. Red flags are respiratory rates less than 20 breaths/min for children younger than 5 years of age, and less than 12 breaths/min for older children. A normal respiratory rate alone never guarantees adequate oxygenation and ventilation. The respiratory rate must be interpreted along with appearance, work of breathing, and air movement.

Auscultation. Listen with a stethoscope over the mid-clavicular and <u>midaxillary lines</u> during inhalation and exhalation to hear abnormal lung sounds, such as <u>crackles</u> and wheezing (**Figure 1-10**). <u>Inspiratory</u> crackles indicate disease in the alveoli (air sacs) themselves. Often crackles are not heard on auscultation, even when the child has a pathologic condition, such as pneumonia. The younger the child, the more difficult it is to appreciate abnormal sounds during auscultation. Expiratory wheezing indicates lower airway obstruction. Auscultation also helps evaluate the volume of air movement and effectiveness of work of breathing. A child with increased work of breathing and poor air movement may be in impending respiratory failure.

Table 1-5 lists abnormal breath sounds, their causes, and common examples of associated disease processes.

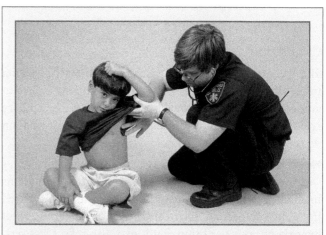

Figure 1-10 Listen for air movement over the mid-axillary line.
© Jones & Bartlett Learning

Table 1-5 Interpretation of Abnormal Breath Sounds

Sound	Cause	Examples
Stridor	Upper airway obstruction	Croup, foreign body aspiration, retropharyngeal abscess
Wheezing	Lower airway obstruction	Asthma, foreign body, bronchiolitis
Expiratory grunting	Inadequate oxygenation	Pulmonary contusion, pneumonia, drowning
Inspiratory crackles	Fluid, mucus, or blood in airway	Pneumonia, pulmonary contusion
Absent breath sounds despite increased work of breathing	Severe airway obstruction (upper or lower airway)	Physical barrier to transmission of breath sounds, foreign body, severe asthma, haemothorax, pneumothorax, pleural fluid, pneumonia, pneumothorax

Table 1-6 Normal Child Heart Rate for Age

Age	Heart Rate (beats/min)
Birth to 11 mos	110–160
12 mos to 2 years	110–150
2 –4 years	95–140
5–11 years	80–120
12 years plus	60–100

Source: JRCALC, 2016.

Circulation

The PAT provides important visual clues about circulation to the skin. Information obtained from the hands-on evaluation of heart rate, pulse quality, skin temperature, capillary refill time, and blood pressure provide further information on the adequacy of perfusion.

Heart Rate. Methods used to assess adult circulatory status (heart rate and blood pressure) have important limitations in children. First, normal heart rate varies with age, as noted in **Table 1-6**. Second, tachycardia may be an early sign of hypoxia or poor perfusion, but it may also reflect less serious conditions, such as fever, anxiety, pain, and excitement. Like respiratory rate, interpret heart rate within the context of the overall history, PAT, and primary assessment. Obtain

an accurate heart rate for all children, either by palpating for a pulse, utilising a pulse oximeter, listening for heart sounds or using a lead II trace. A trend of increasing or decreasing heart rate may be quite useful, and may suggest worsening hypoxia or shock, or improvement after treatment. When hypoxia or shock becomes critical, the heart rate falls, leading to frank bradycardia. Bradycardia indicates critical hypoxia or ischaemia. With tachycardia greater than 180 beats/min, an electronic monitor is necessary to accurately determine heart rate.

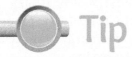

Tip

A rapid initial respiratory rate may simply reflect high fever, anxiety, pain, excitement, and not any real physiological or anatomical problem. Noting a trend of an abnormal respiratory rate is more useful for indicating true pathology.

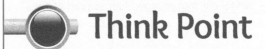

Think Point

Be careful not to underestimate respiratory distress in a child with a pulse oximetry reading above 94%. This child may be using increased work of breathing and tachypnoea to compensate for serious hypoxic stress.

Pulse Quality. Feel the pulse to ascertain pulse quality. Normally, the brachial pulse is palpable medial to the biceps in the antecubital fossa (**Figure 1-11**). Note the quality as either weak or strong. If the brachial pulse is strong, the child is probably not hypotensive. If a peripheral pulse

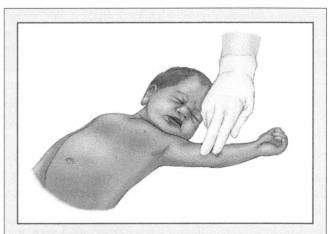

Figure 1–11 The anatomical position of the brachial pulse is medial to the biceps muscle.
© Jones & Bartlett Learning

Case Study 2

A 2-year-old boy was found face down in the family swimming pool. He was under water for no more than 1 minute but required cardiopulmonary resuscitation by the mother to get him breathing again. On arrival of the clinician, the child is alert, pink, and clinging to his mother. Respirations appear regular and non-laboured at 26 breaths/min. When you examine him further, he screams and fights you. You are unable to obtain a blood pressure or heart rate, or assess lung sounds. The mother is sobbing and frightened.

1. How useful is the PAT in evaluating severity of illness and urgency for care?

2. In what ways is the PAT different than the <C>ABCDE in the primary assessment?

cannot be felt, attempt to find a central pulse. Check the femoral pulse in infants and young children, or the carotid pulse in an older child or adolescent. If there is no pulse, or in a cardiac arrest situation the pulse is low (<60 beats/min) and the child is symptomatic with poor perfusion, start cardiopulmonary resuscitation (CPR) (see the *Resuscitation and Dysrhythmias* chapter for more information).

Skin Temperature and Capillary Refill Time. Next, do a hands-on evaluation of circulation to the skin. Although children with normal circulation may have cool hands and feet, the skin should be warm above the wrists and ankles. With decreasing perfusion, the extremities become cooler proximally. Check capillary refill time centrally either on the sternum or forehead as well as peripherally as the value of measuring a peripheral capillary refill time is controversial for several reasons: the peripheral perfusion baseline may vary from child to child; environmental factors, such as cold room temperature, may complicate interpretation; and it may be difficult for the prehospital professional to accurately count seconds under critical circumstances. Normal capillary refill time is less than 2 to 3 seconds. The capillary refill time is just one element in the assessment of circulation. It must be evaluated in the context of the PAT and other perfusion characteristics, such as heart rate, pulse quality, and blood pressure.

Signs of circulation to the skin (skin temperature, capillary refill time, and pulse quality) are helpful tools to assess a child's circulatory status, especially when performed consecutively on a child who is not cold.

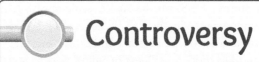

Controversy

The value of capillary refill time is controversial. Peripheral perfusion may be variable in some children, and such environmental factors as ambient temperature may have a strong influence on capillary refill time.

Disability

Assessment of disability, or neurological status, involves quick evaluation of the two main parts of the CNS: the cerebral cortex and the brainstem. First assess neurological status, which is controlled by the cerebral cortex, by looking at appearance as part of the PAT; then assess the level of consciousness using the AVPU scale (**Table 1-7**). Evaluate the brainstem by checking the responses of each pupil to a direct beam of light. A normal pupil constricts after a light stimulus. Pupillary response may be abnormal in the presence of drugs, ongoing seizures, hypoxia, or impending brainstem herniation. Next, evaluate motor activity. Look for symmetric movement of the extremities, seizures, posturing, or flaccidity.

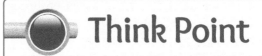

Think Point

Neither the AVPU scale nor the Paediatric GCS allows assessment of restless or agitated behavioural states.

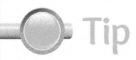

Tip

Interpret heart rate in the context of the overall history, PAT, and entire physical assessment.

AVPU Scale. The AVPU scale is a standardised method of assessing the level of consciousness in all patients. It helps categorise motor response based on simple responses to stimuli. The patient is either alert, responsive to verbal stimuli, responsive only to pain stimuli, or unresponsive.

Table 1-7 AVPU Scale

Category	Stimulus	Response Type	Reaction
Alert	Normal environment	Appropriate	Normal interactiveness for age
Verbal	Simple command or sound stimulus	Appropriate or inappropriate	Responds to name; non-specific or confused
Pain	Pain	Appropriate, inappropriate, or pathological	Withdraws from pain or sound or motion without purpose or localization of pain; posturing
Unresponsive			No perceptible response to any stimulus

Abnormal Appearance and the AVPU Scale. Assessment of appearance using the PAT provides different information than assessment using the AVPU scale. A child with an altered mental status (AMS) on the AVPU scale always has an abnormal appearance in the PAT, because such a child almost always has a serious or critical condition. However, a child with a mild to moderate illness or injury may be alert on the AVPU scale, but have an abnormal appearance in the PAT. Assessing appearance using the PAT may provide an earlier indication of the presence of serious illness and injury.

The accuracy of the AVPU scale is controversial and it has a few important limitations. Its ability to predict the extent of neurological compromise has not been well tested in children. Its scope is limited in the evaluation of children with restless or agitated states. The scale only addresses decreased levels of responsiveness, a problem common to all of the current prehospital methods for disability assessment. However, it is easy to remember (there are no numbers to recall) and to use. The more complicated Paediatric GCS involves memorisation and numerical scoring, tasks that may be hard to remember and apply in critical situations (see the *Trauma* chapter for Paediatric GCS). Recent data suggests that the motor component of the GCS alone is the best predictor of neurological outcome. The much simpler-to-administer motor component of the GCS may be adequate for mental status evaluation on scene. The motor categories of the GCS from lowest point value to highest are (1) no response, (2) extensor posturing (decerebrate), (3) flexor posturing (decorticate), (4) withdrawing, (5) localising, and (6) obeying instructions (as age-appropriate). Like the AVPU scale, the GCS does not address degrees of neurological disability in children who are restless, agitated, or combative.

Exposure

Proper exposure of the child is necessary for completion of the primary physical assessment. The PAT requires that the caregiver remove part of the child's clothing to allow careful observation of the face, chest wall, and skin. Completing the <C>ABCDE components of the primary assessment may require further exposure to fully evaluate physiological function, anatomical abnormalities, and unsuspected injuries. Pay attention to the need for privacy, even for prepubescent children, when possible. Be careful to avoid heat loss, especially in infants, by covering the child up as soon as possible. Infants and younger children have a larger body surface to body weight ratio and are at a greater risk to rapidly lose body heat when left exposed. Cold stress in critically ill or injured patients can increase metabolic demands, worsen the effects of hypoxia and hypoglycaemia, and adversely affect the response to resuscitative efforts.

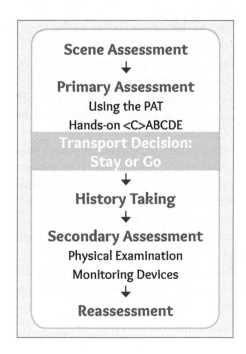

Primary Assessment: The Transport Decision: Treat or Transport?

After completing the PAT and the hands-on <C>ABCDE, and beginning any resuscitation as necessary, the prehospital professional must make a crucial decision: does the child require immediate transport the nearest appropriate hospital, or should they continue with additional assessment and treatment on scene? Should they transport the child, or is there a more appropriate mode of transport available? Should the child be transported to a local district general hospital, for either treatment or stabilisation, or does the child need to go directly to a trauma centre or paediatric specialty hospital? This decision process is different for each child and for each ambulance service.

Clinical Grade and Decision Making

The clinical grade of prehospital professional is an important consideration when making a decision to treat a child at the scene or to transport the child to an appropriate receiving unit. Important points to consider include:

- The mechanism of injury or circumstances of illness
- The history that can be reliably obtained
- Any physiological abnormalities
- Significant pain
- Availability of support, advice and referral pathways
- Local ambulance service discharge and transport policies
- The clinicians comfort and confidence regarding the case
- Transport time and determining what could be provided en route vs what should be provided before leaving the scene

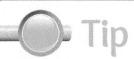

Deciding when to go and when to stay is different for each child and for each ambulance service system. If any grade of clinician does not feel confident or comfortable to discharge a child or to provide assessment and treatment at the scene, they should lower their threshold for admission or referral.

The Clinical Problem

If the 999 call is for trauma, and if the child has a serious mechanism of injury, a physiological abnormality, or a potentially significant anatomical abnormality, or if the scene is unsafe, immediate transport is imperative. In these cases, stop external catastrophic bleeding, manage the airway and breathing with c-spine immobilisation consideration, and then transport. Attempt vascular access as required and where possible you should take the time to establish this before leaving scene. Examples of such patients include a child with an abnormal appearance after a closed head injury from a fall, or a child struck by a car who has a painful, deformed femur.

If the 999 call is for illness, the decision to stay or go is less clear cut and depends on the following factors: expected benefits of treatment, ambulance service regulations, comfort level, and transport time.

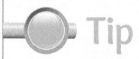

If the child is physiologically unstable, defer or omit history taking and physical examination.

Expected Benefits of Treatment

The time it takes to reach definitive care in the hospital has a major effect on the outcomes of children with serious injuries. Therefore, timely transport after the provision of meaningful interventions is very important. The time it takes to reach hospital care may also significantly affect the outcomes of children with certain medical illnesses. For example, a child in cardiogenic shock benefits most from rapid transport to definitive care, because the hospital is the best place for life-saving treatments of this rare and complex condition.

However, some critically ill children benefit from ALS treatment on scene. For example, for a child who is seizing, early treatment with a benzodiazepine is the best hope to get the seizure under immediate control and avoid additional anticonvulsant administration and endotracheal intubation. Similarly, the risk of brain injury is decreased if glucose is administered to the unconscious diabetic child at the time that the prehospital professional recognises hypoglycaemia with a bedside test.

Ambulance Service Regulations

The decision to treat or transport can often be defined by ambulance service guidelines about treatment and transport. For example, some systems allow prehospital professionals to treat a child in cardiopulmonary arrest with ALS interventions until either the resuscitation is successful or death is declared. Other systems require transport after initial resuscitation is underway, with the decision to discontinue efforts left to the ED staff. It is important that local policy is followed and any clinician should be prepare to undertake timely transport so a hospital if they feel a child would benefit from additional intervention by the hospital team.

Comfort Level

Whenever a prehospital professional believes that the illness or injury requires a higher level of care, it is best to initiate transport to an appropriate receiving unit. Meaningful interventions should be carried out on scene and the clinician should work to their scope of practice. Attempting procedures en route to hospital is not without risk and there is a far greater chance of success if time is taken to do those procedures in a controlled way before leaving the scene (or pulling over on route to hospital and doing those procedures once the vehicle is stationary). For example, a child with hypotensive (decompensated) hypovolemic shock, a paramedic should obtain vascular access and provide the correct dose of fluid (usually Sodium Chloride 0.9%).

Transport Time

The time to the nearest ED is another key factor. A shorter transport time ordinarily supports a shorter scene time. For example, if a child has ingested a potentially lethal poison, immediate transport is prudent if the ED is close by, because of the complications related to delay of definitive care. However, if transport time is long, consider initiating any meaningful treatment on scene.

Summary of Primary Assessment

The components of the paediatric primary assessment include the general impression, the <C>ABCDE, any immediate resuscitation needs, and treat or transport decision. The PAT is the basis for the general impression. It includes evaluation of the characteristics of appearance, work of breathing, and circulation to the skin, and uses clues obtained by looking and listening from across the room. The primary assessment includes a hands-on evaluation of paediatric-specific indicators of cardiopulmonary or neurological abnormalities. Accurate observations are essential for the primary assessment and should be recorded for any child attended by prehospital professionals. They must be interpreted in the context of age and the overall general and primary assessments. Interventions may be necessary at any point in the <C>ABCDE sequence. After the <C>ABCDE, another crucial decision is whether to stay on scene and begin treatment or transport immediately. The type of clinical problem, the expected benefits of earlier transport, the local service policies, the prehospital professional's comfort level, and the transport time are all important elements in the transport decision.

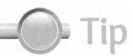

Always perform reassessment to track problems and monitor response to treatment.

History Taking

History taking has two objectives and should be performed on both medical and trauma patients:

1. To obtain a complete description of the main complaint.

2. To determine the mechanism of injury or circumstances of illness.

If the child seems to be physiologically unstable based on the primary assessment, the prehospital professional may decide to transport without delay and perform a focussed history and secondary assessment. If the child is stable and the scene is safe, the prehospital professional should obtain a thorough history and complete the secondary assessment on the scene before making the decision to transport or refer. As opposed to the primary assessment, which focuses on physiological problems that may be immediately life-threatening, this secondary assessment focuses on anatomical abnormalities, which are rarely life-threatening.

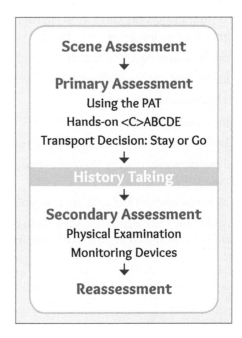

Scene Assessment
↓
Primary Assessment
Using the PAT
Hands-on <C>ABCDE
Transport Decision: Stay or Go
↓
History Taking
↓
Secondary Assessment
Physical Examination
Monitoring Devices
↓
Reassessment

A history should be obtained from the child whenever that is possible. Caregivers can of course support this process and may need to provide support to their child. It is important to make sure that the child who is at an appropriate stage in their development is involved in their care. In some cases, it may be helpful to interview the adolescent separate from the caregiver; many adolescents are hesitant to disclose information about drug use or sexual activity (as it relates to the current illness or injury) in front of their caregiver. The history provides important information that assists the prehospital professional in analysing assessment findings. The SAMPLE mnemonic may be used to elicit information: Signs and Symptoms, Allergies, Medications, Past medical history, Last food or liquid, and Events leading up to this illness or injury (**Table 1-8**).

As well as the SAMPLE mnemonic a more in-depth history can be gathered using a structured history taking framework. Similar in nature to an adults history taking approach there are a few changes specific to paediatrics of various ages. Gathering information on the presenting complaint (PC), past medical history (PMH), birth history, feeding history, vaccination history and infectious illness history, developmental history, family history (FH), social history (SH) both at home and at school and, with older children,

Table 1-8 Paediatric SAMPLE Components

Component	Explanation
Signs and symptoms	Onset and nature of symptoms such as pain or fever Age-appropriate signs of distress
Allergies	Known drug reactions or other allergies
Medications	Exact names and doses of ongoing drugs Timing and amount of last dose Timing and dose of analgesics or antipyretics
Past medical history	History of pregnancy, labour, delivery Previous illness or injuries Immunisations
Last food or liquid	Timing of the child's last food or drink, including bottle or breastfeeding
Events leading to the injury or illness	Key events leading to the current incident Fever history

the psychiatric history is all important in building up the bigger picture. Not all of this information can be gathered from the child themselves so building up a good relationship with caregivers is vital.

Children with special health care needs often require additional history collection, but the type of history necessary is dependent on the underlying illness or condition. The use of patient information passports or personal child health records "the red book" can be extremely helpful in obtaining critical information about these patients. See the *Children with Special Health Care Needs* chapter.

If a child has an apparently minor condition (e.g., fever with no adverse signs, feeding difficulties, fussiness, minor trauma), be careful not to overlook clues to possible serious underlying conditions. Ingestions, metabolic problems, and systemic infections may present with non-specific findings in infants and toddlers. Consider child maltreatment when the physical findings are not logically related to the complaint leading to the call, or if the history is implausible or changes.

At this stage is may be prudent to establish the ideas, concerns and expectations of the child and of any caregiver. Understanding their ideas about what is happening will add important context for your overall decision making. Listening to the concerns of a child or parent ensures that those concerns can be addressed in your advice or treatment. Being aware of a child or caregiver's expectations allows you to plan ahead and make the best decisions for a child's care.

Secondary Assessment: Physical Examination

Often this portion of the assessment is not possible because of transport and treatment priorities. Sometimes it is unnecessary because the problem has been fully evaluated in earlier phases of the assessment, or the complaint and history are minor or medical in origin.

If the child with traumatic injuries is stable on scene and does not need resuscitation after the primary assessment, or if he or she is on the way to the hospital but does not require ongoing treatment, perform a detailed secondary assessment. This physical evaluation must include all anatomical areas affected and builds on the findings of the primary assessment and history taking.

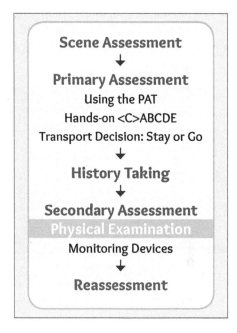

Scene Assessment
↓
Primary Assessment
Using the PAT
Hands-on <C>ABCDE
Transport Decision: Stay or Go
↓
History Taking
↓
Secondary Assessment
Physical Examination
Monitoring Devices
↓
Reassessment

Use the toe-to-head sequence for the detailed secondary assessment of infants, toddlers, and pre-school-aged children. This approach allows the prehospital professional to gain the child's trust and cooperation, and increases the accuracy of the physical findings. Ask for the assistance of the caregiver in the assessment. Note the following special anatomical characteristics of children when performing the secondary assessment.

General Observations

Observe the clothing for any unusual odours or for stains that might suggest a poison. If poisoning is suspected, remove soiled or dirty clothing and save it, and wash the child's skin with soap and water. Observe the demeanour and posture of the child (relate to the Tone in the appearance TICLS mnemonic), is the child an appropriate size for their age?

Skin

Observe the skin carefully for rashes and bruising patterns that may suggest maltreatment, as discussed in the *Child*

Maltreatment chapter. Look for bite marks; straight line marks from cords or straps; pinch marks; or hand, belt, or buckle pattern bruises. Patterned injuries, or those with a geometric shape, are often indicative of abuse. Inspect for non-blanching petechial or purpuric lesions (which may indicate severe infections), and look for any new lesions that develop during transport.

Head

The younger the infant or child, the larger the head is in proportion to the rest of the body (**Figure 1-12**). This disproportionate size increases the risk for head injury with deceleration, such as in motor vehicle crashes. Look for bruising, swelling, and haematomas. Significant blood can be lost between the skull and scalp of a small infant. Assessment of the anterior fontanelle in infants younger than 9–18 months old can provide helpful information (**Figure 1-13**). If possible, the fontanelle should be assessed with the infant in a sitting position. A bulging and nonpulsatile fontanelle

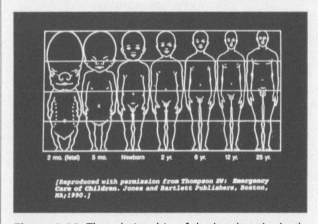

Figure 1-12 The relationship of the head to the body changes with advancing age.
Courtesy of the Health Resources and Services Administration (HRSA), Maternal and Child Health Bureau (MCHB), Emergency Medical Services for Children (EMSC Program.)

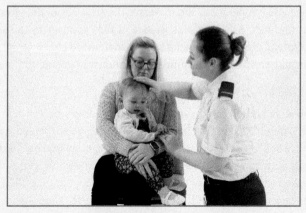

Figure 1-13 The anterior fontanelle of the infant is a window to the CNS.
© Jones & Bartlett Learning

suggests elevated intracranial pressure caused by meningitis, encephalitis, or intracranial bleeding. A sunken fontanelle suggests dehydration.

Eyes

A thorough evaluation of pupil size, reaction to light, and symmetry of extraocular muscle movements may be difficult to perform in infants. Gently rocking infants in the upright position often gets them to open their eyes. A colourful distracting object can then be used to help assess eye movements.

Nose

Young infants preferentially breathe through their noses, so nasal congestion with mucus can cause marked respiratory distress. Gentle suction of the nostrils may bring relief (**Figure 1-14**). Leaking blood (rhinorrhea) or cerebrospinal fluid (CSF) suggests a basilar skull fracture.

Ears

Look for any drainage from the ear canals (otorrhea). Leaking blood or CSF suggests a basilar skull fracture. Check for bruises behind the ear or Battle sign, another indicator of basilar skull fracture. The presence of pus may indicate an ear infection or perforation of the ear drum.

Mouth

In the trauma patient, look for active bleeding and loose teeth. Note the smell of the breath. Some ingestions are associated with identifiable odours, such as hydrocarbons. Acidosis, as in diabetic ketoacidosis, may impart a sweet or "fruity" smell to the breath. Do not routinely use tongue depressors when assessing an infants mouth as this may cause trauma.

Neck

Examine the trachea for oedema or bruising. Listen with a stethoscope over the trachea at the midline (**Figure 1-15**).

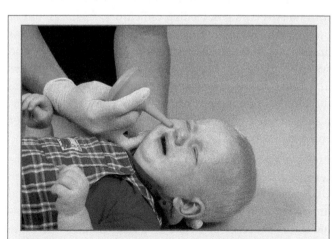

Figure 1-14 Gentle suction may bring relief to the infant.

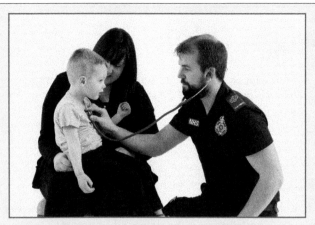

Figure 1-15 Listen at the trachea to distinguish the origin of abnormal airway sounds.
© Jones & Bartlett Learning.

This is a quick and easy way to differentiate between very proximal airway obstruction (usually mucus in the nose) and true wheezing or stridor. The neck should also be assessed for a tracheal shift or jugular vein distention (JVD). These are classic signs of tension pneumothorax, but occur late in the physiological process. JVD may not be present if there are other injuries present that have led to hypovolemia.

Chest

Re-examine the chest for penetrating injuries, lacerations, bruises, or rashes. If the child is injured, feel the clavicles and every rib for tenderness or deformity.

Back

Inspect the back for lacerations, penetrating injuries, bruises, or rashes.

Abdomen

Inspect the abdomen for any bruising, swelling, deformities, or rashes. In the trauma patient, redness or bruising under the site of protective straps, or "seat belt sign", may be apparent. Also, inspect the abdomen for distention. Gently palpate the abdomen and watch closely for guarding or tensing of the abdominal muscles, which may suggest infection, obstruction, or intra-abdominal injury. Note any tenderness or masses. If an infant or toddler has been crying for a prolonged period of time, or if a child's respiratory effort has been supported with a bag-valve-mask, this may also lead to abdominal distention because of air that has been pushed into the stomach.

Extremities

Assess for symmetry. Compare both sides for colour, warmth, size of joints, and tenderness. Put each joint through a full range of motion while watching the eyes of the child for signs of pain; understandably, if there is obvious deformity of the extremity suggesting a fracture, this

technique should not be used. If there is a suspected fracture present, assess for a pulse, capillary refill, motor function, and sensation distal to the injury.

Observations

Although pulse and respirations have been assessed in the primary assessment, they may or may not have been formally counted and recorded because of circumstances of resuscitation or brevity of transportation. It is important to obtain and record these observations to make further assessment of the child's changing condition. When resuscitation is necessary, pulse and respirations should be monitored frequently but additional observations may be deferred until the child has stabilised or the transportation is completed.

Blood Pressure. Blood pressure determination and interpretation may be difficult in children because of the lack of patient cooperation, possessing the proper cuff size, and remembering normal values for age. **Figure 1-16A** illustrates the different sizes of blood pressure cuffs, and **Figure 1-16B** demonstrates the technique for getting a correct blood pressure in the arm or thigh. Always use a cuff with a width of two-thirds the length of the upper arm or thigh. For patients 3 years of age or younger, technical difficulties reduce the value of a blood pressure on scene. When shock is suspected

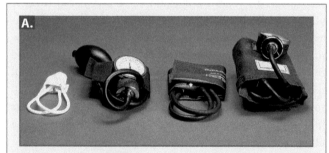

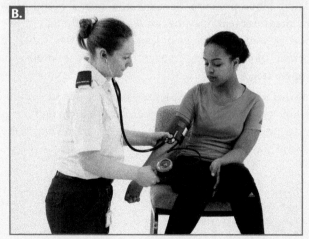

Figure 1-16 A. There are several different blood pressure (BP) cuff sizes: neonatal, infant, child, and adult. **B.** To obtain an accurate BP reading, use a cuff that is two-thirds the length of the child's upper arm.
© Jones & Bartlett Learning.

Table 1-9 Normal Child Blood Pressure by Age

Age	Systolic Blood Pressure (mm Hg)
Birth to 11 mos	70–90
12 – 24 mos	80–95
2 – 4 yrs	80–100
5 yrs	90–100
6 yrs 7 – 11 yrs 12 yrs plus	80–110 90–110 100–120

Source: JRCALC, 2016.

in this age group based on other assessments (e.g., history, mechanism, PAT), do not delay treatment or transport to attempt a blood pressure measurement. For patients older than 3 years of age, try one blood pressure measurement on scene, then move on to the rest of the assessment.

For children older than 1 year of age, an easy formula for determining the lower limit of acceptable blood pressure by age is as follows: minimal systolic blood pressure = 70 + (2 × age, in years). For example, a 2-year-old toddler with a systolic blood pressure of 65 mm Hg is hypotensive. **Table 1-9** shows approximate normal minimal systolic blood pressure values for different ages. High blood pressure is not normally a clinical problem for children on scene. Assume that a blood pressure is within normal limits if an infant or young child is agitated, is crying, has pink skin, and has easily palpable peripheral pulses. In a patient with this clinical profile, do not delay transport to obtain a blood pressure. Remember, a normal blood pressure measurement may be misleading. Although a low blood pressure definitely indicates hypotensive shock, a "normal" blood pressure frequently exists in children with compensated shock.

Note that a widening pulse pressure (systolic pressure minus diastolic pressure) may occur secondary to increased intracranial pressure and early septic shock; a narrowing pulse pressure may be seen early in hypovolemic shock.

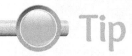 **Tip**

For patients younger than 3 years of age, the value of obtaining a blood pressure on scene may be outweighed by the technical difficulties of getting an accurate measurement.

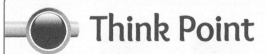 **Think Point**

Do not depend on blood pressure readings to diagnose shock. A "normal" blood pressure frequently exists in compensated shock.

Assessment of Pain: An Additional Observation

It is easy for the prehospital professional to ignore, underestimate, or misinterpret the signs and symptoms of pain in infants and young children. Children are much less likely to receive effective pain medications than adults. Studies have demonstrated reluctance by all levels of emergency care personnel to administer medications to children for control of pain and anxiety. The younger the child, the less likely the child will receive effective analgesia. However, adult and paediatric experience has validated the effectiveness of analgesia in the prehospital setting to decrease pain, without causing respiratory depression or interference with the accuracy of physical assessment.

Pain is present with most types of injury and with many illnesses. Inadequate treatment of pain has many adverse effects on the child and family. Pain itself causes significant morbidity and misery for the child and family or caregivers, and interferes with the prehospital professional's accurate assessment of physiological abnormalities. Children who do not receive appropriate analgesia are more likely to have exaggerated pain responses to subsequent painful procedures. Even neonates have demonstrable chronic changes in pain perception when they are subjected to painful procedures without the benefit of analgesia. Post-traumatic stress is also more common among children who experience pain during acute illness and injury and do not receive pharmacological relief. Hence, just as with adults, it is essential to carefully assess pain in all children and to consider effective methods to provide relief from suffering when appropriate.

It is best practice that prehospital professionals assess and manage pain as a part of the secondary assessment. Indeed, evaluation of pain has become an important observation in all ages, including children. Appropriate pain management relieves distress of the child and family or caregivers, and facilitates communication, physical assessment, and ease of transport.

Assessment of pain must take into consideration the developmental age of the patient. The ability to recognise pain improves as the age of the child increases. For example, in a pre-verbal infant, crying and agitation unrelieved by being held by the caregiver may be caused by hunger, hypoxia, or pain. In infants, further assessment is essential to identify sources of pain before administration of analgesia.

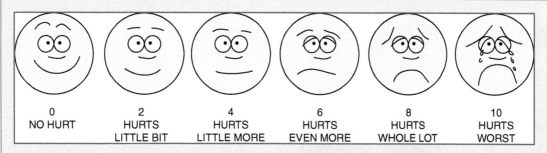

| 0
NO HURT | 2
HURTS
LITTLE BIT | 4
HURTS
LITTLE MORE | 6
HURTS
EVEN MORE | 8
HURTS
WHOLE LOT | 10
HURTS
WORST |

Figure 1-17 Wong-Baker FACES Pain Rating Scale for self-assessment of pain.

From Hockenberry MJ, Wilson D: Wong's essentials of pediatric nursing, ed. 8, St. Louis, 2009, Mosby. Used with permission. Copyright Mosby.

In contrast, verbal children older than 3 years of age are usually quite vocal about pain. Therefore, in older children, pain scales using pictures of facial expressions (Wong-Baker FACES Scale) or visual analogue scores (VAS) may be helpful in assessing the need for pharmacological relief of pain. **Figure 1-17** illustrates the Wong-Baker FACES Scale. Although such "self-report" scales have not yet been extensively used in the prehospital environment, they have been validated in other settings to provide an immediate evaluation of intensity of pain, and to monitor response to treatment.

There is much overlap between the management of fear and anxiety and the management of pain in infants and young children. Many non-pharmacological and pharmacological methods relieve anxiety and reduce the perception of pain, as summarised in **Table 1-10**. Remaining calm and providing quiet professional reassurance to caregivers and child are the first important steps. A calm caregiver helps to make the child calm and more at ease. Distraction techniques may be extremely helpful in reducing pain. Many prehospital professionals learn to use toys, "magic tricks", or engaging stories to provide distraction. Keeping the caregiver with the child and sometimes holding the child are also useful strategies (**Figure 1-18**).

In older children, visual imagery techniques can often be helpful. Ask the child where he or she would most prefer to be at the present time, then assist the child in closing his or her eyes and visualizing a more tranquil or enjoyable environment. Music is also a very effective distraction.

Table 1-10 Methods of Prehospital Analgesia and Anxiolysis

Nonpharmacological	Pharmacological
Calm manner	Paracetamol (Oral and IV)
Caregiver assistance through presence or holding	Ibuprofen
Distraction techniques with "toolbox" of toys	Nitrous oxide
Ice	Oral Morphine
Visual imagery	Morphine
Pacifier	Fentanyl*
Music	Diamorphine*
Splinting of fractures	Ketamine*

*Subject to local policy and availability

Controversy

Although "self-report" pain scales have not yet been extensively used for paediatric patients in the prehospital environment, they have been validated in other clinical settings. They can help provide an immediate evaluation of pain intensity, and they can aid in monitoring response to treatment.

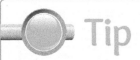

Tip

Pain is often considered an additional observation. Pain management can help relieve distress of the child and family, greatly facilitate communication and physical assessment, assist in timely provision of necessary interventions, and ease the transport process.

Pharmacological methods for reducing pain are also a standard of prehospital care. Opiates, paracetamol and nitrous oxide are available to prehospital professionals in many ambulance services. Intramuscular (IM) medications are less effective because children fear needles, and the injection site pain may last for days. IM administration of pain relief is also rarely used outside of palliative care in UK practice but does remain an option. Analgesic drugs

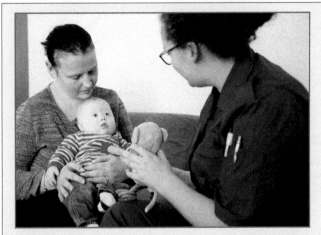

Figure 1-18 Use distraction techniques to help reduce the child's pain.
© Jones & Bartlett Learning

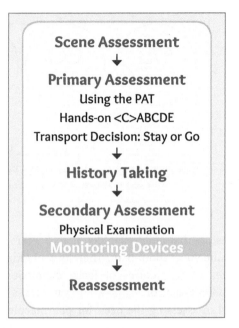

Scene Assessment
↓
Primary Assessment
Using the PAT
Hands-on <C>ABCDE
Transport Decision: Stay or Go
↓
History Taking
↓
Secondary Assessment
Physical Examination
Monitoring Devices
↓
Reassessment

may be easily delivered through inhalation techniques, by the transmucosal (e.g., sublingual, intranasal) route, or by the transdermal route depending on the skill level of the clinician. Techniques, such as inhaled nitrous oxide, have had excellent success in prehospital paediatric care. However, one of the most effective methods for administration of analgesia is by way of the intravenous route. Intravenous (IV) delivery provides the most effective and most controllable or titratable method. A downside is it does involve establishing vascular access, which like the intramuscular (IM) route is usually painful. Also, the child's response to pain medication is sometimes unpredictable and they must be carefully monitored. Medications to reduce pain may also cause sedation and can result in respiratory depression, bradycardia, hypoxemia, hypotension, and even loss of protective airway reflexes, although when administered these side effects are rare.

Assessment of pain has become another observation, and management of paediatric pain must be a routine part of prehospital care in all ambulance services. This entails a thorough understanding of available non-pharmacological techniques, medications, potential medication contraindications and complications, and management of those complications.

Secondary Assessment: Monitoring Devices
Pulse Oximetry

Oxygen Saturation. Pulse oximetry is an excellent tool to assess how well a child is breathing. **Figure 1-19** illustrates the technique of placing a pulse oximetry probe on a young child. In infants and younger children, the patient may tolerate the probe more readily if a wrap-around probe is used and it is placed around the toe or the foot. A pulse oximetry reading above 94% saturation on room air indicates good oxygenation. Be careful not to underestimate respiratory distress in a child with a reading above 94%. Sometimes the child can compensate for hypoxia by significantly increasing work of breathing and respiratory rate, and pulse oximetry may not reflect the true severity or urgency of the respiratory problem. As with any other measurement, interpret pulse oximetry in the context of the "big picture," including work of breathing, appearance, and circulation.

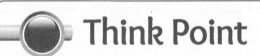

Think Point

Be careful not to underestimate respiratory distress in a child with a pulse oximetry reading above 94%. This child may be using increased work of breathing and tachypnoea to compensate for serious hypoxic stress.

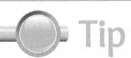

Tip

Analgesic drugs may be easily delivered through inhalation, transmucosal (e.g., sublingual, intranasal) routes, or transdermal routes. Techniques, such as inhaled nitrous oxide, have had excellent success in prehospital paediatric care.

Although pulse oximetry is quite helpful in identifying a child with moderate respiratory distress, it can also help identify the child in respiratory failure. When the pulse oximetry reading is below 90% saturation in a child on 100%

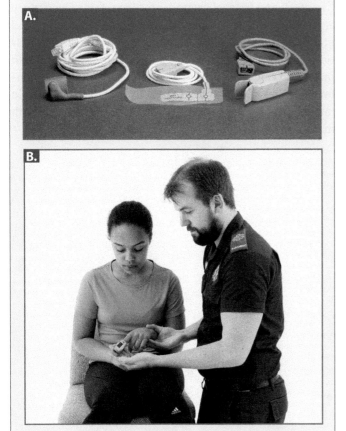

Figure 1-19 A. Various pulse oximeter probes wrap around or clip onto digits or earlobes. **B.** Pulse oximetry is an excellent tool for assessing the effectiveness of breathing.

© Jones & Bartlett Learning; © Jones & Bartlett Learning.

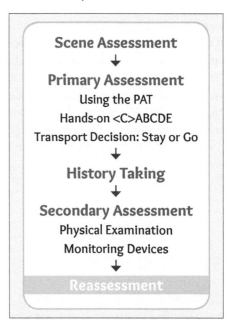

oxygen by a non-rebreathing mask, this usually represents respiratory failure requiring assisted ventilation. However, sometimes a child in severe respiratory distress or early respiratory failure may maintain measured oxygen saturation by increasing work of breathing and respiratory rate. This child may not appear to be critically ill by pulse oximetry alone. Again, interpret pulse oximetry together with the rest of the assessment to accurately evaluate the degree of respiratory distress or failure.

Additional Monitoring Devices

The prehospital professional can perform some types of specific testing on scene, such as blood glucose measurement, 12-lead ECG monitoring, capnography, and other specialty testing available in local service areas.

Diagnostic Testing

The diagnostic testing portion of the assessment frequently requires ancillary testing, such as laboratory and radiographic evaluations. Diagnostic testing is usually part of in-patient assessment in the ED, the hospital paediatric ward, or the paediatric intensive care unit.

Reassessment

Perform reassessment of all patients to gauge the response to treatment and to track the progression of identified physiological and anatomical problems. New problems may also be identified on reassessment. Data from the reassessment will guide ongoing treatment. The elements in the reassessment are:

1. The PAT
2. The <C>ABCDE with repeat observations
3. Assessment of positive anatomical findings
4. Review of the effectiveness and safety of treatment

The elements in the reassessment are also the basis for determination of an appropriate transport destination and for accurate, paediatric-specific radio or telephone communications with the ED.

Pre-alert

Structured prehospital pre-alert messages promote a seamless transfer of care from the prehospital to the ED setting, maximising the ability of all clinicians to provide efficient and effective care. A good pre-alert transmits vital data completely and concisely, highlighting paediatric-specific information to allow the ED team to best prepare for the patient's arrival. If available, provide the ED with a patient weight, as reported by the caregiver.For a step-by-step explanation, see **Pre-alert, Procedure 1**.

Summary

After the primary assessment, and beginning any necessary resuscitative efforts, the prehospital professional must determine the severity of the illness or injury and make a decision to provide treatment on scene, to transport to hospital or to refer to another service. If additional evaluation is appropriate, perform a detailed history and secondary assessment either on scene or on the way to the ED. These additional phases of assessment are not indicated if there is a child who is critically unwell and requires resuscitation. The secondary assessment is more for the detection of anatomical problems than for evaluation of physiological abnormalities. Always perform reassessments to observe the patient's response to interventions, and to guide changes in treatment, transport, and triage. Diagnostic testing refers to laboratory and radiographical evaluation to determine causation, and mainly occurs after arrival in the ED and during hospitalisation for admitted patients. Prehospital professionals should make every effort to record a complete set of observations for any child and should be ready to lower their threshold for admission if they are unsure or feel uncomfortable with managing a paediatric patient at the scene.

Case Study 3

You are called to the home of a 2-month-old boy who stopped breathing and turned blue according to his babysitter. He reportedly had a fever all day. The infant is lying supine; his skin is pale and mottled. When touched, the infant becomes extremely irritable and exhibits a high-pitched, screeching cry. When left alone, he appears lethargic and poorly responsive. There is no abnormal positioning, and no abnormal airway sounds, stridor, nasal flaring, or grunting. The respiratory rate is 60 breaths/min and unlaboured. The heart rate is 200 beats/min. His peripheral pulses are weak and his extremities are cool to the touch. Capillary refill time is approximately 5 seconds.

1. Does this infant's appearance suggest a serious problem?
2. Is this infant in shock?

CASE STUDY ANSWERS

Case Study 1 — page 4

Beware of the pale child! Consider any child who has experienced significant trauma and is pale at the scene to have significant blood loss until proven otherwise. Children are able to compensate for blood loss and hypovolemia through catecholamine surges, which cause tachycardia and peripheral vasoconstriction. These reflexes inhibit the circulation to the skin and result in a pale patient. Although this child could have had a significant head injury based on mechanism of injury, his level of consciousness is reasonably normal; therefore, the initial issue needing emergent attention is haemorrhagic shock. Abdominal injuries with blunt trauma to the liver or spleen can result in significant internal bleeding without external signs of injury. Many children with internal bleeding do not always have abdominal tenderness. Indicators of suspected haemorrhagic shock are mild tachycardia, weak pulses, delayed capillary refill, and a borderline low blood pressure (80 mm Hg/palp). This child requires timely transport to a trauma centre with paediatric capabilities. Delay vascular access until the child is en route to the hospital.

This child is also clearly in pain. However, weigh the benefits of pharmacological therapy to relieve pain against the potential for circulatory collapse, delay in transport, and the need to effectively assess appearance. Use opiate analgesics, such as morphine, in patients with suspected compensated haemorrhagic shock cautiously because of morphine's vasodilatory effect.

Case Study 2 — page 15

The PAT is an accurate tool to evaluate severity of illness or injury, and to determine the urgency for providing life-saving care. Upon arrival at the scene of this patient, it is quite reassuring to find the toddler alert, pink, and with non-laboured respirations. His vigorous responses make it difficult to perform the conventional <C>ABCDE assessment. Since this child clearly has no serious immediate cardiorespiratory problems, is alert and awake, and fights your examination, history taking and secondary assessment can occur. However, the prehospital professional should transport every infant or child who has had a submersion injury to a hospital for observation of progression of symptoms. Still, the findings on the PAT allow the prehospital professional to slow the pace and get more information while on the scene. There is no need for immediate resuscitative interventions, and the prehospital professional can avoid the risk of "lights and siren" transport.

Anytime there is an unwitnessed submersion event, consider that a traumatic injury may be present. The usual mechanism of a toddler pool drowning involves falling less than 3 ft (1 m) into a body of water. In this scenario, it is unlikely that he has sustained a significant head or spinal injury. Furthermore, if he is moving his neck without apparent discomfort while in his mother's arms, but then vigorously screams and fights when you attempt to examine him, it is unlikely that spinal immobilisation will be helpful (and may prove more harmful and distressing than not). Local protocols govern this decision. Although treatment and transport of this patient are not emergent, ongoing assessment during transport is necessary. Pulmonary complications of submersion, primarily hypoxia, may have a delayed presentation.

Case Study 3 — page 26

Any infant who has an acute life-threatening event, who reportedly stopped breathing or turned blue, deserves ambulance transport, regardless of his or her appearance on your arrival. In this case, the need for urgent treatment and transport is obvious. One of the PAT indicators of shock in this infant is altered appearance. Although that finding could be due to causes other than poor brain perfusion (e.g., infection, trauma, toxins, hypoxia), the presence of effortless tachypnoea and pale, mottled skin supports the diagnosis of shock. Alternating lethargy and irritability may progress to unresponsiveness as perfusion worsens.

The hands-on examination confirms the suspicion of shock. This patient's heart rate is rapid at 200 beats/min, with weak peripheral pulses, cool extremities, and delayed capillary refill. Even without a blood pressure, the abnormal appearance and skin findings suggest that he should be treated for hypotensive shock. Although the cause of shock is unknown, treatment of any type of hypotensive shock includes vascular access and 20-ml/kg boluses of crystalloid fluid. Rapidly transport this patient to definitive care. Reassess his response to therapy frequently en route.

SUGGESTED READINGS

Textbooks

Advanced Life Support Group. *Advanced Paediatric Life Support*. Oxford: Wiley-Blackwell; 2016

Aehlert B. *Mosby's Comprehensive Pediatric Emergency Care*. Sudbury, MA: Elsevier; 2006.

American Academy of Pediatrics and the American College of Emergency Physicians. *APLS: The Pediatric Emergency Medicine Resource*. 5th ed. Burlington, MA: Jones & Bartlett Learning; 2012.

Chameides L, Samson RA, Schexnayder SM, Hazinski MF. *PALS Provider Manual*. Dallas, TX: American Heart Association; 2011.

College of Paramedics, Association of American Orthopedic Surgeons. *Nancy Caroline's Emergency Care In the Streets, United Kingdom*. Boston, MA: Jones & Bartlett Learning; 2016.

Douglas G, Nicol R, Robertson C (eds). *Macleod's Clinical Examination*. London: Churchill Livingstone; 2013.

Joint Royal Colleges Ambulance Liaison Committee. *UK Ambulance Services Clinical Practice Guidelines 2016*. Bridgwater: Class Professional Publishing; 2016.

Lissauer, T, Claydon, G. *Illustrated Textbook of Paediatrics*. 4th ed. London: Mosby; 2011.

Qureshi Z. *The Unofficial Guide to Paediatrics*. London: Zeshan Qureshi; 2017.

Resuscitation Council UK. *Emergency Paediatric Advanced Life Support Manual*. 4th ed. London: Resuscitation Council UK; 2016.

Tasker R, McClure R, Acerini C (eds). *Oxford Handbook of Paediatrics*. Oxford: Oxford University Press; 2013.

Articles

American Academy of Pediatrics. Emergency information forms and emergency preparedness for children with special health care needs (policy statement). *Pediatrics*. 2010;125:829–837.

Gausche M, Lewis R J, Stratton SJ et al. Effect of out-of-hospital pediatric endotracheal intubation on survival and neurological outcome: a controlled clinical trial. *JAMA*. 2000;283(6):783–90.

Gausche M. Out-of-hospital care of pediatric patients. *Pediatr Clin North Am*. 1999;46(6):1305–1327.

Green SM. Cheerio Laddie! Bidding farewell to the Glasgow Coma Score. *Ann Emerg Med*. 2011;58:427–430.

Maconochie I, Bingham R, Eich C et al. European Resuscitation Council Guidelines for Resuscitation 2015. Section 6. Paediatric life support. *Resuscitation*. 2015; 233–248.

Thompson DO, Hurtado TR, Liao MM, Byyny RL, Gravitz C, Haukoos JS. Validation of the Simplified Motor Score in the out-of-hospital setting for the prediction of outcomes after traumatic brain injury. *Ann Emerg Med*. 2011;58:417–425.

Tijssen JA, Prince DK, Morrison LJ, et al. Time on the scene and interventions are associated with improved survival in pediatric out-of-hospital cardiac arrest. *Resuscitation*. 2015;94:1–7.

Warren J. Guidelines for the inter- and intrahospital transport of critically ill patients. *Crit Care Med*. 2004;32(1):256–262.

Other Resources

National Institute for Clinical Excellence. *Fever in Under 5s.* London: NICE, 2013. https://www.nice.org.uk/guidance/cg160. Accessed May 30, 2018.

Nieman CT, Manacii CF, Super DM, Mancuso C, Fallon WF Jr. Use of Broselow tape may result in the under resuscitation of children. *Acad Emerg Med.* 2006;(10):1011–1019.

Proehl JA. Initial assessment and resuscitation. In: Hoyt KS, Selfridge-Thomas J, eds. *Emergency Nursing Core Curriculum.* 6th ed. St. Louis, MO: Saunders Elsevier; 2007:125.

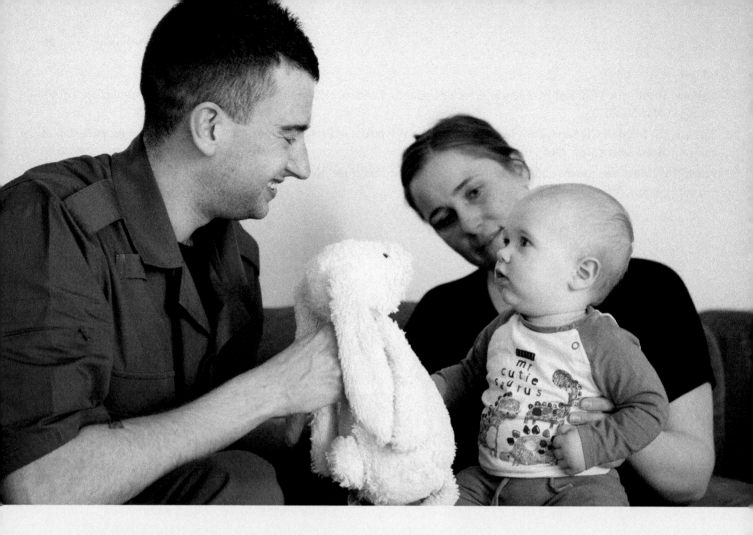

Learning Objectives

1. Discuss the communication challenges in handling the emotional responses of a family with a child who is ill or injured.

2. List the expected changes in vital signs with advancing age.

3. Describe key growth and development characteristics for the following groups: infants, toddlers, pre-school-aged children, school-aged children, adolescents, and children with special health care needs.

4. Explain unique anatomical and physiological characteristics that influence assessment of children in each group.

Using a Developmental Approach

Introduction

Infants and children constitute a small percentage of all patients seen in ambulance services. An even smaller percentage requires advanced life support (ALS). Clinicians must become comfortable with paediatric-specific information to promote success while interacting with this special patient population. Because of the unique anatomical, physiological, and developmental differences in children, clinicians must be well versed in normal developmental changes in infants and children. To successfully complete a paediatric patient assessment, the clinician must be able to incorporate an understanding of how a child's physical growth and psychosocial development relate to his or her condition.

In addition to knowing the growth and developmental characteristics of the different age groups, the prehospital professional must be aware of special considerations when assessing a child with special health care needs (CSHCN). Sometimes the chronological age of the CSHCN does not correspond with his or her developmental stage, and physical growth may not reflect emotional maturity.

Caring for a child also includes caring for the family. In addition to parents, caregivers, friends, and siblings may be present. Each person may have a different response to the child who is ill or injured, and the prehospital professional must be prepared to care for the entire "extended" family of friends and relatives. Communication skills are often as important as assessment and treatment skills in establishing an atmosphere of trust and comfort. Creating such an atmosphere requires that the prehospital clinician has a confident and professional attitude toward children's care, and uses age-appropriate paediatric skills. Communication skills become especially important in the event of a mass-casualty incident or natural disaster (see the *Children in Disasters* chapter).

This chapter addresses age-specific growth characteristics and assessment techniques for physiologically stable children from infancy to adolescence, and for CSHCN. The *Paediatric Assessment* chapter addresses general assessment techniques for the acutely ill or injured child, and the *Children with Special Health Care Needs* chapter expands the discussion on CSHCN.

Case Study 1

You have received a 999 call about a distressed infant. On your arrival, a frantic mother meets you at the door with her 4-week-old daughter in her arms. The infant is crying inconsolably. She has no retractions, but her skin is mottled on both the trunk and the extremities. Her arms and legs are cool. The mother tells you that the baby has been irritable all day, vomiting all her feeds, and the mother thinks her stomach looks swollen. She had a brief episode of floppiness and pallor, and the mother gave her several rescue breaths before calling 999.

1. What are the steps to assess and treat this child, and how will you address the mother's concerns?

2. What are the worrisome findings in this infant?

Paediatric Calls and Response From Family and Providers

Every family responds differently when a child is ill (**Figure 2-1**). Having an ill child places immense pressure on the family unit. Common responses are reviewed in **Table 2-1**. Although some parents' or caregivers' responses may seem too emotional or illogical, listen to their concerns. Acting as an advocate for proper care allows the clinician to care optimally for the paediatric patient. Parent or caregivers usually know the patient best and can provide vital information that allows the interaction with clinicians to be successful. Children, even infants, can quickly sense emotions in adults.

Just as a family may respond emotionally to a paediatric patient, so too may clinicians. Clinicians may also experience any of the emotional responses as outlined in Table 2-1.

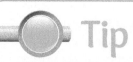

A family's response to a child's illness or injury is influenced by the child's developmental level, previous experience with the healthcare system, coping strategies, culture, availability of support systems, and nature of the emergency.

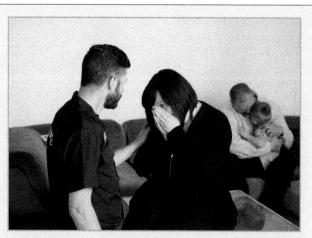

Figure 2-1 Every family responds differently to a child's illness or injury.
© Jones & Bartlett Learning.

Table 2-1 Common Responses of Caregivers to Acute Illness or Injury in a Child

Response	Description
Disbelief	Parents or caregivers may be struggling with the child's illness or injury. They may seem too calm or unconcerned.
Guilt	Parents or caregivers may be horrified that they are unable to recognise the serious nature of their child's condition or that they have been unable to prevent an injury. They may focus their attention on what should have been done, rather than on the child's immediate situation.
Anger	Parents or caregivers may show their concern as anger, and they may direct their anger at the prehospital professional. Caregivers may become hostile when the prehospital professional makes efforts to stabilise their child. They may attempt to refuse transport.
Physical symptoms	Parents or caregivers may have tachycardia, nausea, headache, chest pain, sweaty palms, dry mouth, or hyperventilation.

© Jones & Bartlett Learning

Acting in a calm, professional manner gains trust from the family or caregivers and also helps the prehospital professional to establish control of a potentially emotional situation. This approach also allows the providers to gain as much valuable information as possible from the family or caregivers, which ultimately helps triage the patient to the correct emergency department or include the most accurate differential diagnosis as part of the patient assessment.

The best way to reduce clinician's stress related to patient interactions is to remain up-to-date with paediatric treatment standards. Being familiar with the location of paediatric equipment, currently stocked equipment, and medications also decreases stress while interacting with an ill child. Because of the limited number of paediatric calls, being well versed with the paediatric devices on an ambulance becomes increasingly important.

Often providers feel guilt after interacting with an ill or injured infant or child. It is common for clinicians to think about the paediatric situation after the call. Depending on the situation, a single patient interaction can cause reflection for days, weeks, or months. Any clinician can experience difficult emotions after a stressful paediatric call. Clinicians should seek professional help from official sources of support such as counselling services and mental health support offered by both employers and professional services when unresolved stress results from these interactions.

Communication With the Child and Family or Caregiver

To approach infants and children effectively, clinicians should account for developmental information as it relates to the patient assessment at hand. Similar to interaction with adults, each paediatric patient is unique with a distinct personality that can impact the clinician's ability to obtain pertinent assessment information. Calling 999 is often a stressful situation for the patient and family. Approaching the patient gently and at his or her eye level is important in initiating communication with the child. The best policy is to be honest with a child, because mistrust can interfere with effectively finding important information about the situation at hand. Observing the patient's behaviour can provide clues to age-specific actions.

In addition to communication with the paediatric patient, communication with the caregiver or family is also important. Children seek clues from their parents regarding safety. Infants and children are never a single-patient 999 call. The family and caregivers must be treated as potential patients in the situation, because their involvement can provide necessary information to properly handle the situation. Whenever possible, the paediatric patient and family or caregiver should be kept together. A successful paediatric patient interaction includes information gathering from family and primary caregivers. Effective communication is the cornerstone of all effective healthcare.

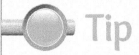

Communication skills are often as important as assessment and treatment skills.

Vital Signs Through the Ages

A common challenge in evaluating infants and children is determining when vital signs are normal based on the age of the patient. Respiratory rate, heart rate, blood pressure, and temperature all change with age. The presence or absence of fever, anxiety, or pain and the child's activity level also affect vital signs. In ill or injured children, the prehospital clinician must distinguish the impact of these outside influences on vital signs from changes caused by pathological processes. JRCALC gives approximate values but these are very dependent on other influences as mentioned above. The *Paediatric Assessment* chapter presents key physical characteristics and assessment techniques that assist the prehospital professional in separating a "sick" child from a "not sick" child.

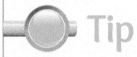

In infants, observe abdominal excursions and count rate for 30–60 seconds to obtain an accurate respiratory rate.

Respiratory Rate

Although normal values for vital signs vary with age, there are a number of physiological or anatomical bases for these changes. The normal range of respiratory rate slows with age because of an increase in the number of alveoli and increasing lung volume and lung compliance with physical growth. **Table 2-2** lists the normal respiratory rate for age.

Table 2-2 Normal Respiratory Rates of Age

Age	Respiratory Rate (breaths/min)
Birth to 11 months	30–40
12 to 24 months	25–35
2 to 4 years	25–30
5 to 11 years	20–25
12 years plus	15–20

Source: JRCALC 2016

At times it may be difficult to record the respiratory rate; it is best to count for at least 30 seconds (infants 30–60 seconds) to improve accuracy, especially in infants and younger children. In infants, observe and count abdominal excursions to obtain an accurate respiratory rate. As a child grows, breathing becomes less dependent on abdominal muscles and the diaphragm and more dependent on the chest muscles. Observing thoracic excursions provides an accurate respiratory rate in an older child.

Heart Rate

The baseline heart rate of infants and children slows with age, reflecting increasing control of the heart rate by the vagus nerve. The vagus nerve transmits cholinergic impulses, which slow the beating of the heart. **Table 2-3** lists normal heart rates for age. In addition, by 2 years of age a circadian rhythm in heart rate is present, seen in a fall of 10–20 beats/min, while the child is asleep. One confusing factor in assessing a child's heart rate during different phases of the sleep–wake cycle, or during different phases of respiration, is that the child's rhythm is more irregular than an adult's. This sinus arrhythmia is more prominent in toddlers to school-aged children and is caused by immature vagus nerve control (**Figure 2-2**).

Table 2-3 Normal Heart Rates for Age

Age	Heart Rate (beats/min)
Birth to 11 months	110–160
12 months to 2 years	110–150
2 to 4 years	95–140
5 to 11 years	80–120
12 years plus	60–100

Source: JRCALC 2016.

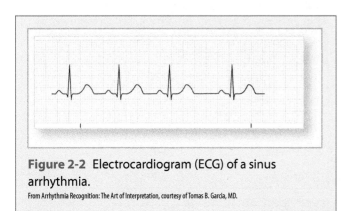

Figure 2-2 Electrocardiogram (ECG) of a sinus arrhythmia.
From Arrhythmia Recognition: The Art of Interpretation, courtesy of Tomas B. Garcia, MD.

Table 2-4 Normal Blood Pressure Values for Age

Age	Systolic Blood Pressure (mm Hg)
Birth to 11 months	70–90
12 to 24 months	80–95
2 to 4 years	80–100
5 years	90–100
6 years	80–110
7 to 11 years	90–110
12 years plus	100–120

Source: JRCALC 2016.

Blood Pressure

A child's blood pressure increases with age (**Table 2-4** lists normal systolic blood pressure values for age). The measured blood pressure is affected by equipment size. A cuff that is too small gives falsely elevated readings, whereas one that is too large gives readings that are too low. If diastolic pressure cannot be auscultated, a systolic pressure can be obtained by palpating the pulse. This value may be approximately 10 mm Hg lower than an auscultated pressure because of the relative insensitivity of palpation in appreciating initial pulsations as the cuff is deflated.

Temperature

Body temperature also varies with age and site of measurement. Newborn temperatures are often higher than those of older children, averaging 37.5°C during the first 6 months of life. After 3 years of age, the temperature falls to below 37.2°C, and finally to 36.7°C by 11 years of age. There is also a circadian rhythm to body temperature that develops by 5 years of age. This results in a lower temperature at night and a higher temperature during the day. A rectal temperature is the accepted as the most accurate but may not be practicable. A tympanic thermometer will provide good accuracy but may not be suitable for very small babies (under 6 months) due to the relatively small size of the ear canal. Temperature may also be obtained with temporal artery thermometers. These devices use infrared technology to measure temperature in the superficial temporal artery. If obtained with good technique, these are quite accurate. An axillary temperature is approximately 1°C lower than the rectal temperature. Normal body temperature decreases with increasing distance from the central circulation. Whichever method is used, follow any contemporary guidelines in place in the service you work for.

Growth Rates

Physical growth of infants and children includes body (somatic) growth and organ system growth. Skeletal and muscular growth has two spurts, the first from birth to 4 years of age and the second in adolescence (ages 9–14 for girls, ages 10–16 for boys). Brain, spinal cord, and nerve growth occurs maximally in the first few years of life and reaches adult proportions by 10 years of age.

The presence or absence of key secondary sex characteristics, especially pubic hair, marks a physiological turning point for children. Genital growth begins about 8 years of age in girls and 9 years of age in boys, but there is significant variation. When children have visible pubic hair, they have usually attained adult physiology and clinical care may then be given according to adult guidelines.

Anatomical Changes
Neck and Airway

The neck is short in infancy and elongates during childhood because of vertebral growth. As this occurs, anatomical landmarks also change in shape, size, and location. The epiglottis changes from a U-shape to the longer and thinner adult structure (**Figure 2-3**). It also moves in location from the level of the C1 vertebra to the C3 vertebra as the child's height increases. At birth, the larynx is only one-third the adult size. It becomes wider and longer until 3 years of age, and undergoes another growth spurt during puberty. At birth, the trachea is one-third the adult length, and increases 300% in circumference by puberty.

Chest and Lungs

At birth, the chest wall is round (anteroposterior, or AP, diameter equals lateral diameter). As the infant grows, it flattens out (lateral growth exceeds AP growth). Because an infant's chest wall is thin, heart and lung sounds are transmitted throughout the chest. Breath sounds are often audible on inspiration and expiration (bronchovesicular). In addition, secretions present anywhere in the respiratory tract are often heard throughout the chest. In an infant, respirations are mainly abdominal, because of the greater role of the diaphragm in breathing mechanics. By 6 years of age, breathing becomes more thoracic in origin, because of the development of chest wall musculature.

The lung tissue itself also changes with age. At birth, an infant has only 8% of the adult number of alveoli. The number of alveoli increases until 8 years of age, after which they increase in size but not number.

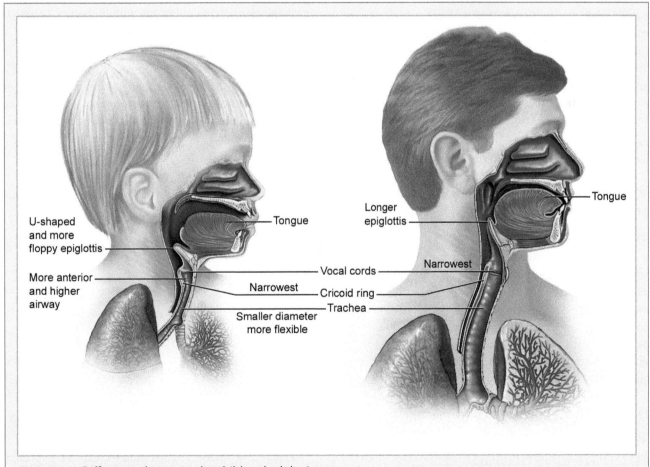

Figure 2-3 Differences between the child and adult airways.
© Jones & Bartlett Learning

Heart

At birth, the right ventricle is the same size as the left ventricle, a function of the demands of foetal circulation. This accounts for a right axis deviation seen on electrocardiograms (ECGs) in infants. However, the left ventricle quickly grows in size and muscle mass, and greatly outsizes the right ventricle with age. The left ventricle reaches adult proportions of 2:1 by 1 year of age.

Abdomen

A newborn infant has a protuberant abdomen for numerous reasons. The liver is relatively large, the stomach is more horizontal, and the lungs expand downward with movement of the diaphragm. The stomach capacity increases from 30–90 ml at birth, to 210–360 ml by 1 year of age, and 500 ml by 2 years of age. It assumes a more vertical position during childhood and reaches an adult volume of 750–900 ml. The abdomen also seems protuberant in toddlers because of a normal lumbar lordosis (curvature) of the spine. The abdomen becomes more scaphoid (flat) in school-aged children.

Musculoskeletal System

In infants and young children, new longitudinal bone growth occurs in secondary centres of ossification at the end of the long bones, vertebral bodies, and the cranium (physeal plates). These cartilaginous growth plates are relatively weak and are vulnerable to fractures exclusive to childhood. Bone growth ends with the ossification of the growth cartilage and union of the epiphysis and diaphysis. Growth in children is asymmetric, with the lower extremities, especially the distal extremities (e.g., feet), growing before puberty and the trunk during puberty.

Muscle growth includes an increase in the size of muscle cells. There is a growth spurt in the number of muscle cells at 2 years of age, with a maximal increase during puberty. The proportion of muscle mass to body weight changes during childhood, going from 1:5 at birth to 1:3 in adolescence.

Nervous System

The growth of the nervous system occurs rapidly during infancy. It is 25% the adult size at birth, 50% by 1 year of age, 80% by 3 years of age, and 90% by 7 years of age. This includes growth of glial cells, dendrites, and synaptic connections. This growth is associated with rapid increase in fine motor, gross motor, and language skills of infants and toddlers. These changing competencies impact the type of assessment techniques appropriate for evaluating children of different ages.

Summary of Changes in Vital Signs and Anatomy Through Childhood

Vital signs are useful for assessment but are sometimes difficult to obtain and difficult to interpret. Not only do normal vital signs change significantly with age, but respiratory and heart rates are especially sensitive to adrenaline release because of fear, pain, anxiety, cold, or high activity level. Other anatomical changes in the airway, chest, heart, abdomen, musculoskeletal system, and nervous system occur throughout childhood and require adaptations in assessment techniques.

Infants
Developmental Characteristics

Infants are vulnerable and have a limited number of behaviours (**Figure 2-4**). Infants less than 2 months of age spend most of their time sleeping or eating. They are not yet able to tell the difference between parents and other caregivers or strangers. They need to be kept warm, dry, and fed. They experience the world through their bodies. Being held, cuddled, or rocked soothes the infant. Hearing is also well developed at birth, and calm and reassuring talk is often helpful.

Infants between 2 and 6 months of age are more active, which makes them easier to evaluate. They spend more time awake, they begin to make eye contact, and they recognise caregivers. Healthy infants in this age group have a strong suck, active extremity movement, and a vigorous cry. They may follow a bright light or toy with their eyes, or turn their heads toward a loud sound or the caregiver's voice.

Between the ages of 6 and 12 months, most infants learn to say two or three words with meaning or 'babble', sit unsupported, reach for toys, move objects from one hand to another, and put things in their mouths. At approximately 1 year of age, most infants start to crawl, pull themselves to a standing position, use furniture to stand, and possibly start to walk.

At 7–8 months, infants show a clear preference for their parents or caregivers, and by the age of 9–10 months

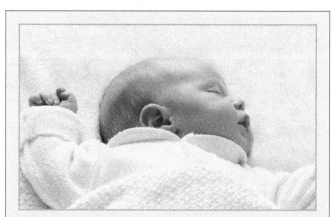

Figure 2-4 Infants are vulnerable creatures, with a limited number of behaviours.

demonstrate stranger anxiety, making separation of the child and parent or caregiver for the purposes of assessment or transport especially problematic. They are most easily comforted by their parent or by a familiar adult. **Table 2-5** summarises anatomical and physiological differences that are important in the assessment and care of the infant.

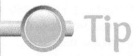

Tip

An infant less than 3 months of age who is reported to be irritable, feeding poorly, or sleeping excessively, or who has a temperature greater than 38°C must be seen by a doctor.

The infant's capacity to interact with the environment is limited, and signs and symptoms of illness are not always easy to appreciate. Because of these factors, always take the parent or caregiver's perception that "something is wrong" seriously. *An infant in the first 3 months of life who is reported to be irritable, feeding poorly, or sleeping excessively, or who has a temperature greater than 38°C must be seen by a doctor.* It is important to find out if there has been a recent history of trauma, how the infant was acting before the event, and if the infant has been healthy since birth. Find out if the infant was born at term and if there were any problems during pregnancy, labour, delivery, or immediately after the birth. The Personal Child Health Record (also known as the PCHR or 'red book') will provide useful information about

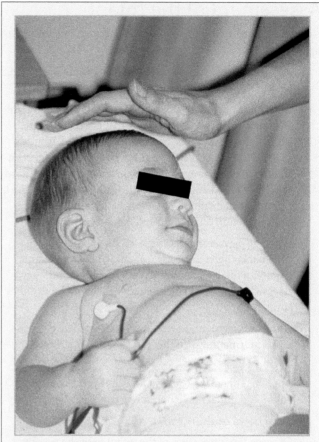

Figure 2-5 The infant's head is disproportionately large compared to older children and adults. The head may be a source of significant heat loss.
Courtesy of Ron Deickmann, MD

a child and should always be taken with you to hospital. In the UK, it is a national standard book forming the main record of a child's health and development and is updated each time the child has contact with any healthcare professional. In the first few months of life, excessive irritability or sleeping, fever, and poor feeding may be symptoms of a very serious illness, such as sepsis or congenital heart disease. Apnoea is a common presenting complaint in the infant. Periods of apnoea may be a sign of infection, heart disease, seizure activity, head injury, or a metabolic problem, such as hypoglycaemia. As the infant grows older and the behavioural repertoire expands, making the "sick" versus "not sick" decision becomes easier.

Important Conditions in Infants

- Viral syndromes (vomiting and diarrhoea)
- Respiratory problems
- Fever
- Ear infections
- Sudden unexpected death in infancy (SUDI)
- Child abuse

Table 2-5 Anatomical and Physiological Features of Infants

- Infants are nose breathers for the first several months of life. Obstruction of the nose from secretions, blood, or oedema may cause respiratory distress.

- The muscles of the infant's chest wall are not yet developed, and the abdominal muscles are the main muscles used for breathing. "Belly breathing" is normal in infants and may become exaggerated as breathing becomes more rapid.

- Retractions are easily seen in the infant with respiratory distress.

- A faster metabolic rate increases the need for oxygen and nutrients.

- Because of immature temperature regulation and high body surface-to-mass ratio, infants are at risk for heat loss and hypothermia if left undressed.

- The head is large in proportion to the body (**Figure 2-5**) and may be a potential source of significant heat loss.

Assessment of the Infant

Conduct the assessment of the infant using the following principles:

- Obtain the name of the child and use it while interacting with the child.

- Obtain the normal disposition of the child and compare it to the current behaviour being displayed; in other words establish what is 'normal' for that child, bearing in mind the variability in developmental stages between children of similar ages. Any acute change in disposition should be noted and relayed during the handover report. Communicate with the infant using a confident but smiling face directed at the infant.

- Have the parent or caregiver hold the infant while the clinician completes the assessment. Unless the infant requires a life-saving intervention, the infant is better assessed in the arms of someone with whom he or she is familiar.

- Observe, auscultate, and palpate in this order to get the most information with the least amount of stress to the infant (**Figure 2-6**).

- Approach the infant slowly and calmly, because loud voices and quick movements may frighten him or her.

- Squat down or sit at "baby level".

- Observe the interaction of the infant with the caregiver. At 7–8 months, infants may begin to show stranger anxiety.

- A comfortable environment is important. An infant who is happily snuggled in a parent or caregiver's arms may become irritable and cry when unwrapped and placed on cold sheets.

- If the infant begins to cry, a pacifier, blanket, or favourite toy may help to calm him or her. Avoid feeding the infant who is seriously ill or injured.

- Perform the assessment based on the infant's activity level. For example, if the infant is calm, get the respiratory rate and auscultate lung sounds at the beginning of the assessment.

- Make non-threatening physical contact first, such as touching an extremity to assess warmth and capillary refill. Perform the most upsetting parts of the examination last.

- Use a warmed stethoscope and warm hands and handle the infant gently. Avoid doing anything potentially painful or distressing until near completion of the assessment. It is difficult to assess heart and lung sounds or to palpate the abdomen when the infant is crying.

- In the older infant who may have stranger anxiety, have the caregiver remove the baby's clothing. Remove one item of clothing at a time and then replace it, if possible, to avoid heat loss and hypothermia.

 Think Point

The older infant is fearful of separation and develops stranger anxiety. Approach slowly and assess the infant while he or she is being held by the caregiver.

Toddlers
Developmental Characteristics

Toddlers (ages 1–3 years) experience rapid changes in growth and development. By approximately 18 months of age, the toddlers are able to run, feed themselves, play with toys, and communicate with others. They begin making their own decisions and asserting their independence. The "terrible two" stage actually begins at about 1 year of age and often lasts into the third year. Toddlers are mobile and opinionated, and may be terrified of strangers. They are illogical by nature and are intensely curious but lack a sense of danger. Problem solving is concrete because toddlers cannot reason abstractly. Learning is done by trial and error, with little anticipation of consequences. Toddlers are playful, imaginative thinkers and are tremendously self-centred. They understand ownership and label things (e.g., toys) as "mine".

Language capabilities vary widely. Some toddlers utter only single words, whereas others may speak in paragraphs. They often understand what is said, even if they cannot respond with words. Older toddlers may remember earlier experiences with doctors or nurses, such as vaccinations or stitches, and be fearful about being examined.

The toddler's anatomy and physiology are much like the infant's, notably a large head and use of abdominal muscles to breathe. Thermoregulation is better, and limb muscles are more developed.

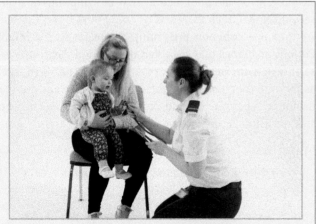

Figure 2-6 Approaching an infant: observe the infant in the caregiver's arms before palpating or auscultating.
© Jones & Bartlett Learning.

Case Study 2

You respond to a call for a 2-year-old who is having respiratory difficulty. On your arrival, you hear a barking cough from the child's room. When you enter, the child is sitting up in bed, starts to cry, and hides behind his mother. With crying, his breathing becomes noisier, and he becomes more anxious. Even though he has pyjamas on, you can see suprasternal retractions. His skin is pink. His mother states he was fine today, but suddenly woke up during the night "gasping for air".

1. Is this appropriate behaviour for this child?

2. How can you assess this child without making him more upset?

Common Ailments in Toddlers

- Viral syndromes (vomiting and diarrhoea)
- Respiratory problems
- Febrile seizures
- Ear infections
- Child abuse
- Unintentional ingestions
- Open wounds

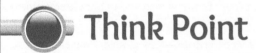

Think Point

Do not separate the older infant or toddler from the parent or caregiver.

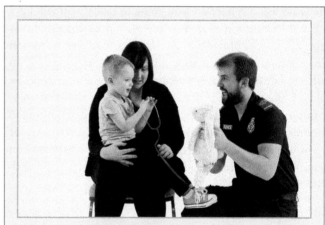

Figure 2-7 Approaching a toddler: offer a toy or distraction tool to help with the assessment.
© Jones & Bartlett Learning.

Assessment of the Toddler

Conduct the assessment of the toddler using the following principles:

- Obtain the name of the child and use it while interacting with the patient.
- Obtain the normal disposition of the child and compare it to the current behaviour being displayed. Any acute change in disposition should be noted and relayed during the handover report.
- Approach the toddler slowly and keep physical contact to a minimum until he or she is familiar with you. Watch the toddler's activity level and behaviour as you approach.
- Communicate with the toddler using a confident but friendly tone of voice.
- Sit or squat and use a quiet, soothing voice. Allow the toddler to remain on the parent or caregiver's lap.
- Use play and distraction tools, such as a penlight or teddy bear, to help with the assessment (**Figure 2-7**).

Introduce equipment slowly and encourage the toddler to hold it.

- Talk to the toddler, preferably about himself or herself. Admire his or her clothes; ask about pets or recent events. A toddler is the centre of his or her universe.
- Give the toddler limited choices, such as "Do you want me to listen to your tummy or your heart first?" This provides the toddler with a sense of control.
- Avoid questions that the toddler can answer with "no".
- Use simple, concrete terms. Provide a lot of reassurance and praise.
- Perform the most critical parts of the assessment first, working from toe to head, with the head and neck last.
- Ask for caregiver assistance with the assessment. The toddler is often less upset if the caregiver removes the toddler's clothes or administers oxygen.
- If necessary, ask the caregiver to gently palpate the toddler's extremity to test for pain.
- Do not expect toddlers to sit still and cooperate. Be flexible but thorough.

- In certain situations, the toddler may be extremely difficult to examine. If he or she is alert but resists the examination, determine the care plan based on history. Use of lights and sirens during transport may increase the toddler's level of fear.

Pre-school-Aged Children
Developmental Characteristics

Pre-school-aged children (ages 3–5 years) are creative and illogical thinkers (**Figure 2-8**). They are not always able to distinguish between fantasy and reality, and they have many misconceptions about illness, injury, and bodily functions. For example, a pre-school-aged child might think of a cut as "my insides leaking out". If you tell a pre-school-aged child you are going to take his or her pulse, they may ask, "Where are you going to take it and will I get it back?" Common fears for this age group include body mutilation, loss of control, death, darkness, and being left alone. Attention span is short. It is always best to maintain honesty about painful procedures. Information should be told as close to the procedure as possible to avoid miscommunication and increased anxiety. Pre-school-aged patients can be easily distracted by parents, caregivers or friendly clinicians. Positively rewarding these patients can help them maintain a good memory about interacting with clinicians.

Common Ailments in Pre-school-Aged Children

- Unintentional ingestions
- Respiratory problems
- Febrile seizures
- Viral syndromes (vomiting and diarrhoea)
- Open wounds
- Child abuse

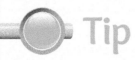

Tip

Pre-school-aged children are creative thinkers who fear loss of control. Explain procedures in simple terms, allow them to handle equipment, and assess from toe to head.

Assessment of the Pre-school-Aged Child

Conduct the assessment of the pre-school-aged child using the following principles:

- Obtain the name of the child, and use it while interacting with the child.
- Obtain the normal disposition of the child and compare it to the current behaviour being displayed. Any acute change in disposition should be noted and relayed during the handover report.
- Use simple terms to explain procedures.
- Choose words carefully, using language that is age-appropriate and that does not induce fear.
- Clarify any apparent misconceptions.
- Use dolls or puppets, if available, to explain what you are doing.
- When appropriate, allow the child to handle equipment (**Figure 2-9**). Allow the patient to help.
- Set limits on behaviour—for example, "You can cry or scream, but don't bite or kick".
- Praise good behaviour.
- Use games or distraction tools.
- Use dressings or bandages freely.
- Focus and carry out one thing at a time.

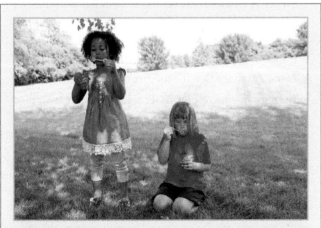

Figure 2-8 Pre-school-aged children are creative and illogical thinkers.
© Jones & Bartlett Learning. Courtesy of Glen Ellman.

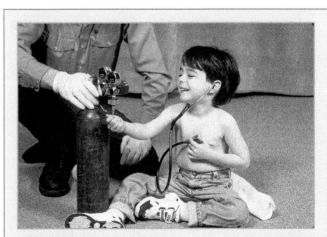

Figure 2-9 When approaching a pre-school-aged child, allow the child to handle the equipment.
© Jones & Bartlett Learning. Courtesy of Glen Ellman.

School-Aged Children
Development Characteristics

School-aged children are talkative, analytical, and able to understand the concept of cause and effect (**Figure 2-10**). They feel a sense of accomplishment as they acquire new skills. Their knowledge of how bodies work may be unclear, and they have limited ability to gauge the seriousness of a particular illness or injury. With careful choice of words, they can understand simple explanations about their bodies, and they like to be involved in their own care.

Common fears include separation from parents and friends, loss of control, pain, and physical disability. They are often afraid to talk about their feelings and may be unable to put their feelings into words. As they become more mobile and more independent, they begin to take more risks. They live in the present. Belonging and peer group support are important.

The anatomy and physiology of a child is similar to an adult's by about 8 years of age.

Common Conditions in School-Aged Children

- Poisonings/ingestion
- Respiratory problems
- Fractures (e.g., sports injuries)
- Open wounds
- Viral syndromes (vomiting and diarrhoea)

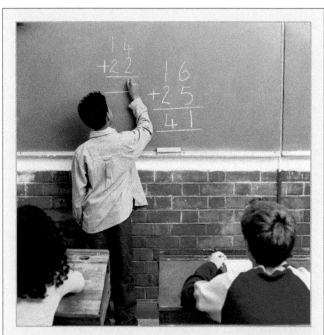

Figure 2-10 School-aged children are talkative, analytical, and able to understand the concept of cause and effect.
© Stockbyte/Creatas

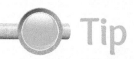

Tip

School-aged children fear separation from caregivers, loss of control, pain, and physical disability. Explain procedures and anticipate questions, provide privacy, and conduct assessment from head to toe.

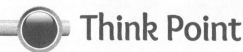

Think Point

Offering choices that are not real violates the child's sense of trust. Tell the school-aged child what you are going to do, and do it!

Assessment of the School-Aged Child

Conduct the assessment of the school-aged child using the following principles:

- Obtain the name of the child, and use it while interacting with the child.
- Obtain the normal disposition of the child and compare it to the current behaviour being displayed. Any acute change in disposition should be noted and relayed during the handover report.
- Speak directly to the child, and then include the parent or caregiver. Be careful not to offer too much information.
- Anticipate the child's questions and fears, and discuss them immediately.
- Explain in simple terms what is wrong and how it will affect them. For example, when speaking to a 5-year-old, you may explain, "Your arm bone is broken, but the doctor will be able to make it better. We'll give you some medicine in your arm to help stop it from hurting so much".
- Explain procedures immediately before doing them. Never lie to a child, telling the child that something will not hurt or that you are almost finished if this is not true. Remember that the child may not ask questions, even if he or she has real concerns.
- Ask the older school-aged child if he or she would like to have the parent or caregiver present.
- Provide privacy. Children in this age group are modest. Expose the child for physical assessment as necessary and cover him or her up when done.
- If physical restraint is necessary to complete a procedure or to guarantee the safety of the child or crew, tell the

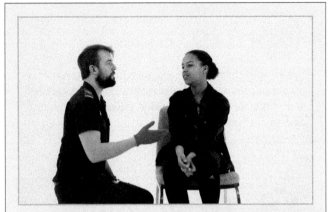

Figure 2-11 Approaching a school-aged child: let the child be involved in his or her own care.
© Jones & Bartlett Learning.

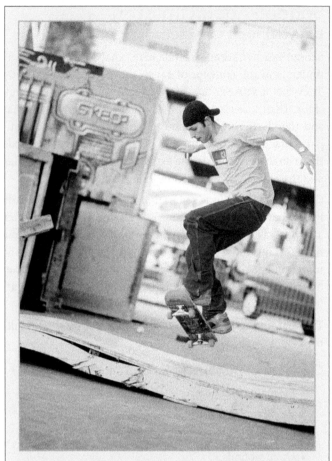

Figure 2-12 Adolescence is a time of experimentation and risk-taking behaviours.
© Photos.com

child what is going to happen and then do it. Great care should be taken in doing this.

- Do not negotiate unless the child really has a choice. For example, it is okay to ask the child if he or she would like the intravenous (IV) line in the right or left hand but not to ask if it is okay to start an IV when it must be done.

- Let the child be involved in his or her own care. Children in this age group are afraid of being out of control (**Figure 2-11**).

- Reassure the child that being ill or injured is not a punishment.

- Praise the child for cooperating. Be careful not to be irritable if the child does not cooperate.

- The physical assessment can usually be done in the head-to-toe format.

Adolescents
Growth and Development Characteristics

Although they are going through a range of differing emotions (and at times behaviours), adolescents are rational, understand cause and effect, and are able to express themselves with words. Adolescence is a time of experimentation and risk-taking behaviours (**Figure 2-12**). Adolescents may believe they are immune to danger, that they are "indestructible". They gradually shift from relying on family to relying on friends for psychological support and social development.

Adolescents struggle with independence, loss of control, body image, sexuality, and peer pressure. Anything that makes them different from their peers may cause anxiety. Psychosomatic complaints are common in this age group. They may have mood swings or depression, and when ill or injured may act younger than their age, leaving a scared child in an adult body.

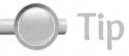

Tip

Adolescents struggle with independence, loss of control, body image, sexuality, and peer pressure. Provide concrete information, respect their privacy, and speak to them directly.

Common Conditions in Adolescents

- Poisonings/drug ingestion
- Respiratory problems
- Fractures (e.g., sports injuries)
- Open wounds

Assessment of the Adolescent

Conduct the assessment of the adolescent using the following principles:

- Obtain the name of the child, and use it while interacting with the child.

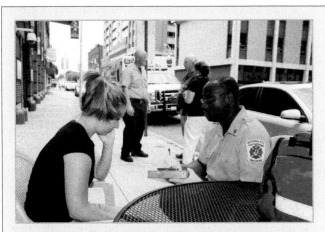

Figure 2-13 When approaching an adolescent, speak to him or her directly.
© Jones & Bartlett Learning. Courtesy of MIEMSS.

- Obtain the normal disposition of the child and compare it to the current behaviour being displayed. Any acute change in disposition should be noted and relayed during the handover report.
- Provide accurate information about the illness or injury, normal body functions, and interventions. Explain what you are doing and why.
- Encourage the patient to ask questions and to be involved in his or her own care.
- Show respect. Speak directly to the adolescent. Do not turn to the caregiver for initial information (**Figure 2-13**).
- Respect the adolescent's modesty, privacy, and confidentiality unless it places him or her at risk.
- Be honest and non-judgmental.
- Do not be misled by the adolescent's size or make assumptions about his or her comprehension of events. Adolescents may misinterpret the seriousness of the situation. They may also have many fears about permanent injury, disfigurement, or "being different" as a result of the illness or injury. Give adolescents accurate information and anticipate their questions or fears.
- Avoid becoming frustrated or angry if the adolescent does not talk or is uncooperative.
- Enlist the adolescent's friends to help persuade the adolescent to cooperate with the assessment or treatment, if he or she resists.

Children With Special Health Care Needs
Growth and Development Characteristics

When working with children with special health care needs (CSHCN), it is important to consider developmental age, rather than chronological age. Information about the patient should be obtained from caregivers. If a clinician does not fully understand the child's medical or developmental history, it is better to be honest than to feign understanding and potentially place the patient at risk. CSHCN may have any type of chronic condition that affects health, normal growth, or development. This may include physical disability, developmental or learning disability, technological dependency, or chronic illness. The developmental or learning disability may include mental impairment, difficulties in communication, sensory impairment, or limitations in physical activity. The child who is technology dependent may have a home ventilator, tracheostomy, gastric feeding tube, or long-term IV device. Specific categories of patients and methods of assessment and treatment are discussed in the *Children with Special Health Care Needs* chapter.

The number of children in the community with special needs is growing. Prehospital clinicians must be familiar with the conditions and types of technology used in assessing and treating CSHCN. These children may require transport and care for exacerbation of their illness or for an unrelated illness or injury.

Unique aspects related to children with special needs include:

- Baseline vital signs may be outside the age-appropriate values.
- Weight may be significantly higher or lower than expected.
- Standard prehospital quick reference guides may be inaccurate.
- The child may have a limited ability to endure respiratory distress or shock.
- Be alert for a latex allergy.

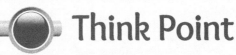 **Think Point**

Do not assume that a child with a physical disability is cognitively impaired. Always ask the parent or caregiver to clarify the child's normal level of functioning and interaction.

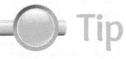 Tip

Even if a disabled child cannot talk or interact, show your respect by introducing yourself, explaining what you are doing, and providing verbal reassurance.

Assessment of a CSHCN

Conduct the assessment of the CSHCN using the following principles:

- Obtain the name of the child, and use it while interacting with the child.

- Obtain the normal disposition of the child and compare it to the current behaviour being displayed. Any acute change in disposition should be noted and relayed during the handover report. Include the impressions of the caregiver in chart documentation. Ask the parent or caregiver what he or she thinks of the child's condition, activity, and behaviours. Find out if the parent or caregiver believes that the child is "not acting right".

- Get a careful history. The parent or caregiver can provide detailed information about the child's medical history, medications, and current complaints. He or she is also aware of how best to approach the child, and of typical responses and behaviours.

- Approach the child with a developmental delay gently and using techniques appropriate to his or her developmental level, not chronological age. Use language and techniques tailored to the child's cognitive level to communicate.

- Do not assume that the child with a physical disability is mentally impaired (**Figure 2-14**). Ask the caregiver about the child's level of function and interaction with others. To get at baseline functional level you might query, "What would Johnny be doing right now, if he were feeling well?"

- Use polite, professional behaviour; acknowledge the caregivers' expertise; and take their concerns seriously. Families of chronically ill children usually have had extensive experience with the medical system. If most of their experiences have been good, they will very likely perceive the prehospital clinician as an ally. However,

if they have had bad experiences, they may feel a need to be very vigilant in protecting their child and be perceived as difficult or controlling.

- Keep in mind the amount of stress that the caregiver of a CSHCN may be experiencing and be empathic. It is often helpful to acknowledge their stress about the care being provided.

Tips for the Clinician

Infant (0–11 months):

- Be diligent about keeping infants warm and dry to limit hypothermia.

- This is a particularly stressful time for parents adjusting to the eating, sleeping, and crying cycle; sometimes this is complicated by postpartum depression, which can be a risk factor for abuse.

- Persistent crying or irritability can be a symptom of serious illness.

- Although infants sleep a lot, they should rouse easily; inability to rouse a baby should be considered an emergency.

- Head control is limited until closer to 6 months, so when handling a baby, make sure to support the head and neck well.

- By 6 months, babies should make eye contact; lack of eye contact in a sick infant could be a sign of significant illness, depressed mental status, or delayed development.

- By 6–12 months, infants are at risk for foreign body aspiration and poisoning because of exploration of the environment with their mouths.

- Reduce separation anxiety by keeping the child and parent together during evaluation and involving the parent in the treatment if appropriate.

- Crawling and walking can increase exposure to physical dangers and injuries.

Toddlers (12–24 months):

- Persistent crying or irritability can be a symptom of serious illness.

- Due to a lack of molars, there is an increased risk of choking, because children may not be able to grind up food before swallowing.

- Increased mobility increases exposure to physical dangers and injury.

- Distracting a child with a flashlight or toy may aid in physical examination.

- Allow a child to hold objects of importance to him or her (e.g., blanket).

- Try to make the interaction as positive as possible; painful procedures make for lasting impressions.

Pre-school-aged children (2–4 years):

- The rapid increase in language means they understand much of what is said if simple terms are used.

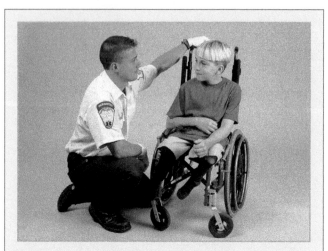

Figure 2-14 Approaching the CSHCN: obtain a thorough history and identify developmentally appropriate approaches that work best with the child.

© Jones & Bartlett Learning

- Respect the patient's modesty and cover him or her up after the physical examination.

- Foreign body airway obstruction risk continues to be high.

- Offer choices to the patient if appropriate (e.g., "Should I listen to your front first or the back?").

- Do not waste time trying to use logic to convince pre-school-aged children; they are concrete thinkers. Avoid frightening or misleading comments.

- Appealing to their magical thinking may allow you to do more (e.g., "This magic mist will help you breathe better (nebuliser)".).

- Communicate about procedures as close to doing them as possible.

- Respect modesty.

School-aged children (5–11 years):

- Provide simple explanations for illness and treatments.

- Be honest about painful procedures.

- If possible, provide sense of control by giving choices.

- Respect the patient's modesty.

- Ask about school/sports/activities or interests to allow patients to warm up to you faster.

Adolescents (12–18 years):

- Explain things as clearly and honestly as you would to an adult.

- Give choices when appropriate.

- Respect modesty.

- Be honest about procedures that will cause discomfort.

- Address concerns and fears about the lasting effects of their injuries.

- Adolescence includes hormonal surges, emotions, and peer pressure; there is increased risk for substance abuse, self-endangerment, pregnancy, and dangerous sexual practices.

Summary

Understanding the developmental characteristics for each age group is essential for accurate assessment and treatment of the child in the prehospital environment. Good field care requires good communication with the child and family. The family may include a large number of people, all of whom become "patients". CSHCN pose additional challenges in assessment, but their parents and caregivers can be a great asset in guiding prehospital evaluation and management.

Every call experience offers the ability for a clinician to learn something. With paediatric patients, the opportunities are larger than with adults. Post-incident self-evaluation and call analysis can offer clinicians an opportunity to identify ways to improve for the next paediatric patient interaction.

Case Study 3

You respond to the scene of a car versus cycle road traffic collision. The rider is a 14-year-old boy, who is now walking around the scene. He was wearing a helmet and denies any loss of consciousness. His only complaints are that his wrist hurts, the front wheel of his bike is bent, and he will be late to meet his friends. He does not want to be examined, definitely does not want to go to the hospital, and starts to leave the scene as you approach him.

1. Is this teenager's reaction normal?

2. What techniques can help you adequately assess his injuries?

CASE STUDY ANSWERS

Case Study 1 — page 32

Even though the mother is distressed, it is important to get additional history: Was the infant full-term? Did she have any problems with delivery or after birth? Has she had feeding problems or vomiting in the past? Any fever or diarrhoea?

Infants in the first few months of life have a limited range of behaviours, so anything out of the ordinary in the child's feeding, sleeping, or basic activity level is concerning for serious underlying illness or injury. Any infant who reportedly had an apnoeic episode that resulted in colour change (pallor, cyanosis) or unresponsiveness may have had a critical illness. Causes of critical illness include sepsis, congenital heart disease, metabolic abnormalities, seizures, oesophageal reflux, and brain injury. These diagnoses are impossible to establish in the pre-hospital setting and require emergency department evaluation.

Reassuring the mother is important, but this baby may be critically ill, and requires rapid assessment and transport. Although an infant's extremities may be mottled because of cold, mottling of the trunk is an extremely worrying sign, reflecting poor perfusion. The possibility of hypovolaemic shock is supported by the baby's cool extremities and history of vomiting. Furthermore, although infants can develop abdominal distention because of crying and swallowing air, abdominal distention in association with vomiting and signs of shock (abnormal appearance and abnormal circulation to skin) suggest serious pathology, such as intestinal obstruction.

Move the baby quickly into the ambulance, explaining what you are doing and why to the mother. Where permissible allow the mother to travel with you to the hospital. Treatment of this infant includes administration of oxygen by a face mask and rapid transport to an emergency department. Prevention of heat loss by swaddling the baby and applying a hat is important, because hypothermia is a risk for a small infant. Consider vascular access en route, with a bolus of 20 ml/kg of crystalloid fluid.

Case Study 2 — page 39

Toddlers are often fearful of strangers, so enlisting the help of parents or caregivers makes patient assessment much easier. Allow the child to remain with the parent. Sit on the bed or crouch down to the child's eye level, and use a calm soothing voice. You can use distractions, such as a penlight, or ask about a stuffed animal on the bed, to gain the child's attention and to evaluate interactivity. Ask the parent to remove the child's pyjamas and observe the work of breathing, including suprasternal, subcostal, or intercostal retractions, and respiratory rate. Although your main concern is the child's respiratory status, you may have to perform other portions of the hands-on examination, such as touching or tickling the child's toes before you get to the chest. When listening to breath sounds, warm the stethoscope beforehand, and explain what you are doing. If the child resists, you may be able to listen to a stuffed animal first, and allow the child to do the same, before resuming your examination.

Your assessment reveals the child's respiratory rate is 32 breaths/min and heart rate is 128 beats/min. You decide to give the child oxygen, but he refuses to keep the oxygen mask in place even with his mother's help, a response you recognise is typical of a toddler who is not seriously ill. For transport to the hospital, you secure the child in a suitable child seat in the ambulance, allowing his mother to accompany you in the ambulance, and direct blow-by oxygen in his direction.

Case Study 3 — page 45

This teenager is asserting his independence. Under the Children Act 1989, a child's competence to consent to treatment should be assessed, appropriate to the patient's age; in the case of a 14 year old, this would be more usual compared with much younger children. This is based on 'Gillick competence'. He may not realise the risks of occult injury. Show respect, be honest and non-judgmental, and speak directly to him. Explain why it is important to check him for potentially serious injuries, and offer him the privacy of the ambulance to conduct the examination. Encourage him as far as possible to allow care to be given, but if he still refuses care, attempt to contact his parents or caregivers or enlist the assistance of police. This area of law in the UK is less than straightforward and varies between, for example, Scotland and England. If in doubt, seek advice from more senior colleagues and act in accordance with any contemporary guidelines that apply.

SUGGESTED READINGS

Textbooks

American Academy of Pediatrics, American College of Emergency Physicians. *APLS: The Pediatric Emergency Medicine Resource*. 5th ed. Burlington, MA: Jones & Bartlett Learning; 2012.

Behrman R, Kliegman R, Jenson H. *Nelson Textbook of Pediatrics*. 20th ed. Philadelphia, PA: Elsevier; 2015.

Cowie H. *From Birth to Sixteen: Children's Health, Social, Emotional and Linguistic Development*. Abingdon: Routledge; 2012.

Joint Royal Colleges Ambulance Liaison Committee, Association of Ambulance Chief Executives. *UK Ambulance Services Clinical Practice Guidelines 2016*. Bridgwater: Class Professional Publishing; 2016.

Marx JA, Hockberger RS, Walls RM. *Rosen's Emergency Medicine Concepts and Clinical Practice*. 7th ed. Philadelphia, PA: Mosby; 2009.

Samuels M and Wieteska S. *Advanced Paediatric Life Support A Practical Approach to Emergencies*. 6th ed. Chichester: Wiley Blackwell; 2016

Sharma A & Cockerill H. *Mary Sheridan's from birth to five years*. 4th ed. Abington, Oxon: Routledge; 2014.

Tintinalli J. *Emergency Medicine: A Comprehensive Study Guide*. 8th ed. Columbus, OH: McGraw Hill; 2016.

Zitelli B, McIntire S, Nowalk AJ. *Zitelli and Davis' Atlas of Pediatric Physical Diagnosis*. 7th ed. Philadelphia, PA: Elsevier; 2017.

Legislation

Gillick v. West Norfolk and Wisbech AHA and the DHSS (1985) 3 All ER 402.

UK Government. *Children Act 1989*. Available at: https://www.legislation.gov.uk/ukpga/1989/41/contents. Accessed 30th May 2018.

Further Resources

Further information, evidence and research are available from the Royal College of Paediatrics and Child Health and the National Institute for Health and Care Excellence.

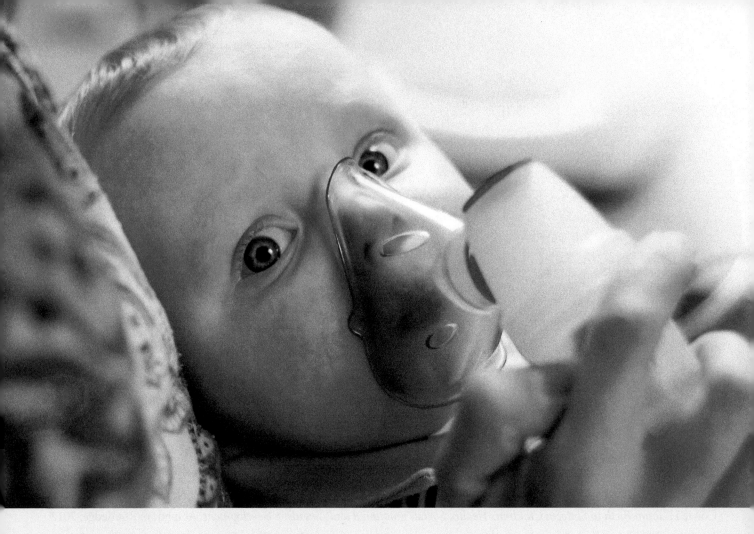

Learning Objectives

1. Describe how to assess airway and breathing, including interpreting information from the Paediatric Assessment Triangle and the <C>ABCDEs.

2. Differentiate between respiratory distress, respiratory failure, and respiratory arrest based on history, physical examination, and physiological monitoring.

3. Define the physiological information provided by pulse oximetry and capnometry, recognise situations in which each should be used, and recognise appropriate management responses to abnormal measurements.

4. Outline a general treatment strategy, going from the least to the most invasive, for children with respiratory compromise.

5. Contrast the key signs, symptoms, and management of upper airway obstruction versus lower airway obstruction.

6. Discuss possible complications of assisted ventilation, and outline strategies to identify and correct these complications.

Respiratory Emergencies

Introduction

Respiratory disease is the most frequent paediatric prehospital medical problem. Of all conditions causing respiratory disease in children, asthma is the most common. However, many other illnesses, foreign bodies, and trauma cause respiratory problems in children. Good assessment and early intervention for paediatric respiratory problems can avert serious illness and preventable death, and may shorten treatment time in the emergency department (ED).

Focusing on certain key physical signs and symptoms allows the prehospital professional to rapidly assess the effectiveness of gas exchange in the airways and lung alveoli. Using the Paediatric Assessment Triangle (PAT) is an important first step in determining the severity of disease, localising the physiological problem, and beginning treatment. Appearance reflects the overall state of ventilation and oxygenation. Increased work of breathing indicates either airway obstruction at some level or a problem in gas exchange at the alveolar level; it is often an early sign of hypoxia or hypercapnia. Fading respiratory effort is a sign of severe hypoxia or hypercapnia. Cyanosis of the skin or mucous membranes also indicates severe hypoxia.

In addition to the PAT, the primary assessment includes counting the respiratory rate; appropriately exposing all paediatric patients to ascertain work of breathing as part of the examination (this can be done in a non-threatening manner by asking the parent or caregiver to lift the child's shirt or clothing to reveal retractions); performing hands-on chest auscultation; evaluating the heart rate; and obtaining pulse oximetry. This assessment not only provides a picture of respiratory function, but also helps prioritise general and specific treatments, and interventions and timing of transport.

Respiratory Distress and Failure

Respiratory distress, failure, and arrest are three points on a continuum of physiological response to different types of hypoxic and/or hypercarbic stressors. Causes of these stressors are variable and include asthma, bronchiolitis, croup, pneumonia, and chest wall injury. Although these three points in the continuum (respiratory distress, failure, and arrest) have different clinical characteristics in theory, in reality they are part of a spectrum that is not black or white. Respiratory distress is an abnormal physiological condition identified by increased work of breathing. Increased respiratory rate; supraclavicular, suprasternal, intercostal, or subcostal retractions; use of accessory muscles; and nasal flaring are signs that alone or together indicate increased work of breathing. These physical signs represent the patient's attempt to make up for decreased gas exchange in the lungs and airways and to maintain oxygenation and ventilation. The brain is still getting enough oxygen, and the child's appearance is relatively normal.

Case Study 1

You are dispatched to the home of a 22-month-old boy who is having difficulty breathing. His mother says that for 2 days he has had a slight fever and has been "wheezing", especially when he cries or becomes more active. He suddenly awoke tonight acutely short of breath and now is making a very loud noise each time he breathes in. The child has no prior history of wheezing or respiratory illness.

The child is sitting on his mother's lap looking anxious, but makes eye contact and cries weakly when you approach. He makes loud, harsh noises with each inspiration. His colour is pink, but he has marked supraclavicular and suprasternal retractions and nasal flaring. Respiratory rate is 42 breaths/min and the heart rate is 180 beats/min. The blood pressure is not obtained. His skin is warm, and he has strong pulses and normal capillary refill time. He has good air movement with loud, harsh breath sounds heard on each inspiration. Lower airway sounds are obscured by these loud inspiratory noises.

1. How sick is this child?

2. Are this child's findings more likely to be caused by upper airway or lower airway obstruction, and how will you manage him in the field?

Respiratory failure occurs when the infant or child exhausts his or her energy reserves or can no longer maintain oxygenation and ventilation. When the effects of the respiratory insult begin to overwhelm the child's ability to respond, he or she begins to decompensate. Respiratory failure may occur when chest wall muscles get tired after a long period of increased work of breathing (e.g., a child with severe asthma who is very tight and has been working hard to breathe for several hours); when the insult is severe and progressive (e.g., fulminant pneumonia); or when there is a failure of central respiratory drive (e.g., a child with a severe closed-head injury). An abnormal appearance (agitation or lethargy) or cyanosis in a child with an increased work of breathing indicates respiratory failure. An abnormally low respiratory rate and decreased respiratory effort, usually with bradycardia, also indicates respiratory failure. Respiratory failure must be treated immediately to restore good oxygenation and ventilation, and to prevent respiratory arrest.

Signs of failure are decreased level of consciousness, slow to agonal respirations, grunting, decreasing pulse oximetry, and bradycardia or inappropriate slowing of the heart rate. It is known that tachypnoea and tachycardia may also be present in a child with respiratory failure.

Respiratory arrest means absence of effective breathing. If ventilation and oxygenation are not immediately supported, respiratory arrest rapidly progresses to full cardiopulmonary arrest. Most episodes of cardiac arrest in paediatric patients begin as respiratory arrest. Intervening at this point often prevents cardiac arrest. Early intervention in respiratory failure and arrest have a far better chance of producing neurologically intact survivors than treatment of cardiac arrest, which has an extremely low probability of survival.

Pre-arrival Preparation

Based on dispatch information and while en route to the scene, prepare mentally for management of respiratory distress and failure by reviewing the appropriate assessment techniques and treatment options for the child's age. This includes recalling an age-based approach to assessment as outlined in the *Paediatric Assessment* chapter, equipment needs, and the likely treatment and transport options. Also, anticipate the determinants of whether to stay on scene and treat or to manage the airway and transport immediately to the ED.

Scene Assessment

Be sure the scene is safe, and there are no obvious illness or injury threats. Assess the environment for foreign body risks, medications, noxious gases, fumes, chemicals, or smoke. Document scene conditions if environmental factors may be contributing to anticipated respiratory problems. If indicated, make sure to wear personal protective equipment (PPE), question how many patients are in the home or facility, determine if additional resources are needed, and attempt to determine mechanism of injury (MOI), nature of illness (NOI), and the need for cervical spine precautions or immobilisation.

General Assessment: The PAT
Evaluating the Presenting Complaint

Find out the nature of the presenting complaint by asking several directed questions, as suggested in **Table 3-1**. After the primary assessment, in patients with mild distress, there is time to get a more complete SAMPLE history (see Table

Table 3-1 Key Questions About the Presenting Complaint

Key Question	Possible Medical Problem
Has your child ever had this kind of problem before?	Asthma, chronic lung disease
Is this the first time that your child has had trouble breathing?	Asthma, chronic lung disease
Is your child taking any medications?	Asthma, chronic lung disease, congenital heart disease
Has your child had a fever?	Pneumonia, bronchiolitis, croup
Did your child suddenly start coughing/choking/gagging?	Foreign body aspiration or ingestion
Has your child had an injury to his or her chest?	Pulmonary contusion, pneumothorax

© Jones & Bartlett Learning

3-9) on scene as part of the focused history. If the child is in respiratory failure, do this later, while en route to the ED.

Assessment of Respiratory Status

Using the PAT

Begin the assessment with the PAT, as discussed in the *Paediatric Assessment* chapter. Carefully evaluate appearance, work of breathing, and skin circulation. The PAT helps establish how sick the child is, the type of physiological abnormality (respiratory distress or respiratory failure), the level of obstruction if present (upper or lower airway), and the urgency for treatment. Table 1-2 in the *Paediatric Assessment* chapter lists physical features in the child to help make these clinical distinctions by simple observation and listening.

Appearance

Appearance reflects the adequacy of oxygenation and ventilation in a child with difficulty breathing. If the child is compensating effectively for the respiratory insult, the appearance is fairly normal, and the TICLS mnemonic (see Table 1-1 in the *Paediatric Assessment* chapter) shows an interactive child with good tone and colour, and normal vocalisations, who looks or gazes at someone. If the child is not compensating, the appearance is abnormal, and the child has abnormal findings in the TICLS mnemonic because his or her brain is impaired from hypoxia or hypercapnia. Abnormal appearance is a spectrum of clinical states, so that the severity of respiratory failure determines how abnormal the child appears. Also, assessing appearance guides urgency of basic

life support (BLS) versus advanced life support (ALS) treatment. Even if ALS procedures are required, start with BLS procedures while preparing to implement ALS procedures based on local protocol.

Example 1: A 3-year-old child who has stridor and retractions, but is running around the room and has a normal appearance, requires general non-invasive treatment and transport. The child is compensating effectively and is only in respiratory distress.

Example 2: An 8-year-old child who is agitated or inconsolable, with wheezing and increased work of breathing, has an abnormal appearance, and is probably hypoxic. The child is beginning to decompensate and is in early respiratory failure. In addition to general non-invasive treatment, this child requires immediate specific treatment on scene with a **bronchodilator**, then rapid transport to an ED.

Example 3: A 3-year-old child who has been working hard to breathe for hours and is now sleepy or poorly responsive has an abnormal appearance. The altered mental status is the result of severe hypoxia or hypercapnia, reflecting late respiratory failure, and impending respiratory arrest. These patients require immediate **assisted ventilations** with airway adjuncts, such as **oropharyngeal airway (OPA)** or **nasopharyngeal airway (NPA)** using a bag-valve-mask device on scene and possibly advanced airway procedures. This may include endotracheal intubation, supraglottic airways, or dual lumen airway.

Work of Breathing

To assess for adequate breathing, sometimes the patient needs to be appropriately exposed. Attempt to visualise the thorax in a non-threatening manner while keeping the child warm. Look for signs of increased work of breathing:

1. Abnormal positioning (tripoding, "sniffing" position)
2. Abnormal airway sounds (e.g., snoring, stridor, wheezing, or grunting)
3. Retractions (or head bobbing in infants)
4. Nasal flaring

The significance of each of these findings is discussed in the *Paediatric Assessment* chapter. These indicators of breathing effort help to identify the anatomical location of the problem (upper airway, lower airway, or lung alveoli), the severity of the physiological dysfunction (respiratory distress, failure, or arrest), and the urgency for treatment (immediate resuscitation, general treatment only on scene with specific treatment en route, general and specific treatment on scene). In addition to abnormal airway sounds (stridor, wheezing, and grunting), retractions and the use of accessory muscles may help localise the site of airway problems. Use of the accessory muscles of the neck and suprasternal and supraclavicular retractions occurs more often with upper airway obstruction. Predominant subcostal and intercostal retractions and the use of abdominal muscles tend to localise an obstructive process to the lower airways. It is difficult to recognise some of these signs when the child has on clothing; if needed, appropriately remove clothing to ascertain these other clinical signs.

Circulation to Skin

Finally, evaluate skin colour. Cyanosis is an ominous sign, signalling profound hypoxia and the need for assisted ventilation. However, a child may have severe hypoxia without an obvious change in skin colour. Pulse oximetry is very helpful; use it whenever available in a child with respiratory distress or respiratory failure.

Primary Assessment: The <C>ABCDEs

After the PAT, perform the second portion of the primary assessment, the hands-on <C>ABCDEs. There are three parts to the "B" or breathing evaluation:

1. Respiratory rate
2. Auscultation for air movement and abnormal breath sounds
3. Pulse oximetry
4. Peak expiratory flow for asthma (age and situation dependant)

Respiratory Rate

In the non-critical patient, determine respiratory rate by sitting the child in the caregiver's lap and exposing the patient's chest. Count the rise and fall of the abdomen over 30 seconds, and then double that number. Normal respiratory rates vary in children of different ages (see Table 1-4 in the *Paediatric Assessment* chapter). Always think about respiratory rates in the context of the PAT and the overall clinical assessment. Respiratory rate may be affected by level of activity, fever, anxiety, and metabolic state.

A respiratory rate of greater than 60 breaths/min is abnormal in a child of any age and should be a signal for careful evaluation for other signs of respiratory or circulatory problems. Even more dangerous is a rate that is too slow for age. A respiratory rate of less than 20 breaths/min in a sick child younger than 6 years of age, or a rate of less than 12 breaths/min in a sick child younger than 15 years of age may be a sign of respiratory failure, and immediate intervention is required.

Auscultation for Air Movement and Abnormal Breath Sounds

Assess air movement by placing the stethoscope and listening for the amount of air movement with each breath (**Figure 3-1**). Poor air movement may exist in children with respiratory problems for many reasons, as outlined in **Table 3-2**.

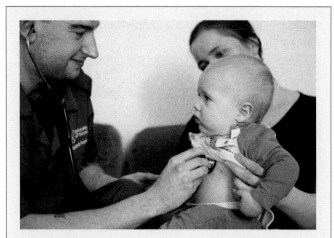

Figure 3-1 Assess air movement by placing the stethoscope and listening for the amount of movement with each breath.
© Jones & Bartlett Learning.

Table 3-2 Causes of Poor Air Movement in Children

Functional Problem	Possible Causes
Obstruction of airway	Asthma, bronchiolitis, croup, foreign body
Restriction of chest wall movement	Chest wall injury, severe **scoliosis** or kyphosis
Chest wall muscle fatigue	Prolonged increased work of breathing, muscular dystrophy
Decreased central respiratory drive	Head injury, intoxication
Chest injury	Rib fractures, pulmonary contusion, pneumothorax
Reduced functional residual capacity and diaphragmatic splinting	Significant abdominal distention (e.g., ascites, organomegaly, necrotising enterocolitis (NEC) in neonates)

© Jones & Bartlett Learning

Assessing air movement, or the volume of air exchanged with each breath, allows clinical estimation of tidal volume. Tidal volume is one of two factors that determine minute ventilation: the volume of air exchanged per minute. Minute ventilation is the basis for gas exchange in the lungs.

Minute Ventilation = Tidal Volume × Respiratory Rate

This equation shows the connection between tidal volume and respiratory rate. A child may not have enough gas exchange if tidal volume is low, even with a normal or fast respiratory rate. Also, a normal or increased tidal volume does not mean there is enough gas exchange if the respiratory rate is too slow.

While listening for air movement, also listen for abnormal breath sounds. Table 1-5 in the *Paediatric Assessment* chapter summarises the types and causes of abnormal breath sounds. Stridor, which is usually inspiratory in nature at least initially, is indicative of upper airway obstruction, whereas wheezes are associated with lower airway processes and crackles or rhonchi are most often associated with issues within the lung parynchema.

Pulse Oximetry

Pulse oximetry is a useful tool for detecting and measuring hypoxia. **Figure 3-2** illustrates possible sites for placement of the oximetry probe. **Pulse Oximetry, Procedure 8**, explains how to use a pulse oximeter. The pulse oximeter emits red light of two different wavelengths. These are absorbed differently by saturated and desaturated haemoglobin. The sensor on the pulse oximeter measures the transmission of the two wavelengths of red light, and a computer in the machine then determines the percentage of haemoglobin saturated

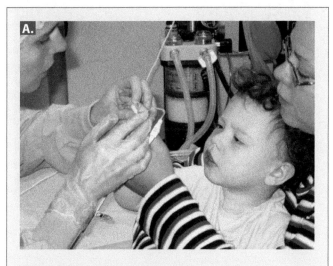
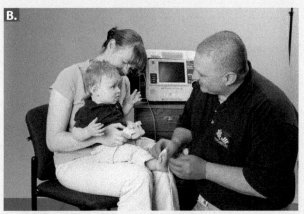

Figure 3-2 Possible sites for placement of the oximetry probe.
© Jones & Bartlett Learning

with oxygen. When properly applied, *and if there is a good arterial tracing*, a reading of 95% or higher means normal blood oxygen saturation. *A value of 94% or less on room air is abnormal and is a signal to give supplemental oxygen.* A reading of less than 90%, with the patient on 100% oxygen, usually indicates respiratory failure in a previously healthy individual.

Patients with uncorrected cyanotic heart disease and some patients with chronic respiratory problems (e.g., bronchopulmonary dysplasia, or cystic fibrosis) may have a low oxygen saturation at baseline. In this type of patient, obtain the baseline value from the caregiver and attempt to provide enough oxygen to get the child to his or her baseline pulse oximetry level. Providing more oxygen than is needed to achieve the baseline pulse oximetry level may actually suppress ventilation by reducing the child's hypoxic drive to breathe. In normal children, hypercapnia or increased carbon dioxide pressure stimulates the drive to breathe, but in some children with chronic respiratory disease, hypercapnia is a constant state. In such cases, hypoxia becomes the stimulus to breathe. Over-treating hypoxia disturbs this regulatory function, and may paradoxically decrease the drive to breathe and make the child worse. The preferred saturation rate is between 94% and 98%.

One must be careful not to over-interpret low oxygen saturation. Pulse oximetry is an adjunct to physical assessment. Falsely low readings are common with pulse oximetry. Movement by the child, cold extremities or a cold ambient temperature, and interference by light in the child's surroundings all may cause inaccurate pulse oximetry readings. Check probe placement, the quality of the tracing, and the child's clinical state before treating. Inaccurate readings or the inability to obtain a reading may also occur in children in shock with poor perfusion. However, give these children oxygen even if they do not have respiratory distress and regardless of pulse oximeter readings. There are also some exposures like carbon monoxide or cyanide poisoning that may affect the pulse oximeter reading. It is also important not to under-interpret a normal pulse oximetry reading. *Sometimes an apparently normal oxygen saturation above 94% may be present in a child with significant respiratory distress, who*

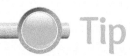

Remember, the pulse oximeter does not detect the adequacy of ventilation. A patient who is receiving supplemental oxygen may have a normal pulse oximeter reading but not have adequate ventilation. Capnometry, which quantitatively measures exhaled carbon dioxide, monitors carbon dioxide levels and adequacy of ventilation.

is compensating by increased work of breathing. Always use pulse oximetry in combination with physical assessment to ensure accurate interpretation of adequacy of breathing.

Peak Expiratory Flow

Where possible, gaining a peak expiratory flow reading can give an indication of the severity of an asthma attack. Measuring the percentage of the actual peak flow against the patient's best normal level, if known, or against the expected level based on a predicted peak flow chart can assist in determining whether the attack should be treated as moderate, severe or life threatening. Moderate asthma is categorised as a peak flow of 50% or above predicted, severe asthma is categorised as between 33% and 50% of predicted, and life-threatening asthma is categorised as presenting with a peak flow of less than 33% of best or predicted.

In some cases, it may not be possible for the patient to provide a peak flow reading. In these cases, do not distress the patient by continued attempts to gain a reading, instead treat for the presentation and gain a peak flow reading if and when possible.

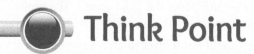

Think Point

Be careful not to over-interpret low oxygen saturation. Match with the physical findings.

General Non-invasive Treatment

For every child in respiratory distress, begin general non-invasive treatment. *The general non-invasive treatment of every non-critical patient is the same—allow patient to assume a position of comfort and supply oxygen, if tolerated* (**Figure 3-3**). This is the only treatment for patients in respiratory distress without upper or lower airway obstruction. If the child is in respiratory failure or arrest, perform assisted ventilation immediately with airway adjuncts and consider advanced airways based on local protocols.

Positioning

A child in respiratory distress naturally moves into the position that provides the best air exchange, called the "position of comfort". For example, a child with severe upper airway obstruction may get into the "sniffing position" to straighten the airway and open the air passages (**Figure 3-4**). A child with severe lower airway obstruction may voluntarily take the "tripod" posture (sitting up and leaning forward on outstretched arms) to help accessory muscles (**Figure 3-5**). Infants and toddlers may be most comfortable in their caregiver's arms or lap. Do not move a child from his or her position of comfort. This might worsen the respiratory distress. In the ambulance, keep the child with dyspnoea safely

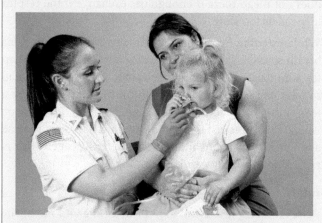

Figure 3-3 Always keep a child with respiratory distress in his or her position of comfort.
© Jones & Bartlett Learning. Courtesy of Glen Ellman.

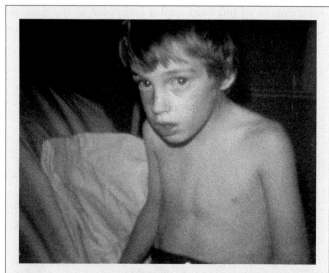

Figure 3-4 Sniffing position.

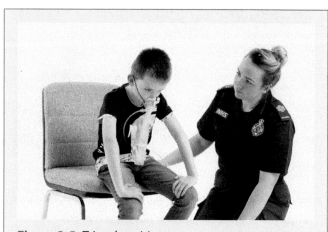

Figure 3-5 Tripod position.
© Jones & Bartlett Learning

restrained in an upright position, unless the child requires assisted ventilations or has other physiological problems that require treatment in a supine position.

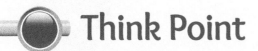

Think Point

Do not move a child from his or her position of comfort.

Oxygen

Treatment with high-flow oxygen is usually safe. If the child has chronic respiratory illness, be careful not to administer too much oxygen. The prehospital professional must weigh the possible benefits of giving oxygen against the risks of agitating the child and worsening the respiratory distress. This is a special concern in a child with an unstable airway. Oxygen toxicity in newborns, especially premature newborns, is occasionally an issue in the prehospital setting. Newborns with respiratory distress, cyanosis, or other signs of respiratory disease require high-flow, 100% oxygen. Newborns without signs of hypoxia no longer require 100% oxygen as explained in the *Emergency Delivery and Newborn Stabilisation* chapter.

Most children accept oxygen therapy, especially if the prehospital professional is creative in the approach. This often means getting the help of the caregiver. If a child resists the use of a mask or nasal cannula, have the caregiver give blow-by oxygen from the end of the oxygen tubing or from tubing inserted into a cup (**Figure 3-6**).

Oxygen Delivery

Give oxygen to any child with clinical signs of cardiopulmonary distress or failure, or with a history suggesting possible

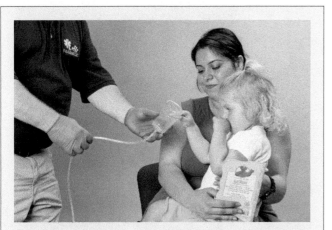

Figure 3-6 If the child resists application of a mask or nasal cannula, administer oxygen through a non-threatening object, such as a cup.

© Jones & Bartlett Learning. Courtesy of Glen Ellman.

abnormalities in gas exchange. The delivery method should provide the concentration of oxygen most appropriate for the child's condition, degree of cooperation, respiratory effort, and age. For a step-by-step explanation of this procedure, see **Oxygen Delivery, Procedure 2**.

Summary of General and Initial Respiratory Assessment and General Non-invasive Treatment

The PAT is a good tool for determining the effectiveness of gas exchange, based on observation of appearance and work of breathing. If the PAT suggests respiratory distress, begin general non-invasive treatment with oxygen and keep the child in his or her position of comfort. The PAT also identifies the critical child in respiratory failure who requires immediate assisted ventilation. Obtaining respiratory rate, listening for air movement, and determining oxygen saturation by pulse oximetry work in concert with the PAT. The primary assessment should allow an evaluation of severity and urgency for treatment and should establish if specific treatment for upper or lower airway obstruction is indicated.

Specific Treatment for Respiratory Distress

After completing the primary assessment, consider specific treatment. The PAT and <C>ABCDE assessment help determine whether the child has upper or lower airway obstruction, lung disease, or disordered control of breathing (from such conditions as brain or nerve injury, poisoning, or sepsis). Snoring or stridor indicates upper airway obstruction; wheezing indicates lower airway obstruction. It can be difficult to separate true stridor from upper airway noise because of nasal congestion. Breath sounds may also make it difficult to tell the difference between upper airway noise and true wheezing. Listen for breath sounds in the second or third intercostal space at the mid-axillary line bilaterally (**Figure 3-7**). Consider the auscultation of breath sounds posteriorly between the scapula and spine bilaterally and lower lobes directly above the kidneys. At this location, it is easier to distinguish upper airway congestion from lower airway obstruction. When abnormal airway sounds are loudest with the stethoscope held near the child's nose rather than over the lungs, nasal congestion is the likely cause.

The absence of abnormal airway sounds in a child with hypoxia and increased work of breathing suggests lung disease, such as pneumonia. Lastly, a child with hypoxia and *decreased* work of breathing may have either respiratory failure from airway obstruction or lung disease or disordered control of breathing from another insult to the brain or metabolic system.

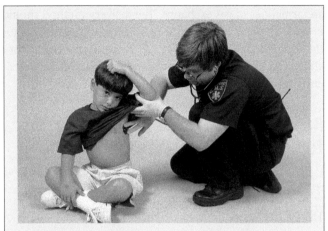

Figure 3-7 Listen for breath sounds in the second or third intercostal space at the mid-axillary line bilaterally.
© Jones & Bartlett Learning

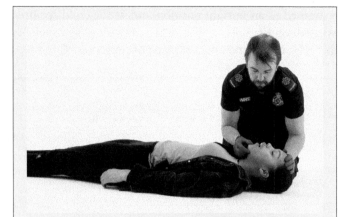

Figure 3-8 Use the head-tilt/chin-lift manoeuvre to place the airway in a neutral position.
© Jones & Bartlett Learning

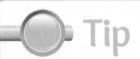
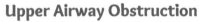

Tip

When abnormal airway sounds are loudest with the stethoscope held near the child's nose rather than over the lungs, nasal congestion is the likely cause.

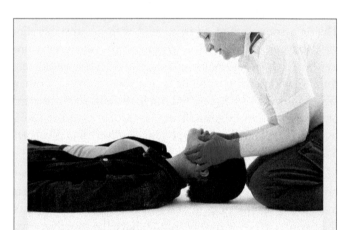

Figure 3-9 Use the jaw-thrust manoeuvre in a child with possible spinal injury.
© Jones & Bartlett Learning

Upper Airway Obstruction
Proximal Airway Obstruction

In a patient with neurological impairment, loss of oropharyngeal muscle tone may cause upper airway obstruction and stridor because of the tongue and mandible falling back and partially blocking the pharynx. This is a common problem in children during and after seizures. The head-tilt/chin-lift manoeuvre (**Figure 3-8**) or jaw-thrust manoeuvre (**Figure 3-9**) may relieve this proximal airway obstruction. At times it may be helpful or even necessary to have two clinicians assist with the jaw-thrust manoeuvre. The use of airway adjuncts based on level of consciousness may help with keeping the airway open, especially in larger children, children who are actively seizing, or children receiving positive-pressure ventilation (**Figure 3-10**).

Sometimes secretions, blood, or foreign bodies block the proximal upper airway. This is an important concern in the child with closed-head injury or seizures. Suctioning alone often relieves the upper airway obstruction caused by fluids or occluding objects in the mouth, pharynx, or nose.

Maintenance of an adequate airway may require placement of an OPA, an NPA, an endotracheal tube, or other approved advanced airways. An OPA should not be used in a conscious patient as there is risk of gagging, vomiting, and aspiration.

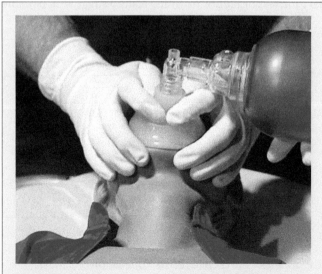

Figure 3-10 Two-rescuer technique for the jaw-thrust manoeuvre and positive-pressure ventilation.
© Jones & Bartlett Learning

The role of endotracheal intubation of children in the pre-hospital setting has been brought into question by data demonstrating significant failure rates, induced hypoxia, airway injury, and endotracheal tube dislodgement. *Bag-valve-mask ventilation is the key life-saving technique that should be mastered by all prehospital providers and provides adequate airway management for most paediatric patients.*

Alternative advanced airways including supraglottic airways and dual lumen airways can be considered in the early treatment of the child in respiratory failure or arrest. The particular type and brand is based on local ambulance service protocols.

Airway Obstruction Above the Thoracic Inlet

Upper airway obstruction beyond the proximal upper airway may result from a variety of causes. It is not necessary to make an exact diagnosis to provide appropriate management to children with upper airway obstruction. In most of these cases, simply allow the child to maintain his or her position of comfort and provide supplemental oxygen by the least invasive and least threatening means possible. Causing the child to become more agitated or struggle may worsen the airway obstruction and precipitate the onset of a severe airway obstruction, leading to respiratory failure or respiratory arrest.

In an awake, alert child, upper airway obstruction and stridor are usually caused by croup, a viral disease with inflammation, oedema, and narrowing of the larynx or trachea. Croup usually affects infants and toddlers. Most children with croup have had several days of cold symptoms. The cold symptoms are followed by the development of a barking or "seal-like" cough, stridor, and various levels of respiratory distress. There is usually a low-grade fever, and symptoms are often worse at night. The severity of symptoms varies widely among patients, but they usually progress over days, rather than hours.

Treatment of Croup. Any intervention that may upset the child should be avoided because this may result in an acute deterioration and, potentially, complete airway obstruction. Interventions to be avoided would include examination of the ears, nose, and throat, cannulation or blood glucose measurement. The use of nebulisation in the pre-hospital setting should also be avoided due to the likelihood of precipitating airway deterioration. All children with stridor must be transferred to hospital. Very few children with croup require assisted ventilation in the prehospital setting. In the rare case of a child with croup and respiratory failure, begin assisted ventilation and reassess. Two-person bag-valve-mask ventilation technique may be necessary.

Pharmacological Treatment of Croup. Steroid treatment is the principle pre-hospital pharmacological intervention in cases of croup. Oral dexamethasone should be administered to relieve subglottic inflammation. In-hospital treatment may include the administration of nebulised budesonide. In severe cases of croup that are not effectively relieved by steroid treatment, the in-hospital administration of nebulised adrenaline may be undertaken.

Invasive Airway Management for Croup. Perform endotracheal intubation only in the unusual case of the child with respiratory failure who does not respond to bag-valve-mask ventilation. Preparation for intubation includes choosing an endotracheal tube that is one or two sizes smaller than normal for age or length. Inflammation of the trachea at the subglottic level makes it difficult or impossible to use an endotracheal tube of normal size. Do not use paralytics when attempting endotracheal intubation for upper airway obstruction. Refer to local protocols when making the decision for rapid sequence intubation (RSI). Other advanced airways should also be considered based on local protocols and availability.

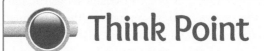

Think Point

Stridor is often mistaken for wheezing. Stridor is an inspiratory sign of upper airway obstruction.

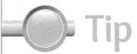

Tip

Position of comfort and avoiding any agitation are the best treatments for suspected croup.

Bacterial Upper Airway Infections

Bacterial infections may also cause upper airway obstruction in children. Unlike viral croup, these infections tend to progress rapidly with severe respiratory compromise developing over hours. The child with a bacterial upper airway infection usually is older than 12 months, appears ill or toxic, has pain on swallowing, and may drool. Stridor may be present, but the child does not have the barking cough that is common with croup.

There are several possible causes of bacterial upper airway infections. Epiglottitis, inflammation of the epiglottis, is now extremely rare because of widespread vaccination of infants against the bacteria *Haemophilus influenzae* type b (Hib). A retropharyngeal abscess involves swelling of the retropharyngeal nodes that are located between the cervical vertebrae and oesophagus. It usually occurs in children younger than 4 years and can mimic the presentation of epiglottitis. The child may have torticollis, and there may be swollen cervical lymph nodes. A peritonsillar abscess is a collection of pus adjacent to the tonsil. It tends to occur more often in adolescents and is often caused by group A streptococcus (Strep A) (so the child may be on antibiotics for a strep throat). The child complains of trouble speaking, is unable to open his or her mouth fully, and often drools. Tracheitis can occur in two forms. In the child without a tracheostomy, it can mimic the presentation of epiglottitis. In a child with a tracheostomy, it results in increased thick airway secretions.

Treatment. When a bacterial upper airway infection is suspected, give only general non-invasive treatment with high-flow oxygen in a position of comfort. Avoid agitating the child by trying to place an intravenous (IV) line or attempting another manoeuvre, and quickly transport. If the child is in respiratory failure, initiate bag-valve-mask ventilation and consider endotracheal intubation.

Foreign Body Aspiration

Foreign body aspiration may cause mechanical obstruction anywhere in the airway, from the pharynx to the bronchus. A retained oesophageal foreign body can also cause respiratory distress in an infant or young child. This happens because the trachea is pliable and can be compressed by the adjacent distended oesophagus. A typical history of foreign body aspiration includes the sudden onset of coughing, choking, gagging, and shortness of breath in a previously well child without a fever or other symptoms of upper respiratory tract infection. Older infants and toddlers, who explore their world by placing things in their mouths, are at highest risk.

Treatment. If the child can still cough, cry, or speak, the airway is only partially obstructed. Stridor may be present. Immediately transport such children, who have mild upper airway obstruction. Use only general non-invasive treatment, avoid agitating the child, and keep the child in a position of comfort.

If the child has severe respiratory distress and is at risk for getting worse during transport, be prepared to perform foreign body airway obstruction (FBAO) manoeuvres for severe airway obstruction, as illustrated in **Figures 3-11** and **3-12**. **Table 3-3** summarises these manoeuvres. Consider these FBAO manoeuvres if the child cannot cough, cry, or speak. *Never perform FBAO procedures if the child has mild airway obstruction (i.e., can cough, cry, or speak).*

Airway Obstruction and Foreign Body Removal

In the setting of severe airway obstruction, prehospital professionals can make the difference between life and death. Immediate removal of an airway foreign body can often be achieved using BLS procedures while the child is still conscious. Sometimes basic manoeuvres are unsuccessful. In such cases, paediatric Magill forceps along with direct laryngoscopy may be the only option for removal. For a

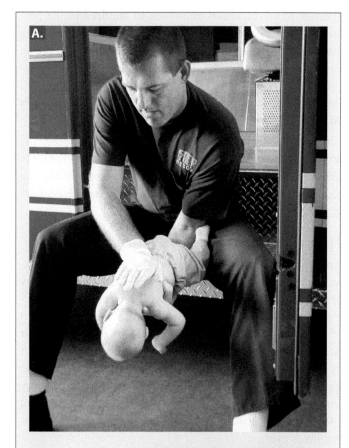

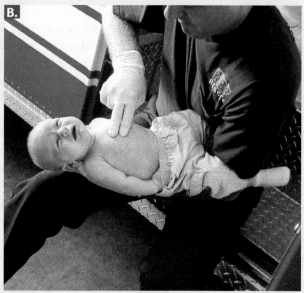

Figure 3-11 Foreign body airway manoeuvres for a conscious infant. **A.** Use five back blows (slaps), followed by **B.** five chest compressions in infants with severe airway obstruction.
© Jones & Bartlett Learning

step-by-step explanation of this procedure, see **Foreign Body Obstruction, Procedure 5**.

Foreign Body Airway Obstruction Manoeuvres. If the child has severe airway obstruction and BLS manoeuvres

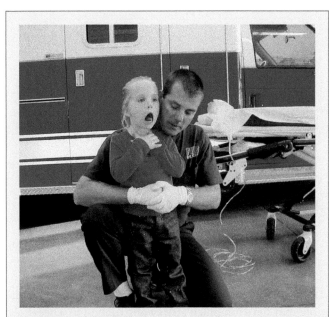

Figure 3-12 Foreign body airway manoeuvres for a conscious child. Use abdominal thrusts to treat severe airway obstruction in the conscious child in the standing position.
© Jones & Bartlett Learning

Table 3-3 Foreign Body Airway Obstruction Manoeuvres

Age	Technique
Infant (<12 months)	Five back blows (slaps) followed by five chest compressions until unresponsive, then start CPR
Child (>1 year)	Abdominal thrusts until unresponsive, then start CPR

fail to dislodge the foreign body to the mouth where it can be easily removed, and the patient loses consciousness, begin cardiopulmonary resuscitation (CPR) with chest compressions, then open the airway. If the foreign body can be seen at or above the level of the larynx, and if local policies allow, remove it using paediatric Magill forceps. If the use of Magill forceps is not permitted, continue CPR and look for airway obstruction before delivering ventilations. Finger sweep FBAO only if the object is seen. If the child has severe airway obstruction and neither FBAO manoeuvres nor direct laryngoscopy relieve the obstruction, attempt bag-valve-mask ventilation, using the two-person technique whenever possible (**Figure 3-13**). If bag-valve-mask ventilation fails to achieve chest rise, consider endotracheal intubation. Suction should be readily available when performing unconscious airway manoeuvres.

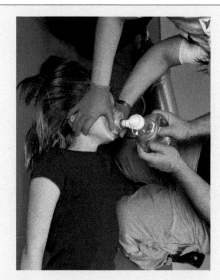

Figure 3-13 Two-person bag-valve-mask ventilation technique.
© Jones & Bartlett Learning. Courtesy of Glen Ellman.

Based on local protocols and skill levels, needle or surgical cricothyroidotomy might be considered in cases where obstructions that cannot be removed.

Specific Treatment of Upper Airway Obstruction

When transporting any child with suspected mild upper airway obstruction, have airway equipment immediately available. Consider transporting the caregiver with any conscious child with airway obstruction, because this may keep the child calm. Also, the caregiver can help administer oxygen.

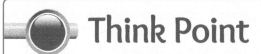 **Think Point**

Never perform airway obstruction procedures if the child has only mild airway obstruction and can still cough, cry, or speak.

Lower Airway Obstruction

Bronchiolitis and asthma are the most common conditions causing lower airway obstruction in children. Foreign body aspiration is much less common and usually occurs in toddlers who have been otherwise well, and then suddenly start choking, coughing, or wheezing. *Wheezing is the clinical hallmark of lower airway obstruction of any cause.* Pneumonia can also cause lower airway disease but usually without obstruction. A prehospital specific diagnosis of lower airway obstruction is not necessary, and many times it is impossible to tell which of the three main conditions

Case Study 2

You are dispatched to a childcare centre for a child in respiratory distress. On arrival you and your crewmate find a 23-month-old girl very cyanotic in colour grasping her throat. The childcare worker states that she believes that the child has a history of asthma and tried giving her an inhaler treatment but the child would not tolerate it. The child is making no audible noises and seems desperate for help.

1. What is the most important thing for you to do at this time?

2. What would you do if your initial steps failed? What would you do next?

the child is experiencing: (1) bronchiolitis, (2) asthma, or (3) foreign body aspiration. Treatment for all forms of bronchoconstriction is similar, but asthma is much more likely to respond to bronchodilators than bronchiolitis.

Asthma

Asthma is the most common chronic disease of childhood, affecting almost 1.1 million children in the United Kingdom, among the highest prevalence rates worldwide. Preventable factors have been identified in 90% of childhood deaths from asthma where earlier intervention could have been undertaken. The severity of asthma can be classified as mild/moderate, severe or life-threatening. Common reasons for an asthma attack include upper respiratory infection and exercise. Exposure to cold air, emotional stress, environmental allergen exposure, and passive exposure to smoke also may trigger attacks.

Asthma is a chronic inflammatory condition of the distal airways. The inflammatory reaction leads to bronchoconstriction, mucosal oedema, and profuse secretions. These three factors in combination cause airflow obstruction and ventilation-perfusion mismatch. Clinically, children having an asthma attack show different degrees of tachypnoea, tachycardia, increased work of breathing, and wheezing, which tends to be worse on exhalation. Pulse oximetry may be normal or low.

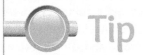 Tip

Attempt BLS manoeuvres first in a child with suspected foreign body aspiration and critical airway obstruction.

Carefully assess air movement by auscultation both anteriorly and posteriorly; this helps to distinguish not only sounds but also tidal volume. The person with asthma complaining of shortness of breath, but without wheezing on auscultation, may have too much airway obstruction to wheeze. Aggressive bronchodilator treatment may improve airflow and increase audible wheezing. Beware of the following features of the primary assessment, which suggest severe bronchospasm and respiratory failure:

- Altered appearance
- Exhaustion
- Inability to recline
- Interrupted speech
- Severe retractions
- Decreased air movement

In the focused history, several things suggest that a severe or potentially life-threatening attack may occur. These include:

- Prior intensive care unit admissions or intubation
- More than three ED visits in a year
- More than two hospital admissions in past year
- Use of more than one metered dose inhaler canister in the last month
- Use of steroids for asthma in the past
- Use of bronchodilators more frequently than every 4 hours
- Progressive symptoms despite aggressive home therapy

Home therapy of asthma has several goals: preventing and controlling asthma symptoms, reducing the number and severity of attacks, and reversing existing airflow obstruction. Some children with a history of severe or frequent asthma attacks are on daily medications, but most children receive treatment only during serious attacks. **Table 3-4** lists the medications frequently used in home asthma therapy for quick relief. Some patients may think they will obtain quick relief from medications that do not have a quick onset of action, e.g., "preventer" inhalers, and delay calling for help.

Table 3-4 Asthma: Common Home Therapy Quick-Relief Medications for Acute Asthma Attacks

Class of Medication	Medication	Mechanism of Action
β₂ agonists	Inhaled bronchodilators (salbutamol, terbutaline sulfate)	Relax bronchiole smooth muscle; prevent bronchospasm; rapid onset of action
Anticholinergics	Inhaled anticholinergics (ipratropium)	Relax bronchiole smooth muscle; decrease secretions; rapid onset of action

© Jones & Bartlett Learning

Treatment of Lower Airway Obstruction

For all children with lower airway obstruction, give general non-invasive treatment in the first instance.

Asthma Treatment. Specific pre-hospital treatment of asthma includes inhaled bronchodilators and hydrocortisone or intramuscular (IM) adrenaline, depending on the severity of the attack. See **Figure 3-14** for further details on assessing and managing asthma in children.

Figures 3-15 and **3-16** illustrate administration of inhaled bronchodilators.

Bronchodilators

Early bronchodilator therapy, on the scene and on the way to the ED, helps immediately open airways, relieve respiratory distress, and improve oxygen delivery in asthma. In unstable or critical patients, continuous inhaled treatment with a β agonist is the preferred approach. For a step-by-step explanation of this procedure, see **Bronchodilator Therapy, Procedure 6**. In-line bronchodilator used with continuous positive airway pressure (CPAP) can be used on older children based on local protocols.

Pharmacological Treatment of Wheezing. Salbutamol is the most popular inhaled bronchodilator. Because of its selective action on the bronchiole smooth muscles and its minimal effect on cardiac rate, the drug has a high margin of safety.

Depending on local protocols, in cases of severe or life-threatening asthma ipratropium bromide should be given after salbutamol. Ipratropium is an anticholinergic that may provide additional bronchodilatation in addition to β agonists. Precautions include sensitivity to the effects of ipratropium or atropine. Adverse reactions include dry mouth, headache, cough, hoarseness, blurred vision, tachycardia, and occasionally flushing.

If a child is moving air so poorly that life-threatening asthma has been diagnosed, IM adrenaline 1 in 1,000 should be administered. Transport with cardiac monitoring if frequent nebulised treatments or IM adrenaline is necessary. **Table 3-5** summarises the drugs and doses for prehospital bronchodilator therapy.

In most cases of known asthma, begin a bronchodilator on scene before transport, and then give additional doses en route, as indicated.

In critical patients, salbutamol doses may be repeated continuously en route to the ED.

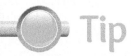
Tip

When a child has a history of increased work of breathing, but now has altered appearance and a slow or normal respiratory rate without retractions, THINK RESPIRATORY FAILURE.

IM Injections. IM is the preferred route of administration for adrenaline in patients with severe respiratory distress due to asthma. SQ absorption is slow and unreliable. The IM route may result in nerve damage, particularly if the injection is in the buttocks of infants and small children. For a step-by-step explanation of this procedure, see **Intramuscular Injections, Procedure 12**.

Assisted Ventilation. Because of the severe air trapping associated with bronchospasm, assisted ventilation may be associated with many complications and death. Positive-pressure ventilation requires very high inspiratory pressures and may result in pneumothorax or pneumomediastinum. Consider bag-valve-mask ventilation and endotracheal intubation of a wheezing child only if the child is in respiratory failure and has failed to respond to high-flow oxygen and maximal bronchodilator therapy. While assisting ventilation in any patient with lower airway obstruction, slow rates (12–15 breaths/min in older children and adolescents, and a maximum rate of 20–30 breaths/min in infants) with long expiratory times are useful in minimising barotrauma and complications.

Bronchiolitis

Bronchiolitis is a viral lower respiratory infection, which usually affects infants and children younger than 2 years of age. Often caused by respiratory syncytial virus (RSV), this disease is widespread in the winter months. The infection leads to destruction of the lining of the bronchioles, profuse secretions, and bronchoconstriction. Infants are particularly likely to develop the disease because of their

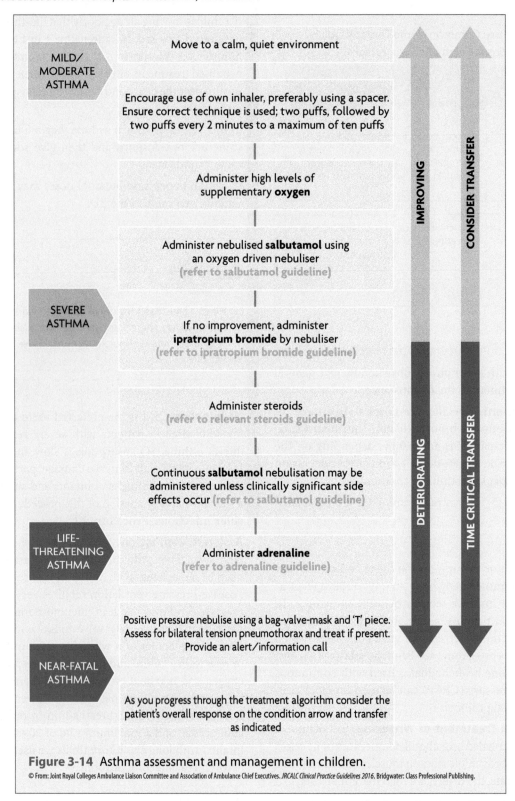

Figure 3-14 Asthma assessment and management in children.

small airway size, high resistance to airflow, and poor airway clearance. Airway oedema and debris from sloughed cells and mucus are much more important in the pathophysiology of this disease than bronchospasm and smooth muscle contraction.

Presenting complaints of bronchiolitis include upper respiratory infection symptoms, fever, cough, vomiting, poor feeding, poor sleep, significant nasal congestion and trouble breathing. Assessment shows variable degrees of increased work of breathing, tachypnoea, diffuse wheezing, inspiratory crackles, and tachycardia.

Historical risk factors for respiratory failure in infants with suspected bronchiolitis include age younger than 2 months, history of prematurity, underlying lung disease, congenital heart disease, and immune deficiency. **Table 3-6** lists important clinical predictors of respiratory failure in

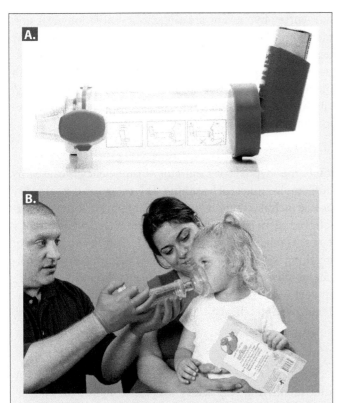

Figure 3-15 A. A metered dose inhaler and spacer can be used with or without a mask. **B.** A metered dose inhaler with spacer and mask can be used in children as young as 6 months old.

© Jones & Bartlett Learning

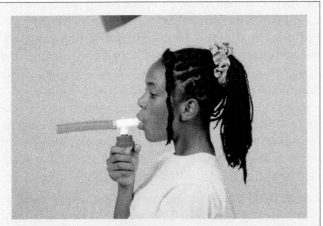

Figure 3-16 One method for delivering a bronchodilator is with an oxygen-powered nebuliser.

© Jones and Bartlett Publishers. Photographed by Kimberly Potvin

children with suspected bronchiolitis. Initial treatment can include nasopharyngeal suctioning with a bulb syringe.

It is often difficult to distinguish new-onset reactive airway disease from viral bronchiolitis.

Table 3-5 Management of Wheezing: Bronchodilator Treatment

Bronchodilator	Dose
Salbutamol	Nebules containing 2.5 mg/2.5 ml. Ages 1 month to 5 years = 2.5 mg repeated every 5 minutes. Ages 6 years and above = 5.0 mg repeated every 5 minutes. There is no limit on repeat doses.
Ipratropium bromide inhalation solution	Nebules containing 250 micrograms in 1 ml or 500 micrograms in 2 ml. *Children* 12 months and below: 125–250 micrograms, single dose only. *Children* between 1 and 12 years: 250 micrograms, single dose only. *Children* >12 years: 500 micrograms, single dose only.

© Jones & Bartlett Learning

Table 3-6 Predictors of Respiratory Failure in Suspected Bronchiolitis

Respiratory rate >60 breaths/min with increased work of breathing
Heart rate >200 beats/min or <100 beats/min
Poor appearance
Blood oxygen saturation <90% on supplemental oxygen

© Jones & Bartlett Learning

Foreign Body Aspiration

Children with lower airway obstruction caused by foreign body aspiration usually are only mildly ill. Unlike foreign bodies in the upper airway, it is rare to develop respiratory failure or severe airway obstruction from a small foreign body in the lower airway. Foreign body aspiration is most common in older infants and toddlers (**Figure 3-17**). Often, there is an abrupt onset of coughing or choking that may be followed by a period of relatively few symptoms. Tachypnoea, increased work of breathing, and wheezing or decreased breath sounds, which are usually unilateral unless the foreign body is in the trachea, may develop rapidly or over a period of hours to days. The absence of a history of asthma or the symptoms of an upper respiratory infection in a child of the right age should suggest the possibility of foreign body aspiration. General non-invasive treatment, including allowing the child to assume a position of comfort and providing oxygen if tolerated, should be given to all patients. Additional diagnostic tests may be done after arrival at the ED.

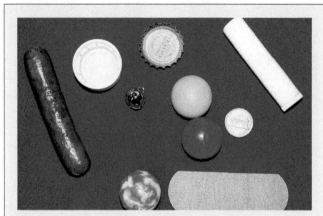

Figure 3-17 Examples of foreign bodies that can obstruct the upper or lower airway.
© Jones & Bartlett Learning. Courtesy of Glen Ellman.

Lung Disease

In children, most lung disease is caused by pneumonia. Other causes, such as pulmonary oedema or pulmonary contusion, are rare. Pneumonia may cause symptoms of lower airway disease and respiratory distress or failure in children. Almost all children with pneumonia have fever or a history of fever at some point in their illness. Most pneumonias in children are caused by viruses. These children generally have less severe symptoms and symptoms of a more gradual onset than children with bacterial pneumonia.

Bacterial pneumonia in children occurs after aspiration or haematogenous seeding of bacteria into the lung. This is followed by an acute inflammatory reaction leading to the accumulation of fluid within the airspaces of the lung. At times, this may be accompanied by the development of a pleural effusion or collection of fluid in the pleural space outside the lung parenchyma. Children with bacterial pneumonia usually have symptoms including fever, chills, tachypnoea, and frequently non-specific complaints including lethargy or irritability, poor appetite, and occasionally chest pain. Cough may not develop until after a period of other more non-specific symptoms.

Physical findings may include fever, tachypnoea, increased work of breathing, decreased breath sounds, and rales. Grunting respirations are relatively common in young children with any form of lung disease. Wheezes may be heard, especially with viral infections, but are not as common as rales or decreased breath sounds. In the absence of underlying illness, disability, or very young age, it is unusual for a child to abruptly develop respiratory failure caused by pneumonia. Respiratory distress is more likely.

Approach children with suspected pneumonia like any patient with symptoms of lower airway disease. Making the diagnosis is not as important as providing good supportive care. Give general, non-invasive treatment to all patients. Nebulised treatments are generally not necessary and in fact

may worsen hypoxia by creating more ventilation perfusion mismatch. Patients with signs of respiratory failure may need assisted ventilation. Respiratory failure from lung disease is more commonly seen in young infants, children with underlying neurological or pulmonary disease, and children who have been ill for several days. There is no specific prehospital therapy for children with pneumonia.

Disordered Control of Breathing

Sometimes hypoxia or respiratory insufficiency is caused by problems in control of breathing. This category of respiratory disease includes brain injury, spinal injury, poisoning, metabolic problems (e.g., botulism, Guillain-Barré syndrome), or sepsis. The hallmark of patients with disordered control of breathing is inadequate minute volume, from poor tidal volume or slow breathing rate. Treatment includes ventilatory support with oxygen, bag-valve-mask ventilation, and occasionally endotracheal intubation or other advanced airways.

Summary of Specific Treatment for Respiratory Distress

After identifying respiratory distress or failure and beginning general supportive measures, assess whether the anatomical level of the respiratory problem is in the upper or lower airway, using the PAT and the hands-on <C>ABCDEs. Stridor is the hallmark of upper airway obstruction; wheezing is the hallmark of lower airway obstruction; grunting is the hallmark of lung disease; and inadequate minute volume and decreased work of breathing are the clinical markers for disordered control of breathing.

The most common cause of upper airway obstruction is croup. Rarely, foreign bodies lodged at or above the vocal cords may be the cause of stridor in infants and toddlers. Frequent causes of lower airway obstruction are asthma and bronchiolitis—a disease of infants. Asthma is the most likely cause of wheezing in all children from infancy to adulthood. A nebulised bronchodilator, delivered continuously if necessary, is the specific treatment for all causes of wheezing. Salbutamol is effective as a bronchodilator, and ipratropium provides added benefit in patients with asthma. Start treatment on scene in those with asthma.

Foreign body aspiration and pneumonia may present as lower airway problems, but there is no specific treatment for these conditions in the prehospital setting other than the general non-invasive measures for respiratory distress. Disordered control of breathing has many causes and often requires general ventilatory support.

Management of Respiratory Failure

Regardless of the cause, initially treat every cooperative child in respiratory failure with general non-invasive measures. If upper or lower airway obstruction is present, attempt specific

Case Study 3

A caregiver calls 999 because a 3-month-old girl has had 3 days of cough, runny nose, and low-grade fever. The caregiver is concerned because the child seems to be working harder to breathe and is having a hard time taking feedings. On arrival, the child is found lying on the caregiver's lap. She appears sleepy and does not make eye contact or respond to examination. She has audible wheezing and a deep subcostal and intercostal retractions. There is nasal flaring. Her skin is mottled. Respiratory rate is 70 breaths/min and heart rate is 180 beats/min. Her breath sounds are tight with only fair air movement, but you hear high-pitched, inspiratory and expiratory wheezes throughout. Pulse oximetry in room air is 74% with a pulse that corresponds to the patient's pulse on examination.

1. Is this child in respiratory distress or respiratory failure, and what is the level of airway obstruction?

2. What are the first steps in the management of this child?

treatment. However, if the child has altered appearance or altered mental status and has signs of increased or decreased work of breathing (e.g., flaring, grunting, gasping, apnoea, or cyanosis), or if the child has a documented blood oxygen saturation of less than 90% on 100% non-rebreathing oxygen mask, the child is in respiratory failure or respiratory arrest. For this child, bypass general non-invasive treatment and consider immediately beginning assisted ventilation.

First, position the patient to maintain an open airway. Then use suction. Suctioning is a basic technique to maintain an open airway. Children have tiny airways that are easily obstructed by secretions, vomitus, pus, blood, or foreign bodies. Children of different ages, with different clinical problems, need different types of suction devices and suctioning procedures. For a step-by-step explanation, see **Suctioning, Procedure 3**.

If the patient is unresponsive, use an airway adjunct. Adjuncts may immediately improve the child's spontaneous ventilation. In addition, they may allow more effective bag-valve-mask ventilation, reduce gastric inflation, and avert the need for endotracheal intubation. For a step-by-step explanation of this procedure, see **Airway Adjuncts, Procedure 4**.

Rarely, standard bag-valve-mask ventilation using basic airway adjuncts fails. Examples of such patients are children with massive head trauma and airway oedema or haematoma of the mouth or upper airway, or infants with significant congenital or acquired airway abnormalities who cannot be easily ventilated. In such circumstances, the use of supraglottic airways or dual lumen airways may be appropriate, utilising a stepwise approach to airway management, prior to considering intubation.

Then deliver assisted ventilation or positive-pressure ventilation using bag-valve-mask. Bag-valve-mask is usually the best method for providing oxygenation and ventilation during stabilisation and transport. Use an age-appropriate rate of 30 breaths/min in infants and 20 breaths/min in

older children. Saying the words, "squeeze, release, release" helps time the ventilations to avoid a rate that is too rapid. Ensure that there is good chest rise. Good bag-valve-mask technique decreases the risk of gastric distention, a common complication leading to elevation of the diaphragm, decreased lung compliance, and increased risk of vomiting and aspiration of gastric contents. With severe, lower airway obstruction, slower rates and longer expiratory times are indicated. Consider placing a nasogastric (NG) tube if local policies allow.

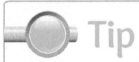

Tip

For an older child in respiratory failure who has increased work of breathing, ventilating at a rate of 20 breaths/min may assist the patient's respiratory effort.

Bag-Valve-Mask Ventilation

Bag-valve-mask ventilation is one of the prehospital professional's most useful skills in paediatric prehospital care. Although the technique does not provide the definitive airway control that endotracheal intubation does, in most cases bag-valve-mask ventilation is the best technique for providing oxygenation and ventilation during resuscitation and transport. For a step-by-step explanation of this procedure, see **Bag-Valve-Mask Ventilation, Procedure 7**.

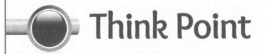

Think Point

Minimise gastric distention during bag-valve-mask ventilation with good bagging technique.

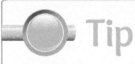

Tip

If the child does not respond to bag-valve-mask ventilation, or if there is a long transport time with a critically ill or injured child who has an unstable airway, consider using airway adjuncts.

Management With Endotracheal Intubation. The indications for endotracheal intubation of a child in the prehospital setting are very limited, meaning that it is a rarely undertaken procedure. Potential advantages of intubation include definitive airway control, decreased risk of aspiration, and ease of assisted ventilation. Potential complications include transient hypoxia and hypercapnia caused by prolonged intubation attempts; unrecognised misplacement of the tube; elevation of intracranial pressure; aspiration of stomach contents; and injury to the teeth, mouth, tongue, palate, larynx, and soft tissues of the pharynx and neck.

Dislodgment of the tube from the trachea during patient movement or transport is common and may be catastrophic. If an intubated patient fails to respond with improved colour, oxygen saturation, heart rate, and appearance, the DOPE mnemonic may help to identify potential technical problems (**Table 3-7**). Paediatric intubation should only be

Table 3-7 Troubleshooting the Endotracheal Tube: DOPE

	Problem	Assessment	Intervention
Dislodgment	oesophageal intubation	End-tidal carbon dioxide monitor or detector reads no or low carbon dioxide or has poor waveform, or no colour change Oxygen saturation <90% Bradycardia Lack of chest rise with ventilation Auscultation of bubbling over the stomach	Extubate Bag-valve-mask ventilation Re-intubate
	Mainstem bronchus intubation	Asymmetric chest rise Asymmetric breath sounds	Pull tube back until breath sounds and chest rise are symmetric
	Accidental extubation	End-tidal carbon dioxide monitor/detector reads no or low carbon dioxide level, or has poor waveform, or no colour change Oxygen saturation <90% Bradycardia Lack of chest rise with ventilation Poor or absent air movement on auscultation	Bag-valve-mask ventilation Re-intubate
Obstruction	Tube blocked with blood, secretions, or kink	Decreased chest rise Decreased breath sounds bilaterally Oxygen saturation <90% Carbon dioxide monitor has abnormal waveform Increased resistance to bagging	Suction, if no improvement extubate Bag-valve-mask ventilation Re-intubate
Pneumothorax	Tension pneumothorax, spontaneous or induced, compromises air exchange and may lead to decreased cardiac output	Asymmetric chest rise Asymmetric breath sounds Shock Oxygen saturation <90% *Jugular venous distention *Tracheal deviation	Needle thoracostomy
Equipment	Big air leak around tube Activated pop-off valve on resuscitator Oxygen tubing disconnected Oxygen tank empty	Oxygen saturation <90%	Check equipment, "patient-to-tank"

*Not always detectable in young children.

© Jones & Bartlett Learning

undertaken by those competent in the procedure and, when it is attempted, there must be constant monitoring of endotracheal tube placement.

Nasogastric and Orogastric Insertion

During positive-pressure ventilation, it is common to inflate the stomach and the lungs with air. Gastric inflation with air slows downward movement of the diaphragm and decreases tidal volume, making ventilation more difficult and necessitating higher inspiratory pressures. In addition, inflation of the stomach with air increases the risk that the patient will vomit and aspirate. Where the clinician is appropriately trained, and local policies allow, gastric intubation with an NG or orogastric (OG) tube can be undertaken in order to take air from the stomach and help positive-pressure ventilation. However, only use this technique if there is difficulty ventilating the patient. Insertion may be painful and frightening to the child and family.

Controversy

The value of nasogastric and orogastric tubes is unknown. Avoid inserting a nasogastric or orogastric tube unless ventilation is impaired by a distended stomach.

Endotracheal Intubation

Successful endotracheal intubation allows optimal oxygenation and ventilation, provides a tube for medication delivery, and decreases the risk of aspiration and loss of airway control. A properly placed and secured endotracheal tube is a good tool for managing critical patients, but the procedure can take a long time, and there can be frequent and serious complications. Every placement of an advanced airway must be confirmed for proper placement of the device. Exhaled carbon dioxide colorimetric devices or in-line capnometry or capnography should be used during the confirmation process. For a step-by-step explanation of this procedure, see **Endotracheal Intubation, Procedure 9**.

Additional adjuncts to assist in endotracheal intubation, where permitted, include the gum-elastic bougie, a lighted stylet, and RSI. Needle cricothyroidotomy is another option, if necessary. None of these techniques have been well evaluated in children in the prehospital setting and maybe of limited use in the very young child..

Table 3-8 summarises the advantages and disadvantages of airway management techniques. For a step-by-step explanation of the LMA, Combitube and its recommended removal, gum-elastic bougie, lighted stylet, and RSI (if permitted by local protocols), see **Advanced Airway Techniques, Procedure 11**.

Confirmation of Endotracheal Tube Placement

Several products are currently available for confirming proper placement of the endotracheal tube. These include quantitative end-tidal carbon dioxide monitors or capnometers, which read out the blood carbon dioxide tension ($Paco_2$) (**Figure 3-18**); colorimetric end-tidal carbon dioxide detectors that give a qualitative reading; and syringe and self-inflating bulb devices that distinguish endotracheal from oesophageal intubation based on positive aspiration of air from the tube (not approved for children <5 years or 20 kg).

The optimal method for tube confirmation in children in the out-of-hospital setting is not known. Because the child's airway is so short, even slight movement of the endotracheal tube can lead to extubation or mainstem intubation. If capnometry shows no carbon dioxide, if the colorimetric detector fails to change colour with ventilation, or if no air is aspirated into the oesophageal bulb or syringe, these are indications that the endotracheal tube may not be in the trachea. In such cases, remove the endotracheal tube, perform bag-valve-mask ventilation, and re-intubate after 1–2 minutes of oxygenation and ventilation.

The only exception to this approach is the patient in full cardiopulmonary arrest, where pulmonary circulation may be too low to generate detectable expired carbon dioxide. In this case, if the capnometer shows a low or absent end-tidal carbon dioxide reading, or if the colorimetric device shows a tan colour (low carbon dioxide), observe for chest rise, auscultate bilaterally for air movement, and attempt to visualise the tube passing through the vocal cords by direct laryngoscopy. If the endotracheal tube seems to be in proper position, leave the tube in place.

Tip

If an oesophageal bulb or syringe is used, cardiac arrest and low pulmonary blood flow should not affect the result.

Controversy

The optimal method for tube confirmation in children in the out-of-hospital setting is not known.

If an oesophageal bulb or syringe is used, cardiac arrest and low pulmonary blood flow should not affect the result. If air is aspirated, the tube is in the trachea. Hence, the oesophageal bulb or syringe technique for confirmation of endotracheal

Table 3-8 Advantages and Disadvantages of Airway Management Techniques

Technique	Advantages	Disadvantages
Supraglottic airway devices (LMA, SALT, King LAD, i-gel)	Simple insertion Good airway seal Adapts to bag-valve-mask equipment	Does not prevent aspiration Fewer size choices
Gum-elastic bougie	May facilitate endotracheal tube insertion	No equipment or data in infants and young children Prolonged attempts may worsen hypoxia
Lighted stylet	Does not require airway visualisation	Poor information in children Unknown accuracy
Dual lumen airway (e.g., Combitube), pharyngeotracheal lumen airway	Effective isolation of the airway Reduced risk of aspiration More reliable ventilation relative to bag-valve-mask ventilation Does not require visualisation of the glottis	Fatal complications may occur if the position of oesophageal-tracheal tube is identified incorrectly Potential for oesophageal trauma
Laryngeal tube/supralaryngeal airway	Effective isolation of the airway Reduced risk of aspiration More reliable ventilation relative to bag-valve-mask ventilation Does not require visualisation of the glottis Less complicated to insert than oesophageal-tracheal tube	Limited data published on the use of the laryngeal tube in children Potential for oesophageal trauma
Rapid sequence intubation	Paralyzes child and eliminates muscle resistance Improves visualisation Allows mild hyperventilation	Drugs remove spontaneous breathing Drugs may decrease blood pressure or respiratory rate Succinylcholine may cause high potassium
Cricothyroidotomy	Provides tiny airway for life-saving oxygenation or ventilation Bypasses obstruction	Technically difficult Bleeding Injury to other neck structures

© Jones & Bartlett Learning

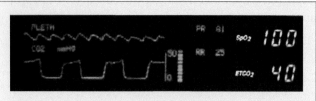

Figure 3-18 Carbon dioxide detector showing normal end-tidal carbon dioxide waveform.

tube placement may offer an advantage over the other two techniques in the setting of cardiac arrest and low pulmonary blood flow.

For a step-by-step explanation of these confirmation procedures, see **Confirmation of Endotracheal Tube Placement, Procedure 10**.

Summary of Management of Respiratory Failure

Respiratory failure or arrest can result from many different insults to the airway, mechanics of breathing, or gas exchange. Infection, trauma, and bronchospasm are important causes in children. Think respiratory failure when primary assessment reveals a child with altered appearance in the setting of significantly increased or decreased work of breathing. Bradycardia, poor air movement, and low oxygen saturation are key findings. In a child with respiratory failure or respiratory arrest, immediately begin assisted ventilation with a bag-valve-mask device at an age-appropriate rate. Avoid gastric insufflation. Add specific treatment for airway obstruction, such as an inhaled bronchodilator, if indicated.

Primary Assessment: The Transport Decision—Stay or Go?

When a child has respiratory distress, begin general non-invasive treatment (position of comfort and oxygen) and consider specific treatment on scene. Never transport a child who is in respiratory failure without assisted ventilations. Also, never transport a child with a severely obstructed airway until after performing FBAO manoeuvres. Immediate on-scene care to support breathing improves the outcomes of children with many respiratory emergencies. After opening the airway and providing assisted ventilation when necessary, or after simply giving general treatment, the prehospital professional must decide whether to stay on scene to assess further and treat specifically, or to go.

If the PAT and <C>ABCDEs are normal and the child has no history of serious breathing problems, the child does not usually require urgent treatment or immediate transport. Take the time to get a focused history and physical examination and perform a detailed physical examination (trauma patient) on the scene if possible.

If the child has respiratory distress and signs of upper airway obstruction, transport is usually indicated after general non-invasive treatment. Consider specific treatment of suspected croup with oral dexamethasone. *If the child has asthma and has lower airway obstruction with wheezing, begin specific treatment with bronchodilators on scene, and continue treatment during transport to the most appropriate receiving hospital with paediatric capabilities.* Place a pre-alert call in accordance with local policy.

For critical children, consider advanced airways or, less commonly, endotracheal intubation, if the child is in respiratory failure and ventilation by bag-valve-mask device is ineffective, or if an airway is difficult to maintain. However, endotracheal intubation increases on scene time and delays the time to definitive care at the ED. There has been a high rate of complications documented in prehospital studies of endotracheal intubation in children. Intubation skills tend to diminish

rapidly because they are used infrequently. In most cases, bag-valve-mask ventilation is the most appropriate option.

Additional Assessment

If the child has minimal respiratory distress and there are no immediate safety concerns for the child or prehospital professional, consider obtaining the focused history and physical examination and performing a detailed physical examination (trauma patient) on scene. Use the SAMPLE mnemonic to find important features of the complete respiratory history. **Table 3-9** gives examples of a focused history in a child with a breathing problem.

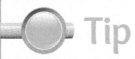 **Tip**

When a child fails to respond to assisted ventilation with improvement in clinical status, quickly assess your equipment—from the oxygen supply to the patient—for mechanical failure.

Perform vigilant ongoing assessment of all children with respiratory distress or failure while on the way to the ED. Use the PAT to recall observational indicators of effective gas exchange, and watch respiratory rate, heart rate, and pulse oximetry. Be prepared to increase the level of respiratory support or to correct complications of therapy if the child worsens or fails to respond.

Table 3-9 SAMPLE Components in a Child With Respiratory Distress

Component	Explanation
Signs and symptoms	Onset and nature of shortness of breath Presence of hoarseness, stridor, or wheezing Presence and quality of cough; chest pain
Allergies	Known allergies: food, medications, environmental Cigarette smoke exposure
Medications	Exact names and doses of ongoing drugs, including metered dose inhalers, and over-the-counter medications Recent use of steroids Timing and amount of last dose Timing and dose of analgesics and antipyretics
Past medical problems	History of asthma, chronic lung disease, or heart problems or prematurity Prior hospitalisations for breathing problems Prior intubations for breathing problems Immunisations
Last food or liquid	Timing of the child's last food or drink, including bottle or breastfeeding
Events leading to the injury or illness	Evidence of increased work of breathing Fever history

© Jones & Bartlett Learning

CASE STUDY ANSWERS

Case Study 1 — page 50

This child is in respiratory distress but does not seem to have progressed to respiratory failure. He is exhibiting many of the signs and symptoms of upper airway obstruction. His loud, harsh inspiratory breath sounds are consistent with stridor. This sound along with the supraclavicular and suprasternal retractions help localise the obstruction to the upper airway. He has increased work of breathing, but does not show any signs of hypoxia or hypercapnia (carbon dioxide retention). Upper airway obstruction and stridor in a young child after a few days of an upper respiratory infection are most consistent with croup, a swelling in the trachea below the area of the vocal cords caused by a viral infection. Other problems that may cause upper airway obstruction include foreign bodies; bacterial infections (e.g., epiglottitis or retropharyngeal abscess); and airway oedema caused by allergic reactions.

Regardless of the cause, the management of children with upper airway obstruction is similar and is based on the severity of the symptoms. Keep this patient in a position of comfort, give oxygen, and transport to an ED for further care.

ALS The child should be closely monitored because his upper airway obstruction may progress and respiratory failure may develop.

Case Study 2 — page 60

This is a choking child who needs first BLS manoeuvres and, if unsuccessful, progression to ALS manoeuvres by removing the FBAO using paediatric Magill forceps. This cannot be accomplished until the patient becomes unconscious. If the level of training prohibits the use of ALS skills, rapid transport to the ED while continuing chest compressions and ventilation is required.

Case Study 3 — page 65

Using the PAT, this child has an increased work of breathing, abnormal appearance, and poor circulation to the skin. She is in respiratory failure. Her wheezes and subcostal and intercostal retractions localise her airway obstruction to her lower airways. In the setting of preceding upper respiratory symptoms, fever, and progressive lower airway obstruction, the child probably has bronchiolitis. Open the child's airway, give high-flow oxygen, and begin bag-valve-mask ventilation. Do not delay transport because the child is not likely to have an easily reversible condition. This is unlike the child with asthma, who will likely benefit from a dose of a bronchodilator begun on scene, before transport.

ALS During transport monitor the child's respiratory status closely. Any evidence of decreased respiratory effort or slowing of the respiratory rate should prompt initiation of positive-pressure ventilation with a relatively slow rate and a long expiratory time.

SUGGESTED READINGS

Textbooks

American Heart Association. *Textbook of Pediatric Advanced Life Support.* Dallas, TX: American Heart Association; 2011.

Gausche M. *Pediatric Airway Management for the Prehospital Professional.* Burlington, MA: Jones & Bartlett Learning; 2004.

Joint Royal Colleges Ambulance Liaison Committee. *UK Ambulance Services Clinical Practice Guidelines 2016.* Bridgwater: Class Professional Publishing; 2016.

Articles

Anders J, Brown K, Simpson J, Gausche-Hill M. Evidence and controversies in pediatric prehospital airway management. *Clin Pediatr Emerg Med.* 2014;15(1):28–37.

Bhende MS, Thompson AE, Orr RA. Evaluation of an end-tidal CO_2 detector during pediatric cardiopulmonary resuscitation. *Pediatrics.* 1995;96(5 Pt 1):983.

Brownstein D, Shugerman R, Cummings P. Prehospital endotracheal intubation of children by paramedics. *Ann Emerg Med.* 1996;28:34–39.

Gausche M, Lewis R, Stratton S, et al. Effect of out-of-emergency department pediatric tracheal intubation on survival and neurologic outcome: controlled clinical trial. *JAMA.* 2000;283:783–790.

Kellner JD, Ohlsson A, Gadomski AM, et al. Efficacy of bronchodilator therapy in bronchiolitis—a meta-analysis. *Arch Pediatr Adolesc Med.* 1999;153(4):430.

Menon K, Sutcliffe T, Klassen T. A randomized trial comparing the efficacy of epinephrine with salbutamol in the treatment of acute bronchiolitis. *J Pediatr.* 1995;126:1004–1007.

Qureshi F, Pestian J, Davis P, et al. Effect of nebulized ipratropium on hospitalization rates of children with asthma. *N Engl J Med.* 1998;339:1030–1035.

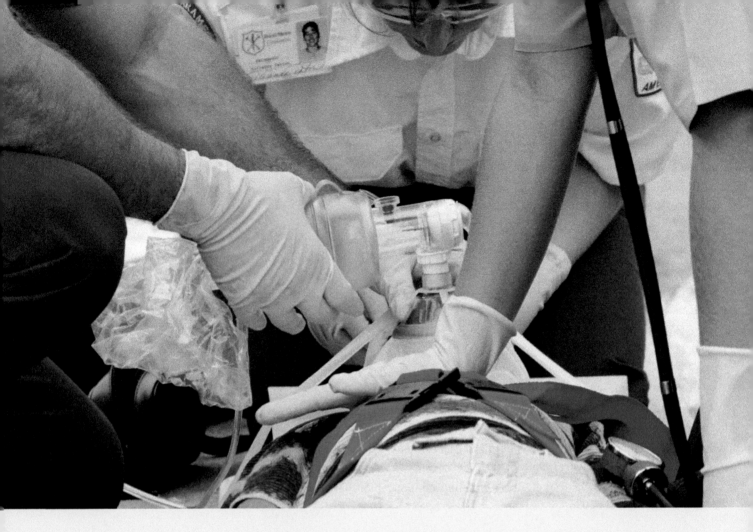

Learning Objectives

1. Describe how to assess circulation using the PAT, <C>ABCDEs, and additional assessment.

2. Explain the relationship between shock and blood pressure.

3. Differentiate between compensated and hypotensive (decompensated) hypovolaemic shock, and discuss appropriate management.

4. Distinguish the types of shock (hypovolaemic, distributive, cardiogenic, and obstructive) and outline treatment.

Shock

Introduction

Shock as a paediatric problem is uncommon in the out-of-hospital setting. Emergencies involving shock, or inadequate perfusion, may be the result of hypovolaemia, increased vascular permeability, cardiac failure, output obstruction, or a combination of any or all of these causes. Hypovolaemia is the usual cause of inadequate perfusion in children, most commonly precipitated by acute gastrointestinal losses from viral illnesses. Traumatic haemorrhage is a less frequent aetiology for severe hypovolaemia in children. Regardless of the type of emergency involving hypoperfusion, early recognition and timely management can reduce the likelihood for serious morbidity or mortality.

Most perfusion problems in children arise from loss of intravascular fluid. The child's young, healthy cardiovascular system compensates for fluid loss by increasing heart rate and reducing blood flow to non-essential anatomical areas through the mechanism of peripheral vasoconstriction, or "clamping down". Vasoconstriction limits blood flow to less essential peripheral sites, such as the skin, and preserves blood flow to the "core" organs, such as the brain, heart, and kidneys. The physiological process of restricting circulation to such areas as the skin and mucous membranes results in important physical signs of hypoperfusion.

Distributive shock is less common in children and is usually caused by sepsis. This type of shock primarily involves loss of vascular tone. Additionally, distributive shock can result from anaphylaxis, spinal cord injury, and exposure to toxins.

Cardiogenic shock is unusual in paediatrics, except in children with congenital heart disease, dysrhythmias, or acquired viral myocarditis. Cardiogenic shock results from heart rates that are either too fast or too slow to support perfusion, or from primary congestive heart failure. Regardless of the underlying cause, cardiac output is insufficient to meet perfusion requirements.

Obstructive shock is the rarest of all shock types in children. It is caused by pericardial tamponade or tension pneumothorax, secondary to injury to the chest. A third cause, pulmonary emboli, is extremely rare in children.

Identifying the type of shock can be difficult, especially when the pathophysiology is mixed. For example, bacterial toxins or ingested poisons may have adverse effects on vascular tone and myocardial function; sepsis may involve a volume deficit from third spacing (loss of plasma from the vascular space because of leaky blood vessels) and loss of vascular tone and myocardial depression. However, a careful history and physical assessment usually identify the cause of shock and drive appropriate management. Shock from any cause, if unrecognised or inadequately treated, may advance to cardiac arrest. After arrest has occurred, successful resuscitation is unlikely.

Case Study 1

A father calls 111 about an 18-month-old boy with a fever of 6 hours duration. The call is transferred to 999 and the EOC dispatches you to the scene. On your arrival, the child is listless. He will not interact and cries inconsolably when held. There is a purplish rash of the face, trunk, and legs. There are no abnormal airway sounds. Breathing is rapid without retractions or flaring. The brachial pulse is faint, the skin is warm to touch, and capillary refill time (CRT) is about 4 seconds. Respiratory rate is 60 breaths/min, and blood pressure is 60 mm Hg by palpation. The cardiac monitor shows a heart rate (HR) of 190 beats/min.

1. What type of shock is present?

2. What differs in the management of this case versus treatment of pure hypovolaemic or cardiogenic shock?

Prearrival Preparation

Based on the dispatch information, prepare mentally for the assessment and management of a child with circulatory problems en route to the scene. Recall appropriate techniques for assessment, the role of vital signs, and the possible equipment, drug, and fluid requirements of the child. Consider when to stay and treat on scene and when to transport immediately.

Scene Assessment

Be sure that the scene is safe. Evaluate the environment and document potentially important features, especially concerns for child maltreatment.

General Assessment: The Paediatric Assessment Triangle

Evaluating the Presenting Complaint

On arrival, determine the child's presenting complaint. Key questions include the onset of illness, presence of fever, frequency and amount of fluid losses (vomiting and diarrhoea), when the child last ate or drank, and prior history of possible congenital or cardiovascular problems. Ask if the child has been injured. In children with mild circulatory compromise who are not in shock, obtain a more complete SAMPLE history (see **Table 4-1**) during the additional assessment.

Assessment of Circulation

Using the Paediatric Assessment Triangle

The Paediatric Assessment Triangle (PAT) is the first step in assessment of perfusion, as outlined in the *Paediatric Assessment* chapter. The PAT evaluates three characteristics: (1) appearance, (2) work of breathing, and (3) circulation to skin. Knowing these characteristics helps to determine whether the child is sick or not sick, the type of physiological abnormality, and the urgency for treatment. Circulatory problems affect each of these characteristics in identifiable patterns.

Appearance

First, assess the child's appearance. A child with decreased core circulation from any shock type may have signs of poor brain perfusion. The abnormality in the child's appearance will be variable, depending on the type of perfusion problem, the degree of circulatory insufficiency, and the presence of associated problems, such as fever, head trauma, or intoxication. Abnormalities in the appearance of a child with decreased core circulation include the following:

- Lethargy or listlessness
- Decreased motor activity
- Diminished interactiveness with caregivers, the prehospital professional, and the environment (**Figure 4-1**)
- Inconsolability
- Poor eye contact
- Weak cry

Sometimes the child in shock is restless and inconsolable. Appearance alone, however, is not a very accurate sign of inadequate perfusion. An abnormal appearance may be caused by many different things, such as poor oxygenation and ventilation, head trauma, hypothermia, drugs, or fever. Assessing appearance is a good way to tell if the child is ill, but not a good way to identify the physiological cause. Assessment tools other than the PAT, such as the hands-on <C>ABCDE assessment, help distinguish the type of physiological problem and the presence or absence of abnormal perfusion.

Work of Breathing

Next, assess the work of breathing. If circulation to vital organs is decreased, the child's respiratory rate increases. "Effortless tachypnoea", sometimes known as "silent tachypnoea", is a

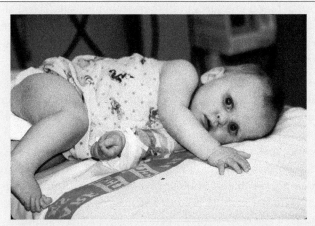

Figure 4-1 A child with decreased core circulation and too little blood and oxygen to the brain has an abnormal appearance. This dehydrated child has listlessness, poor motor activity, and decreased interactiveness.
Courtesy of Ron Dieckmann, MD.

fast respiratory rate without increased work of breathing. Effortless tachypnoea is a common but non-specific sign of shock. It reflects the child's attempt to blow off carbon dioxide and reduce the metabolic acidosis created by decreased perfusion to cells. Signs of increased work of breathing, such as abnormal positioning, retractions, flaring, or abnormal airway sounds, such as grunting, stridor, or wheezing, are not usually present in a child without a corresponding respiratory problem. These signs reflect poor gas exchange and hypoxia, typically from a primary lung problem. Although increased work of breathing is most commonly a function of respiratory disease, these signs may also occur with hypoxia and pulmonary oedema, when cardiogenic shock results from congestive heart failure, or in anaphylaxis when the respiratory system is a target organ often causing stridor and bronchospasm.

Circulation to Skin

After assessing appearance and work of breathing, assess circulation by looking at skin colour. This is difficult to interpret if the environmental temperature is low, because vasoconstriction, as a reflexive effort to preserve heat, falsely alters skin findings, especially in infants. Disrobe the child and look for mottling, pallor, and cyanosis, which reflect peripheral vasoconstriction or clamping down of non-essential skin perfusion to maintain essential core circulation. If a child has abnormal appearance and abnormal skin signs in a warm ambient environment, the child may be in shock.

Primary Assessment: The <C>ABCDEs

After the PAT, perform the hands-on <C>ABCDE assessment. After evaluating airway and breathing, as described in

the previous chapters, assess circulation. There are four parts to the assessment of circulation: (1) HR, (2) pulse quality, (3) skin temperature and CRT, and (4) blood pressure.

Heart Rate

First, measure HR by feeling a pulse for 30 seconds, and then double the number. A normal HR is between 60 and 160 beats/min, depending on the child's age, as noted in Table 2-3. The radial or brachial areas are preferred sites to measure pulse rate in infants and children. The carotid pulse is acceptable in older children and adolescents, but it is hard to locate in infants. If a pulse is difficult to feel, determine HR by listening to the heart sounds directly with a stethoscope placed on the medial side of the child's left nipple. However, be aware that the presence of a "normal" HR by auscultation does not necessarily reflect adequate cardiac output and perfusion.

Interpreting HR may be difficult, as explained in the *Paediatric Assessment* chapter. Ranges of normal HR change inversely with advancing age. Also, many conditions can increase HR, ranging from serious physiological problems to noxious stimuli that are rarely life-threatening. Stimuli that can cause tachycardia include pain, fever, fear, cold, and anger. Interpret HR in the context of overall signs of perfusion, age, presence or absence of noxious stimuli, and observed trends. Although a single measurement of HR is usually of limited value in determining the degree of physiological derangement, a trend of mounting tachycardia, or a HR that is falling below the lower limits of normal, suggests a serious physiological problem. In addition, sustained tachycardia is a worrisome sign. Finally, be extremely vigilant when the child has bradycardia, because this may mean hypoxia or an advanced state of hypoperfusion.

Pulse Quality

Presence of a strong central pulse (carotid or femoral) with a strong peripheral pulse (brachial, radial, or pedal in children) suggests an adequate blood pressure. A strong central pulse with a weak peripheral pulse indicates a shock-like state. If a brachial pulse is not palpable, the child is probably hypotensive and in hypotensive (decompensated) shock.

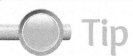 Tip

Tachycardia is often the first sign of shock in a paediatric patient.

Skin Temperature and Capillary Refill Time

The next part of the hands-on cardiovascular assessment involves evaluating skin signs. Check skin temperature for warmth centrally and peripherally, on the head or torso and

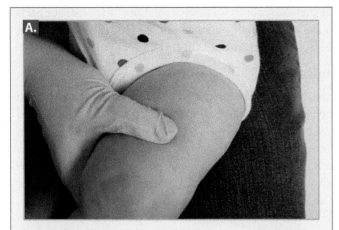

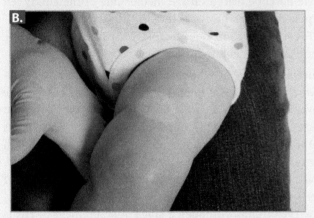

Figure 4-2 To determine CRT, first depress the skin (**A**), and then count the seconds before colour returns (**B**). Capillary refill time should be less than 2–3 seconds in a child who is not cold.

© Jones & Bartlett Learning.

also at the hands, feet, thighs, or forearms. Cool hands and feet may be normal, but cool proximal extremities reflect poor perfusion and shunting of blood to the core. Determine CRT by pressing firmly on the skin. CRT should be less than 2–3 seconds in a child who is not cold (**Figure 4-2**). Again, inadequate core perfusion results in peripheral vasoconstriction, which manifests as cool skin and delayed CRT. Although CRT is a good test of circulation in children, it must be interpreted in the context of overall signs of perfusion. The prehospital professional can become comfortable with the technique and interpretation of the key skin findings by practicing on every child.

Blood Pressure

Last, consider taking a blood pressure. A high blood pressure value is not clinically significant in the field, unless the child has a history of hypertension, known renal disease, or acute head injury. However, a true low blood pressure value is significant and means hypotensive (decompensated) shock. A normal blood pressure does not rule out a shock-like state. Children in significant shock may have

normal blood pressures until they decompensate. The challenges in the out-of-hospital setting include knowing when to get a blood pressure reading, obtaining the blood pressure correctly, and interpreting it accurately.

Systolic blood pressure does not accurately reflect intravascular volume status until the acute volume loss is greater than 25%–35% of normal circulating paediatric blood volume. This is because of the efficiency of compensation in a child, including vasoconstriction and an increase in HR. Therefore, a normal blood pressure does not mean the child has a normal blood volume or normal perfusion. A normal minimal systolic blood pressure in a child older than 1 year of age is 70 + (2 × years of age). Proper equipment, technique, and patience are required to obtain an accurate blood pressure in an infant or toddler. Because this can be a time-consuming process and may not contribute greatly to the clinical assessment of perfusion, in a child 3 years old or younger, attempt a blood pressure measurement only once or skip altogether. Inadequate perfusion is better reflected in the other signs of perfusion described previously (skin colour, HR, pulse quality, CRT, and skin temperature).

In a child older than 3 years of age, make at least one blood pressure attempt in every patient. Use a cuff with a width two-thirds the length of the upper arm. Applying too large a cuff falsely decreases the blood pressure measurement, and too small a cuff falsely increases the measurement.

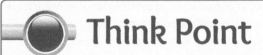

Think Point

A normal blood pressure does not rule out shock.

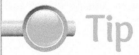

Tip

In children, one can use the combination of tachycardia, poor pulse quality, delayed CRT, and decreased mental status to diagnose shock, even with a normal blood pressure.

Additional Assessment

If the child is stable after the primary assessment and does not require immediate treatment, and if there are no immediate safety concerns for the child or prehospital professional, conduct history taking and physical examination and the detailed physical examination (trauma patient) on scene. Use the SAMPLE mnemonic (**Table 4-1**) to recall important features of the history in a child with inadequate perfusion. Use age-appropriate approaches to gain the child's trust and

Table 4-1 SAMPLE Components in a Child With Hypoperfusion Problems

Component	Features
Signs/Symptoms	Presence of vomiting or diarrhoea Number of episodes of vomiting or diarrhoea Abnormally frequent or reduced frequency of wet nappies (in infants) Vomiting blood or bile External haemorrhage Presence or absence of fever Rash Respiratory distress or shortness of breath (e.g., in cardiogenic shock with congestive heart failure)
Allergies	Known allergies History of anaphylaxis
Medications	Exact names and dosages of ongoing medications Use of laxatives or antidiarrhoeal medications Chronic diuretic therapy Potential exposure to other medications or drugs Timing and doses of analgesic/antipyretics
Past medical history	History of heart problems History of prematurity Prior hospitalisations for cardiovascular problems
Last food or liquid	Timing of the child's last food or drink, including bottle or breastfeedings, in particular any reduced frequency of feeding
Events leading to the injury or illness	Travel Trauma Fever history Symptoms in family members Potential toxic exposure

© Jones & Bartlett Learning.

speak directly to him or her. Ask the caregiver to add to the child's history. Obtain the history from the caregiver if the child is too young to speak or is unable to cooperate.

After the history, perform a focused examination of the heart, peripheral circulation, and the abdomen. Then, do an anatomical examination of the entire body, as outlined in the *Paediatric Assessment* chapter. If the child has a traumatic injury, also do a detailed physical examination, searching for other injuries.

Perform an ongoing assessment of all children with perfusion problems while on the way to the emergency department

(ED). The child's status may change during transport, so observe and document any physiological trends. Use the PAT to monitor effective perfusion and watch respiratory rate, HR, blood pressure, and pulse oximetry. Keep a child who is in shock on a cardiac monitor. Be prepared to increase the level of respiratory and cardiovascular support if the child worsens or fails to respond to treatment.

Summary of Cardiovascular Assessment

The PAT provides a good first-line evaluation of perfusion: Abnormal appearance, normal work of breathing, and poor circulation to skin suggest a perfusion problem. Pallor, mottling, and cyanosis all indicate poor peripheral perfusion. The circulatory portion of the hands-on <C>ABCDEs consists of evaluating HR, pulse quality, skin temperature, CRT, and blood pressure. These physical features complement the PAT and help identify the type and severity of circulatory compromise. Vital signs can sometimes be misleading and must be correctly obtained and interpreted for age. Trends in vital signs or persistence in abnormal vital signs, such as tachycardia, are more accurate indicators of real physiological problems than mild vital sign abnormalities on primary assessment.

Using the Assessment to Identify Shock

Shock is inadequate perfusion at the tissue level, with insufficient oxygen delivery to maintain normal cellular function. Oxygenation and ventilation, HR, intravascular volume, myocardial function, and vascular stability are all determinants of effective systemic cardiovascular function. If any one of these factors is impaired by illness or injury, the body attempts to compensate and normalise perfusion through modification of other physiological components.

In a child, the same physiological components are at work as in an adult. However, there are some differences. The physiological compensatory mechanisms, such as vasoconstriction and tachycardia, are very efficient in a child. Vasoconstriction is so efficient that a line of demarcation can sometimes be seen on extremities and mottling may be evident when circulation to the capillary beds has become stagnant. Sweating as a response to compensation, although common in an adult, does not always occur in a young child. Therefore, most children in shock have cool, dry skin versus, cool, diaphoretic skin. By adolescence, sweating as a response to compensation for shock is consistent. The last difference involves the child's energy reserves. A child does not have the same amount of energy reserves as an adult. The younger the child, the less is the capacity for energy reserves. Infants in particular have high glucose needs with low energy stores. As a result, compensatory mechanisms, although efficient, cannot last as long as those of an adult. This is one of the reasons why a child tends to decompensate quickly. This is also why checking a blood glucose level is important in any child who is under stress or has an altered mental status.

Because of these differences, clinical signs of decreased perfusion include altered mental status, persistent tachycardia as a compensatory mechanism, and changes in skin colour and temperature as a result of vasoconstriction. Do not expect sweating unless the child has increased work of breathing and is building up body heat, as in a congenital cardiac condition. As long as vasoconstriction, increased HR, and increased myocardial contraction are supported by the child's reserves, systolic pressure is maintained and the child compensates. When the body's reserves begin to fail or are exhausted, perfusion to the vital organs, such as the brain, is compromised. Blood pressure falls, mental status is impaired, and organ systems fail.

There are four general classes of shock (hypovolaemic, distributive, cardiogenic, and obstructive) (**Table 4-2**) reflecting impairment of the three major functional components of circulation: (1) the blood volume (hypovolaemic), (2) the vascular system (distributive), and (3) the heart (cardiogenic and obstructive). Studies of hypovolaemia (the most common type of paediatric shock) have allowed researchers to describe the clinical signs that characterise the progression of shock from a compensated state (adequate systolic blood pressure) to an uncompensated state (hypotension). However, the clinical signs characterising the progression of distributive, cardiogenic, or obstructive shock are not as well defined. This reflects the complex physiology of these other forms of shock.

Table 4-2 Summary of Different Types of Shock

Shock Type	Physiological Insult	Common Causes	Treatment
Hypovolaemic	Volume loss	Haemorrhage Gastroenteritis (vomiting, diarrhoea) Burns (extensive) Prolonged poor fluid intake	Rapid transport Intravenous fluid boluses
Distributive	Decreased vascular tone	Sepsis Anaphylaxis Drug overdose Spinal cord injury (neurogenic shock)	Rapid transport Fluid administration Epinephrine for anaphylaxis
Cardiogenic	Heart failure	Congenital heart disease Cardiomyopathy Dysrhythmia Drug overdose	Rapid transport Cautious crystalloid fluid administration, if required give 10 ml/kg
Obstructive	Obstructed blood flow	Pericardial tamponade Pneumothorax	Rapid transport Needle thoracostomy Fluid administration

© Jones & Bartlett Learning.

Case Study 2

The emergency operations centre (EOC) receives a call about a lethargic 12-year-old boy. On your arrival, he is lying in bed and barely notices your entrance. There is no increased work of breathing, but you do notice that he is breathing fast. His colour is pale. Vital signs are as follows: HR, 160 beats/min; RR, 40 breaths/min; BP, 80/40 mm Hg; SpO_2, 99% in room air. His capillary refill is 4 seconds. His mother states that he has been vomiting for 2 days and has had diarrhoea for 1 day.

1. Is this patient in shock?

2. If so, what type of shock is this?

3. What is the prehospital treatment?

Hypovolaemic Shock

Hypovolaemia (loss of fluid) is the most common cause of shock in children in the out-of-hospital setting. Vomiting and diarrhoea from gastroenteritis is the most common cause of hypovolaemic shock. Bleeding from blunt injuries, such as falls or vehicle collisions with the child as a pedestrian, bicyclist, or passenger, is the most common cause of haemorrhagic hypovolaemic shock.

The signs and symptoms of hypovolaemic shock vary with the amount, duration, and timing of fluid loss. As intravascular volume is further compromised by ongoing fluid losses (such as profuse diarrhoea or continued bleeding), the child may progress from compensated to decompensated shock.

Compensated Hypovolaemic Shock

Children who lose bodily fluids through minor blood loss or dehydration from gastroenteritis usually show no clinically significant effects on circulation. However, if fluid losses are more than about 5% of body weight, the body compensates for decreased blood flow by predictable adjustments in cardiovascular physiology. Sympathetic stimulation results in vasoconstriction and an increase in HR or tachycardia. As long as these processes maintain cardiac output to core organ systems, perfusion is maintained. This is compensated shock.

Vasoconstriction causes the following signs of abnormal circulation to the skin: delayed CRT, decreased pulse strength, poor skin colour (pallor or mottling), and dry and cool or cold skin temperature. A cold environment or hypothermia may also cause vasoconstriction as a reflex to maintain body heat, which mimics poor perfusion. Systolic blood pressure is normal in compensated shock.

In the compensated stage of hypovolaemic shock, appearance may be normal, or the child may appear slightly restless or less interactive. In a child with gastroenteritis, the appearance may be abnormal because of fever, which can alter appearance regardless of the circulatory status.

Hypotensive Hypovolaemic Shock

In hypotensive (decompensated) shock, perfusion is profoundly affected because compensatory mechanisms (increased HR and peripheral vasoconstriction) have failed to maintain sufficient circulation to core organs. The clinical signs are those of organ failure. Although a child in hypotensive shock may still be alert on AVPU, assessment of appearance is abnormal because of inadequate brain perfusion. The child may be restless and agitated, or poorly responsive. Hypotension, or low blood pressure for age, develops when there is about a 25% loss of intravascular volume (blood volume). Other late signs are effortless or silent tachypnoea, extreme tachycardia, extreme pallor or presence of mottling, and cold skin temperature.

If not reversed, hypotensive shock leads to cardiac failure, with bradycardia and respiratory failure, and then to cardiac arrest.

Although the course is less predictable, decreasing perfusion in children with distributive, cardiogenic, or obstructive shock results in progressive changes in appearance, skin signs, and work of breathing. For example, a child with cardiogenic shock may present only with tachycardia and diminished peripheral perfusion, and then progress to respiratory distress and lethargy as cardiac output worsens and congestive heart failure develops. In all shock types, hypotension is an ominous sign. More than one type of shock can occur concurrently in the same patient, as previously described.

Distributive Shock

In distributive shock, the child has decreased vascular muscle tone (peripheral vasodilation), impaired vascular integrity, or both in the presence of a normal circulating blood volume. This creates a relative hypovolaemia, and can be thought of as operating with a "less than full" tank. This change in the capacity of the vascular system and relative hypovolaemia leads to hypoperfusion to vital organs because of loss of vascular integrity. Patients with distributive shock may also have a component of hypovolaemia. This is the case in a patient with sepsis, who in addition to loss of vascular tone has "capillary leak" caused by the effect of bacterial toxins, or in the case of anaphylaxis where capillary leak may occur in the lungs or in the target tissues. In these situations, hypovolaemia is the result of "third spacing" of fluid from the vascular space into the surrounding tissues.

The most common cause of distributive shock is sepsis, especially in children younger than 2–3 years of age. In addition to anaphylaxis, chemical intoxication with drugs that decrease vascular tone (e.g., β-blockers, barbiturates) and spinal cord injury (above T6) with interruption of spinal sympathetic nerves to the muscle walls of peripheral arteries can cause distributive shock.

Special Features in Assessment of Distributive Shock

Signs of distributive shock reflect low peripheral vascular resistance (warm skin, bounding pulses, wide pulse pressure, changes in HR, hypotension) and decreased organ perfusion (abnormal appearance and behaviour). These signs may vary with the specific cause, as noted in the descriptions of the three major types of shock. Although the progression of physical signs in distributive shock is not as predictable as that in hypovolaemic shock, the late findings are indistinguishable from those of hypotensive shock from any cause: abnormal appearance from poor brain perfusion and hypotension.

Major Types of Distributive Shock

Sepsis

Sepsis occurs when any type of infection, usually bacterial or viral, overwhelms the body's defence system and causes a generalised breakdown in core organ function. Distinctive signs of early septic shock are warm skin, tachycardia, and bounding pulses. A septic child's appearance is abnormal and may include listlessness, lethargy, decreased interactiveness, restlessness, and poor consolability. Rash, fever, poor feeding, vomiting, diarrhoea, and fussiness may also be present.

Ill children usually like to be held and cuddled. If a child with a fever does not want to be held but is more comfortable when left alone, the child may have paradoxical irritability. This may be a sign of meningitis, where movement irritates the inflamed meninges (membranes covering the spinal cord and brain).

Sometimes, a septic child has a petechial rash or purpura (non-blanching dark red or purple dots or splotches) (**Figure 4-3**). These skin lesions are the result of toxins that cause inflammation of the blood vessels and leakage of blood into the skin. Consider a child with shock in association with a rash and fever to be septic. He or she may require aggressive volume resuscitation in the field, and prehospital professionals should use strict infection-control practices, including masks, to decrease their risk of infection.

Anaphylaxis

Anaphylaxis is a major allergic reaction that involves a generalised, multisystem response to an antigen (foreign protein). The airways and cardiovascular system are important sites of this often life-threatening reaction. Common causes include insect stings by bees, wasps, or fire ants; peanuts; latex; or medication. A child in anaphylactic shock has hypoperfusion and possibly additional signs, such as stridor or wheezing, with increased work of breathing. The child also has altered appearance with restlessness and agitation and sometimes a sense of impending doom. Hives (an intensely itchy skin rash) (**Figure 4-4**) and angioedema (flushed, swollen skin) are also common. Signs and symptoms of anaphylactic shock are dependent on the target organ. This is why some victims of anaphylaxis present with vomiting, diarrhoea, and hives, whereas others have angioedema, wheezing, and stridor.

Shock From Drug Intoxication

There are numerous cardiovascular drugs that can cause loss of vascular tone and hypoperfusion when ingested. **Table 4-3** lists common agents. The mechanism usually involves direct depressant effect on the cardiovascular system (slowing of the HR and decreased strength of contraction, and vasodilation).

Neurogenic Shock

Neurogenic shock is rare in children. It results from a mechanism of injury that involves the back, neck, or both, and interrupts nervous system pathways. There is a loss of the autonomic nervous system's sympathetic control of

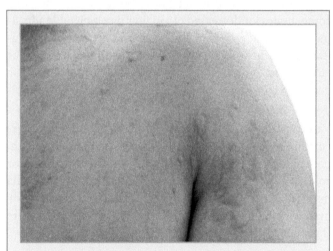

Figure 4-4 Hives suggest an allergic reaction and are usually present with anaphylaxis, the most extreme form of an allergic reaction.
Beth Van Trees/Shutterstock.

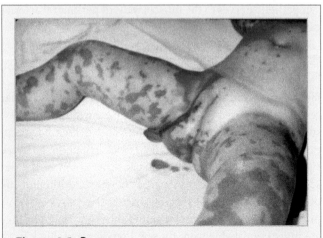

Figure 4-3 Purpura.
Courtesy of Ron Deickmann, MD.

Table 4-3 Drug Intoxications That May Cause Shock

Antihypertensives
β-blockers
Calcium antagonists
Clonidine
Cyclic antidepressants
Iron
Opioids
Phenothiazines

© Jones & Bartlett Learning.

circulation. This is observed when the injury occurs at T6 or above. The result is vasodilation and impaired sympathetic stimulation of the heart. The child has motor paralysis and is hypotensive and bradycardic, with loss of the normal tachycardic response to actual or relative hypovolaemia. With loss of the normal vascular reflex to maintain body heat, the body also loses heat to the environment.

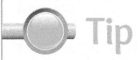

Tip

If a trauma patient has a normal or slow HR and low blood pressure, think spinal cord injury and neurogenic shock.

Cardiogenic Shock

Cardiogenic shock is uncommon in children and is rarely diagnosed in the prehospital setting unless the child has a known cardiac history (**Figure 4-5**). In fact, the child's condition may be misdiagnosed as septic or hypovolaemic shock, resulting in the administration of fluid boluses. The most likely cause is either congenital heart disease, dysrhythmia, or cardiomyopathy from myocarditis. Myocarditis is

a disease of the heart muscle, usually caused by a virus. A dysrhythmia, such as supraventricular tachycardia (SVT) or bradycardia (<60/min), may also cause cardiogenic shock. Overdose with a cardiac medication, such as a calcium channel blocker or β-blocker, is another possible aetiology.

Special Features in Assessment of Cardiogenic Shock

A history from the caregiver usually reveals that the child has had non-specific symptoms, such as loss of appetite, abdominal pain, poor feeding, lethargy, irritability, and inappropriate sweating over a period of days. The sweating is caused by the increased work load (work of breathing or work of the heart) and is an attempt to cool off the body. This is true of children with myocarditis and congenital heart disease. There is often a history of congenital heart disease or the presence of a midline chest scar from heart surgery. **Table 4-4** summarises the common symptoms and signs of cardiogenic shock.

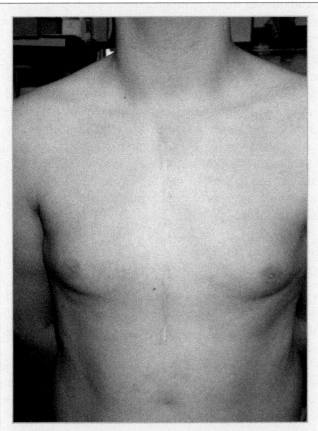

Figure 4-5 A midline sternal scar could be an indicator of a cardiac history.

Courtesy of Lisa Wise.

Table 4-4 Symptoms and Signs of Cardiogenic Shock

Possible historical findings in cardiogenic shock
Preceding history of chest pain
Previous history of flu-like symptoms associated with weakness and fatigue
Difficulty feeding because of fatigue and sweating during feeding in the breast or bottle-fed infant
No history of fever
No history of volume loss (e.g., diarrhoea, vomiting, or blood loss)
Positive history of congenital heart disease
No history of asthma despite wheezing on examination
Persistent wheezing despite the administration of β-agonist (e.g., salbutamol)
History of cyanosis
Recent history of exercise intolerance
Possible physical findings
Tachypnoea or grunting with clear lungs on examination
Unexplained dysrhythmias in the presence of a flu-like illness
Tachycardia disproportionate to the degree of fever
Persistent or worsening tachycardia despite fluid administration
Heart murmur, friction rub, or gallop on examination
Presence of cyanosis that does not improve with the administration of oxygen
Crackles on lung examination
Peripheral oedema or pitting oedema
Hepatomegaly

© Jones & Bartlett Learning.

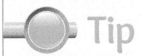

Cardiogenic shock can occur from HRs that are too fast or too slow.

Cardiogenic shock may develop from left heart failure. Impaired left heart function causes decreased core organ perfusion. On physical assessment, the child may appear abnormal: sluggish, irritable, or agitated, and the skin colour mottled or cyanotic. Heart rate is rapid; blood pressure may be high (early), normal, or low (late). The skin is cool and the child may be diaphoretic (not dry as with hypovolaemic shock) related to the increased work load. Pulmonary oedema causes increased work of breathing and inspiratory crackles or wheezing. The increased work load may deplete energy stores resulting in hypoglycaemia. Checking blood glucose levels is recommended.

Increased right-sided cardiac pressures are also present in cardiogenic shock and result in liver enlargement (hepatomegaly). Hepatomegaly is an especially useful finding in infants and toddlers. Peripheral oedema and jugular venous distention are rare in children. Cardiogenic shock can also occur from HRs that are too fast or too slow. Because the origin of a rate-related problem is often congenital, assessment and treatment are discussed under congenital cardiac problems.

Obstructive Shock

Several pathologic conditions may obstruct blood flow from the heart and cause shock. Pericardial tamponade and tension pneumothorax are two acute conditions that cause dramatic development of shock after blunt or penetrating injuries to the chest wall. Haemopericardium develops quickly after a gunshot or sharp object penetrates into a blood-filled heart chamber, usually the right ventricle. Blunt trauma to the chest at just the right time during the cardiac cycle can produce pressures great enough to rupture the tendons stabilizing the cardiac valves or rupture the tissue between the chambers of the heart. The hole in the wall of the heart provides a route for blood to escape into the space between the two pericardial membranes. Because the membranes do not stretch quickly, blood collects and collapses the right ventricle (tamponade). This interrupts venous return to the right heart and produces a profound drop in cardiac output.

Rarely, pericardial tamponade may develop after an infectious or inflammatory process in the chest. Cancer or chronic renal failure causes pericardial fluid accumulation. This type of fluid accumulation is slow and the membranes around the heart stretch. Therefore, obstructive shock caused by infectious or inflammatory processes rarely occurs.

Tension pneumothorax develops after a penetration into the pleural space. Sometimes blunt injury to the chest wall can also rupture alveoli, causing a pneumothorax, which may rapidly progress to a tension pneumothorax when vigorous ventilation with a bag-valve-mask device occurs. Air and sometimes blood (haemothorax) collects in between the two membranes of the pleura. When the pressure increases enough to cause a shift of the mediastinum, venous return to the right heart is impaired. This causes a drop in cardiac output and hypoperfusion.

In children or adolescents with cystic fibrosis, the lung may have blebs that rupture spontaneously, resulting in a pneumothorax, which can progress to a tension pneumothorax.

Special Features in Assessment of Obstructive Shock

Penetrating injuries to the chest wall are often deceptive. The appearance of the wound may be benign and seem superficial. Consider all gunshot wounds or stab wounds to the chest as major penetrations into the heart or pleura. Other types of penetrations from sticks or sharp objects may also cause severe internal injury. Be especially vigilant when the penetration has an entry site in the area between the two nipples and the clavicles, because this is a high-risk location for cardiac injury. Blunt chest injury may also cause a pneumothorax that may progress to a tension pneumothorax. Suspect this condition in a child with a significant blunt mechanism of injury and signs of obstructive shock.

The cardinal features of obstructive shock are signs of decreased circulation in an injured child with increased jugular venous distention. The increased jugular pressures reflect the obstruction to venous return to the right ventricle. Sometimes, however, blood loss into the chest (haemothorax) or other related injuries may be associated with haemorrhage, so that jugular venous distention is not apparent. In the case of a tension pneumothorax, lung sounds are unequal or absent on the affected side, and ventilation is increasingly difficult.

General Non-invasive Treatment of Suspected Shock of All Types

Begin general non-invasive treatment of every child with suspected hypoperfusion after completing the PAT and initiating the hands-on <C>ABCDEs. The general treatment is always the same: allow the child to assume a position of comfort if the cause is medical. In the case of trauma, the child may need spinal stabilisation. Supply oxygen, as required and as tolerated. This is the only management for most patients.

Positioning

Infants and toddlers may be most "comfortable" in their caregiver's arms or lap during assessment. If the primary assessment indicates that the child is physiologically unstable, place the child in a position of comfort that decreases his or her anxiety and activity. This is usually the supine position (**Figure 4-6**). Elevating the legs when the child is in the supine position is not effective. Putting the child in a head-down position is not known to improve outcome. In a head-down position, the internal organs of the abdomen put pressure on the diaphragm, interfering with breathing. The resulting agitation increases oxygen demand and complicates treatment. In the supine position, alignment of the airway is aided by placing a towel under the shoulders and trunk of the child. This helps with ease of breathing. Keep the child warm because children have a high surface-to-volume ratio and can lose body heat rapidly.

Oxygen

Treat all children in shock with high-flow oxygen. The prehospital professional must weigh the potential benefits of oxygen administration against the risk of agitating the child. "Blow-by" may be the only mechanism for delivering supplemental oxygen without upsetting the child and increasing his or her oxygen consumption.

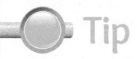

Tip

Provide high-flow oxygen to all children in shock.

Specific Treatment of Hypovolaemia

After the primary assessment and beginning general supportive measures, provide additional specific treatment of shock. If the child has hypovolaemic shock, consider how to stop the child's fluid losses and whether to attempt to replace them. In trauma patients, always look carefully for bleeding sites and assume there may be internal bleeding. Apply direct pressure to stop external bleeding. Consider appropriate immobilisation and splinting of injured extremities, as described in the *Medical Emergencies* chapter.

If the child has severe fluid losses from vomiting or diarrhoea, consider obtaining vascular access to give fluids. If the child has hypotensive shock from illness, do not delay by attempting to gain IV access at the scene. Make up to two attempts to gain IV access during transport, stopping the ambulance for venipuncture attempts if needed. If attempts at IV access fail or a suitable vein is not apparent within a reasonable timeframe then gain IO access.

Intravenous Access

Intravenous (IV) access makes it easier to give medications and provides a way to give fluid therapy in severe blood or fluid loss. IV delivery is the gold standard for giving medication, because it permits rapid drug and fluid treatment and allows titration of important drugs. See **Intravenous Access, Procedure 13**.

IV Fluid Treatment of Compensated Hypovolaemic Shock

If the child has mild-to-moderate volume losses as determined by HR, pulse quality, CRT, and skin temperature, and has a normal blood pressure, he or she is in compensated shock. Do not remain on scene to perform IV insertion and fluid administration. On the way to the hospital, consider obtaining vascular access and giving IV crystalloid fluid at 20 ml/kg boluses to stabilise the patient. The patient may require additional fluid boluses up to a total of 60 ml/kg or until the patient has an appropriate clinical response. In shock caused by trauma reduced dose fluid boluses of 5 ml/kg should be given.

IV Fluid Treatment of Hypotensive (Decompensated) Shock

If the child has decompensated shock from illness, do not delay transport to attempt to gain IV access. Once access

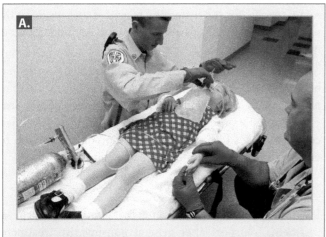

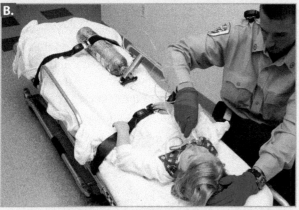

Figure 4-6 A. Treat suspected hypovolaemic shock with high-flow oxygen and supine positioning. **B.** Keep the patient warm.

© Jones & Bartlett Learning.

is established during transport, give 20 ml/kg boluses of IV crystalloid fluid. Consider intraosseous (IO) needle insertion as above, if vascular access cannot be obtained. Repeat boluses (20 ml/kg up to 60 ml/kg) as needed to stabilise perfusion, based on ongoing reassessment of the PAT and vital signs. In trauma patients the fluid bolus volume should be reduced to 5ml/kg.

IO Needle Insertion

Using an IO needle to give drugs or fluids is an excellent alternative to cannulating peripheral veins. The IO space is highly vascularised and functions as a non-collapsible vein. Needle insertion into this space is quick, simple, effective, and usually safe. Complications are infrequent and usually minor. See **Intraosseous Needle Insertion, Procedure 14**.

Think Point

In a child with hypovolaemic shock, crystalloid fluid boluses need to be given as fast as possible. Do not let the fluid just drip in.

Specific Treatment of Distributive Shock

The primary difference between treatment of distributive and hypovolaemic shock is the potential need for a vasopressor agent to improve vascular tone and heart muscle function when the child has distributive shock, which is currently outside of the scope of practice for paramedics in the UK. Treat all shock conditions first with general non-invasive measures. Administer high-flow oxygen and put the poorly responsive child with shock in a supine position.

Treatment of Hypotensive (Decompensated) Distributive Shock

Do not delay transport in order to gain IV access. Deliver fluid boluses, up to 60 ml/kg of a crystalloid fluid solution in 20 ml/kg boluses on the way to the ED.

Treatment of Anaphylaxis

A child with anaphylaxis requires fluid and special treatment with adrenaline, a β-agonist if bronchospasm is present, and may require chlorphenamine and hydrocortisone. Unlike a simple allergic reaction, anaphylaxis has dangerous cardiovascular effects (**Figure 4-7**).

Adrenaline is an excellent drug for treatment of anaphylaxis. It stimulates α- and β-adrenergic receptors, leading to two important effects: (1) constriction of the blood vessels to help counter the vasodilation and increased permeability of anaphylaxis (alpha effect), and (2) opening up the airways to help reverse the bronchospasm of anaphylaxis (beta effect).

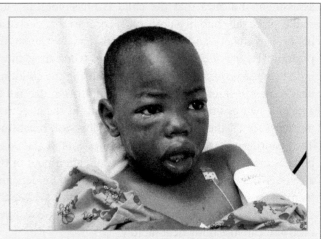

Figure 4-7 An allergic reaction, with oedema of face, lips, and tongue.
Courtesy of Susan Fuchs, MD.

For all children with anaphylaxis, administer adrenaline, 1:1,000 solution intramuscularly (IM).

In cases of severe anaphylaxis or where symptomatic allergic reactions are causing patient distress chlorphenamine may also be necessary. Chlorphenamine works as an antihistamine, specific for the histamine receptors that reside in the walls of the blood vessels and in the skin. Administration of this medication eases itching.

Adrenaline is a short-acting drug and repeated dosing may be necessary. A long-acting steroid, such as hydrocortisone, is given with anaphylaxis to help decrease biphasic anaphylactic reactions. Hydrocortisone acts to stabilise mast cell membranes to prevent perpetuation of the reaction by chemicals triggered by the allergic reaction.

Treatment of Cardiogenic Shock

If cardiogenic shock is suspected by history or physical assessment, transport after general non-invasive treatment. On the way to the ED, consider vascular access. If the diagnosis of cardiogenic shock is uncertain, give a cautious fluid bolus of only 10 ml/kg of crystalloid fluid, and then reassess appearance, work of breathing, CRT, HR, and blood pressure. If the child is known to be in congestive heart failure with cardiogenic shock, avoid fluid boluses.

The major difference between treatment of hypovolaemic, distributive, and cardiogenic shock is the amount of fluid administration.

Think Point

Do not withhold fluid from a child in cardiogenic shock; just give it in boluses of 10 ml/kg and reassess.

Case Study 3

A 6-year-old boy in primary school is having trouble breathing, so the teacher calls 999. On your arrival, the boy has swollen eyes, but answers your questions about his name and age. He has increased work of breathing with audible wheezing. There are hives on his face and arms. The teacher says he has a peanut allergy and may have eaten a birthday cake with nuts. Vital signs are as follows: HR, 150 beats/min; RR, 50 breaths/min; BP, 90/50 mm Hg; Spo$_2$, 90% in room air.

1. Is this child in shock?

2. What is the appropriate prehospital therapy?

Treatment of Obstructive Shock

The additional option for treatment of obstructive shock from a tension pneumothorax is needle thoracostomy to decrease air pressure.

This technique relieves pressure in the pleural space. Rapid transport is an essential feature of field management of chest injury.

Primary Assessment: Transport Decision

After completing the primary assessment and beginning general treatment when appropriate, the prehospital professional must decide whether to go or stay on scene. If the PAT and <C>ABCDEs are normal and the child has no history of serious illness or injury mechanism, no anatomical abnormalities, and no pain, the child does not usually require urgent treatment or immediate transport. Take the time to get a history and physical examination and perform a detailed physical examination (trauma) on the scene if possible.

If the child has a serious mechanism of injury, a physiological or anatomical abnormality, severe pain, or if the scene is not safe, transport immediately. With such patients, do the additional assessment and attempt specific treatment on the way to the hospital, if possible.

The transport decision is sometimes difficult in a child with a suspected cardiovascular problem who needs vascular access. Do not waste time attempting to gain IV or IO access on scene. Obtain access en route unless delay is unavoidable.

Summary of Shock States

There are four major classes of shock seen both in children and adults: (1) hypovolaemic, (2) cardiogenic, (3) distributive, and (4) obstructive. Hypovolaemic shock is commonly the result of trauma and haemorrhage after injury. Vomiting and diarrhoea leading to dehydration is the most common medical cause of hypovolaemia. Distributive shock may result from sepsis, anaphylaxis, drug intoxication, or spinal injury. Always suspect sepsis in the infant or toddler who has fever and abnormal appearance. A petechial or purpuric skin rash is a red flag for sepsis. Cardiogenic shock caused by inadequate left ventricular contraction is rare in children and difficult to identify in the field, unless the child has a known congenital cardiac problem. Obstructive shock sometimes occurs in conjunction with significant chest wall injury. Clinical findings may reflect more than one type of shock pathophysiology. Treatment of all shock types includes general non-invasive interventions, and then specific treatment based on clinical findings. Consider rapid fluid boluses in children who are hypotensive with an abnormal appearance.

CASE STUDY ANSWERS

Case Study 1 — page 74

This child has septic or distributive shock. He has decompensated shock with hypotension. The rash is an ominous sign and aggressive treatment is necessary to save the child's life. The appropriate first interventions are oxygen and bag-valve-mask ventilation.

Attempt IV or IO access en route to hospital and give a 20 ml/kg crystalloid fluid bolus as fast as possible. Deliver additional 20 ml/kg fluid boluses to a maximum of 60 ml/kg while en route to the ED.

This case also requires universal precautions to protect the prehospital professional because the child has a serious communicable disease. Direct specific questions about exposures and prophylactic treatment to your infection control personnel.

Case Study 2 — page 78

This child is in hypotensive (decompensated) shock, because his blood pressure is low. The aetiology is likely hypovolaemia, because of the history of vomiting and diarrhoea. His lethargy can be caused by shock, but could also be caused by hypoglycaemia. Prehospital treatment is to attempt IV or IO access en route to hospital and give a 20 ml/kg normal crystalloid fluid bolus as fast as possible. Give additional 20 ml/kg fluid boluses to a maximum of 60 ml/kg while en route to the ED. A bedside glucose can also be obtained, and if it is low, 10% dextrose given, in addition to the IV fluids. In this case, his glucose is 2 mmol/L, so 50g (100 ml from a 500 ml bag) can be administered.

Case Study 3 — page 85

This is a case of anaphylaxis, and although this child is not in shock at this time, it could still develop. Anaphylaxis requires urgent treatment of adrenaline 1:1,000 IM. Administration of Salbutamol via a nebuliser may help his wheezing. Insertion of an IV now can be useful to give IV Chlorphenamine and Hydrocortisone. If his blood pressure begins to drop a rapid infusion of 20 ml/kg normal crystalloid fluid bolus is indicated.

SUGGESTED READINGS

Textbooks

JRCALC JRCALC Clinical Practice Supplementary Guidelines 2017. Bridgwater: Class Professional Publishing; 2017.

NICE. (2016). Sepsis: recognition, diagnosis and early management NICE Guideline NG51. https://www.nice.org.uk/guidance/ng51.

NICE. (2015). Intravenous fluid therapy in children and young people in hospital NICE Guideline NG29. https://www.nice.org.uk/guidance/ng29.

World Health Organization. *Oxygen therapy for children: a manual for health workers.* Geneva: World Health Organisation; 2016.

American Academy of Pediatrics and the American College of Emergency Physicians. *APLS: The Pediatric Emergency Medicine Resource.* 5th ed. Burlington, MA: Jones and Bartlett Learning; 2012.

Articles

deCaen AR, Maconochie IK, Aickin R, et al. Part 6: Pediatric basic life support and pediatric advanced life support; 2015. International Consensus and Cardiopulmonary Resuscitation and Emergency Cardiovascular Care Science with Treatment Recommendations. *Circulation.* 2015;132 (suppl 1):S177–S203.

Kleinman, ME, Chameides L, Schexnayder SM, et al. Part 14: Pediatric advanced life support: 2010 American Heart Association Guidelines for Cardiopulmonary Resuscitation and Emergency Cardiovascular Care. *Circulation.* 2010;122(suppl 3): S876–S908.

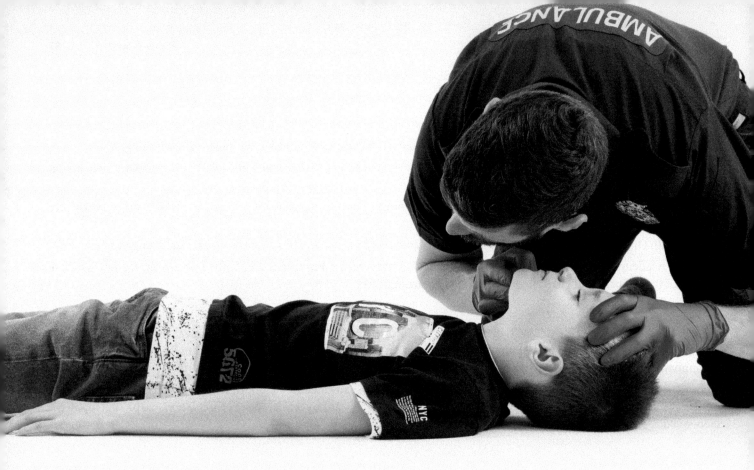

Learning Objectives

1. Describe how to perform an immediate assessment using the Paediatric Assessment Triangle (PAT), <C>ABCDEs, and additional assessment. List the links in the paediatric "Chain of Survival".

2. Order the steps in managing paediatric cardiac arrest caused by asystole, pulseless electrical activity (PEA), ventricular fibrillation (VF), and pulseless ventricular tachycardia (VT).

3. Define indications for the use of defibrillation (manual and automatic) in paediatric patients.

4. Describe the causes of primary cardiac arrest in the paediatric patient.

5. Explain when to treat tachycardia and bradycardia, and discuss management. Discuss medical issues in children with congenital heart disease who may present to the prehospital professional.

Resuscitation and Dysrhythmias

Introduction

Paediatric cardiac arrest is uncommon in the out-of-hospital setting. Survival to discharge from paediatric out-of-hospital cardiac arrest varies depending on age and aetiology. Data from London Ambulance Service shows how survival to discharge rates change according to age: 10.2% for under 1 year, 16.7% for those aged 1–8 and 8.1% for those aged 9–18 (London Ambulance Service Cardiac Arrest Annual Report 2016/17). The primary cause of arrest in children is usually related to a hypoxic situation that deteriorates into cardiac arrest. However, this does not mean that all cardiac arrest in children will have a hypoxic cause and as such all reversible causes must be carefully considered each time you attend an incident of this nature.

While ventricular fibrillation (VF) and pulseless ventricular tachycardia (pVT) may be uncommon in out-of-hospital paediatric cardiac arrest, early monitoring is essential to recognise those few children who do present in a shockable rhythm and provide immediate defibrillation. **Table 5-1** shows data from London Ambulance Service regarding the initial rhythm.

Prearrival Preparation

Based on dispatch information, the clinician needs to be prepared to assess, manage, and make transport decisions for a child exhibiting a symptomatic cardiac dysrhythmia, cardiac event, or cardiac arrest. Recall appropriate techniques for assessment, the role of vital signs (to recognise the deteriorating child), and the possible equipment, medications, fluid requirements and defibrillation a child may require. We will discuss in more detail when to stay and treat on scene and when to transport immediately.

Scene Assessment

All clinicians need to ensure that the scene is safe, and note any significant findings that may be contributing factors to the situation. The clinician must also assess the scene, as appropriate, for signs of non-accidental injury and safeguarding concerns.

General Assessment: The PAT
Evaluating the Presenting Complaint

On arrival, determine the child's presenting complaint. Gathering a complete patient history is a vital component in determining the cardiac event the patient may be experiencing. Attempt to gather a complete SAMPLE history (see **Table 5-2**) during the primary assessment.

Case Study 1

You have been dispatched to a 7-year-old child who is unconscious. You arrive at a residential property and find the child lying in bed. You assess the child and find them to be unresponsive, tachypnoeic (40/min) and tachycardic (160/min). They are centrally warm, but have cold hands and feet. They have been unwell for 5 days. The central capillary refill time is 5 seconds.

1. Based on the information you have so far, what is the most likely cause of deterioration in this child?
2. What intervention may prevent this child from deteriorating into cardiac arrest?

Table 5-1 Initial Rhythm (LAS Cardiac Arrest Annual Report 2016/17)

Initial Rhythm (LAS Cardiac Arrest Annual Report 2016/17)			
	Under 1	1–8	9–18
Number of Patients	66	27	52
Asystole	78.8% (52)	77.8% (21)	63.5% (33)
Pulseless electrical activity (PEA)	12.1% (8)	22.2% (6)	21.2% (11)
VF/Pulseless VT	1.5% (1)	-	13.5% (7)
Not documented	7.6% (5)	-	1.9% (1)

Republished with kind permission of London Ambulance Service.

Table 5-2 SAMPLE Components in a Child With Cardiovascular Problems

Component	Features
Signs/symptoms	Presence of vomiting More cyanotic than usual Lower pulse oximeter reading Number of episodes of vomiting Presence or absence of fever Rash Respiratory distress or shortness of breath (e.g., in cardiogenic shock with CHF)
Allergies	Known allergies and what reaction occurs History of anaphylaxis
Medications	Exact names and dosages of ongoing medications Chronic diuretic therapy Potential exposure to other medications or drugs Timing and doses of analgesics or antipyretics
Past medical history	History of heart problems or heart surgery History of prematurity Prior hospitalisations for cardiovascular problems
Last food or liquid	Timing of the child's last food or drink, including bottle or breastfeedings
Events leading to the injury or illness	Travel Trauma Fever history Symptoms in family members Potential toxic exposure

© Jones & Bartlett Learning.

Assessment of Circulation

Using the PAT

The PAT is the first step in assessment of circulation, as outlined in the *Paediatric Assessment* chapter. The PAT evaluates three characteristics: (1) appearance, (2) work of breathing, and (3) circulation to skin. Knowing these characteristics helps to determine whether the child is sick or not sick, the type of physiological abnormality, and the urgency for treatment. Circulatory problems affect each of these characteristics in identifiable patterns.

Appearance

First, assess the child's appearance. A child with decreased core circulation from any cardiac compromise may have signs of poor brain perfusion. The abnormality in the child's appearance will be variable, depending on the type of perfusion problem and the degree of circulatory insufficiency.

Abnormal features in the appearance of a child with decreased core circulation include the following:

- Lethargy or listlessness
- Decreased motor activity for infants, poor muscle tone
- Diminished interactiveness with caregivers, the prehospital professional, and the environment
- Inconsolability
- Poor eye contact
- Weak cry

Sometimes the child with haemodynamic instability will be restless and inconsolable. *Appearance alone, however, is not a very accurate sign of circulatory problems.* Assessing appearance is a good way to tell if the child is ill, but not a good way to identify the physiological problem. Assessment tools other than the PAT, such as the hands-on <C>ABCDE assessment, will help distinguish the type of physiological problem and the presence or absence of abnormal perfusion.

Work of Breathing

Next, assess the work of breathing. If circulation to vital organs is decreased, the child's respiratory rate will increase. "Effortless tachypnoea", or a fast respiratory rate without increased work of breathing, is a common but non-specific sign of haemodynamic instability. It reflects the child's attempt to blow off carbon dioxide and reduce the metabolic acidosis created by decreased perfusion to cells. Signs of increased work of breathing, such as abnormal positioning, retractions, flaring, or abnormal airway sounds, such as grunting, stridor, or wheezing, are not usually present in a child with a pure circulatory problem. These signs reflect poor gas exchange and hypoxia, typically from a primary lung problem.

Circulation to Skin

After assessing appearance and work of breathing, assess circulation by looking at skin colour. This will be difficult to interpret if the environmental temperature is low, because vasoconstriction, as a reflexive effort to preserve heat, will falsely alter skin findings, especially in infants. Disrobe the child and look for mottling, pallor, and cyanosis, which reflect peripheral vasoconstriction or clamping down of non-essential skin perfusion to maintain essential core circulation. If a child has abnormal appearance and abnormal skin signs in a warm ambient environment, the child may be haemodynamically unstable.

Primary Assessment: The <C>ABCDEs

After the PAT, perform the hands-on <C>ABCDE assessment. After evaluating airway and breathing, as described in the previous chapters, assess the circulation. There are four parts to the assessment of circulation:

1. Heart rate
2. Pulse quality
3. Skin temperature and capillary refill time
4. Blood pressure

Heart Rate

First, measure heart rate by feeling the pulse for 30 seconds, and then double the number. A normal heart rate is between 60 and 160 beats/min, depending on the child's age, as noted in Table 1-6. The radial or brachial areas are preferred sites to measure pulse rate in infants and children. The carotid pulse is acceptable in older children and adolescents, but it is hard to locate in infants. If a pulse is difficult to feel, determine heart rate by listening to the heart sounds directly with a stethoscope placed on the medial side of the child's left nipple. However, be aware that the presence of a "normal" heart rate by auscultation does not necessarily reflect adequate cardiac output and perfusion.

Interpreting heart rate may be difficult, as explained in the *Paediatric Assessment* chapter. Ranges of normal heart rates change inversely with advancing age. Also, many conditions can increase heart rate, ranging from serious physiological problems to noxious stimuli that are rarely life-threatening. Stimuli that can cause tachycardia include pain, fever, fear, cold, and anger. Interpret heart rate in the context of overall signs of perfusion, age, presence or absence of noxious stimuli, and observed trends. Although a single measurement of heart rate is usually of limited value in determining the degree of physiological derangement, *a trend of mounting tachycardia, or a heart rate that is falling below the lower limits of normal, suggests a serious physiological problem.* In addition, sustained tachycardia is a worrisome sign. Finally, be extremely vigilant when the child has bradycardia, because this often indicates hypoxia or may be a sign of profound ischaemia.

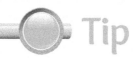

Bradycardia is always a critical sign in a young child and reflects hypoxia or advanced shock.

Pulse Quality

Presence of a strong central pulse (carotid, femoral, or brachial in infants) with a strong peripheral pulse (brachial, radial, or pedal in children) suggests a good blood pressure. A strong central pulse with a weak peripheral pulse indicates compensated shock. If a brachial pulse is not palpable, the child is probably hypotensive and is haemodynamically unstable.

Skin Temperature and Capillary Refill Time

The next part of the hands-on cardiovascular assessment involves evaluating skin signs. Check skin temperature for warmth at the hands, feet, kneecaps, or forearms. Cool

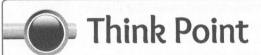

Think Point

The carotid pulse is an acceptable site for measurement of pulse rate in older children and adolescents, but it is hard to locate in infants.

hands and feet may be normal, but cool proximal extremities reflect poor perfusion and shunting of blood to the core. Capillary refill time (CRT) *should be less than 2–3 seconds in a child who is not cold.* Inadequate core perfusion results in peripheral vasoconstriction, which will manifest as cool skin and delayed CRT. Although CRT is a good test of circulation in children, it must be interpreted in the context of overall signs of perfusion. The prehospital professional can become comfortable with the technique and interpretation of the key skin findings by practising on every child.

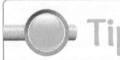

Tip

Practise CRT and pulse quality on every child. This will help you to become comfortable with the technique and interpret key findings accurately.

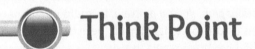

Think Point

CRT is a good test for circulation in children, it should be performed centrally and be recorded for every single child that you attend.

Blood Pressure

Last, consider taking a blood pressure. A high blood pressure value in a child is not clinically significant in the field, unless he or she has a history of hypertension, known renal disease, or acute head injury. However, a true low blood pressure value is significant of haemodynamic instability. The challenges in blood pressure measurement in children in the out-of-hospital setting are: knowing when to get a blood pressure reading; obtaining the blood pressure correctly; and interpreting it accurately.

A normal minimal systolic blood pressure in a child older than 1 year of age is $70 + (2 \times \text{years of age})$. Proper equipment, technique, and patience are required to obtain an accurate blood pressure in an infant or toddler. Because this can be a time-consuming process and may not contribute greatly to the clinical assessment of perfusion, in a child 3 years old or younger attempt a blood pressure measurement only

once or skip altogether. Inadequate perfusion will be better reflected in the other signs of perfusion described previously (heart rate, pulse quality, CRT, and skin temperature).

In a child older than 3 years of age, make at least one blood pressure attempt in every patient to provide a baseline for future assessments. Repeated vital signs provide trends that can yield useful information to determine patient severity. Use a cuff with a width that is two-thirds the length of the upper arm. Applying too large a cuff will falsely decrease the blood pressure measurement, and too small a cuff will falsely increase the measurement.

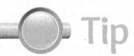

Tip

A normal minimal systolic blood pressure in a child older than 1 year of age is $70 + (2 \times \text{years of age})$.

Additional Assessment

If the child is stable after the primary assessment and does not require immediate treatment, and there are no immediate safety concerns for the child or prehospital professional, conduct the focused history and physical examination and the detailed physical examination on scene. Use the SAMPLE and OPQRST mnemonics (**Table 5-3**) to recall

Table 5-3 The OPQRST of Pain
O—Onset **Key Question:** What were you doing when the pain/discomfort started?
P—Provocation/Palliation **Key Question:** What makes the pain/discomfort better or worse? What have you tried to reduce the symptoms? Did it work? **Support Questions:** Has this ever happened before? If so, when?
Q—Quality **Key Question:** What does the pain feel like?
R—Region/Radiation **Key Question:** Can you point with one finger to the main area of pain/discomfort? **Support Questions:** Do you feel pain anywhere else? If so, can you show me or tell me where it is?
S—Severity **Key Question:** How bad is the pain or chief complaint on a scale of 1 to 10, with 1 being no pain and 10 being extreme pain? You may need to use other methods to determine severity of the pain (e.g. Wong-Baker Faces). **Support Questions:** What is the worst pain you've ever experienced? How does this compare?
T—Time frames **Key Question:** When did you first notice the symptoms? **Support Questions:** Have the symptoms been continuous? If not, has the feeling come and gone?

important features of the focused cardiovascular history. Use age-appropriate approaches to gain the child's trust and speak directly to him or her. Ask the caregiver to add to the child's history. Obtain the history from the caregiver if the child is too young to speak or is unable to cooperate.

After the focused history, perform a focused examination of the heart, peripheral circulation, and abdomen. Then, do an anatomical examination of the entire body, as outlined in the *Paediatric Assessment* chapter. If the child has a traumatic injury, also do a detailed physical examination, searching for other injuries.

Perform an ongoing assessment of all children with cardiovascular problems while on the way to the emergency department, observing for changes on the cardiorespiratory monitor. The child's status may change during transport, so observe and document any physiological trends. Use the PAT to monitor effective perfusion and watch respiratory rate, heart rate, blood pressure, and pulse oximetry. Be prepared to increase the level of respiratory and cardiovascular support if the child worsens or fails to respond to treatment.

Summary of Cardiovascular Assessment

The PAT provides a good first-line cardiovascular evaluation: abnormal appearance, normal work of breathing, and poor circulation to skin suggest a perfusion problem. Pallor, mottling, and cyanosis all indicate poor peripheral perfusion. The circulatory portion of the hands-on <C>ABCDEs consists of evaluating heart rate, pulse quality, skin temperature, CRT, and blood pressure. These physical features complement the PAT and will help identify the type and severity of circulatory compromise. Vital signs can sometimes be misleading and must be correctly obtained and interpreted for age. Trends in vital signs, or persistence in abnormal vital signs, such as tachycardia, are more accurate indicators of real physiological problems than mild vital sign abnormalities on primary assessment.

Cardiac Arrest

The emphasis for patients in cardiac arrest is based on early and excellent compressions (**Figure 5-1**). The new "Chain of Survival" has added a fifth component to enhance the post-resuscitation care for the patient who has suffered a cardiac arrest.

The Paediatric Chain of Survival is as follows:

- Prevention
- Early CPR
- Early access
- Early ALS
- Post-resuscitation care

Survival from cardiac arrest depends on several factors: time to CPR, with airway and breathing support, and presenting rhythm. The shorter the "downtime" before BLS, the better the outcome. As in adults, paediatric patients who present to clinicians in VF are more likely to survive than children who present in asystole, as long as there is early CPR and access to early defibrillation. **Figure 5-2** shows infant CPR.

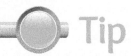

The only intervention associated with survival in paediatric asystolic cardiac arrest is time to onset of CPR, with airway and breathing support.

Causes

In contrast to adults, paediatric cardiac arrest is almost always a secondary event, the result of profound hypoxia or shock. Cardiac arrest in children usually follows a primary respiratory arrest, often from respiratory failure originating from common conditions, such as pneumonia, bronchiolitis, or asthma. Myocardial infarction and a cardiac dysrhythmia, such as hypertrophic cardiomyopathy (HCM), frequent causes of cardiac arrest in adults, are extremely unusual in young children.

Children can present in arrest from conditions from genetic disorders, such as HCM, which has a high incidence of sudden death, and is the leading cause of cardiac death in both preadolescent and adolescent children. Hypertrophic cardiomyopathy is a condition in which a child has profound hypertrophy of the ventricles and intraventricular septum that causes an outflow obstruction. It also has effects on the coronary arteries, leading to a thickening of the lining of the artery causing a narrowing in the vessel and leading to a decrease of flow to the myocardium.

Long QT syndrome is a congenital problem with the electrophysiology of the heart resulting in an increased risk of dysrhythmias including bradycardia and VF. Another cause of cardiac arrest occurs when a child is struck by a non-penetrating object in the anterior chest leading to VF and sudden death. Commotio cordis occurs when a child is hit with a baseball, hockey puck, softball, karate blow, or other similar projectile force from sports. The blow is most likely to be critical if it is over the centre of the left ventricle. Because this results in VF and collapse, the use of a defibrillator is critical.

The primary age group for paediatric cardiac arrest is infancy, when sudden unexpected death in infants, children and adolescents (SUDICA), infection, or child maltreatment precipitates respiratory failure. In toddlers and school-aged children, however, the causes of cardiac arrest change. In

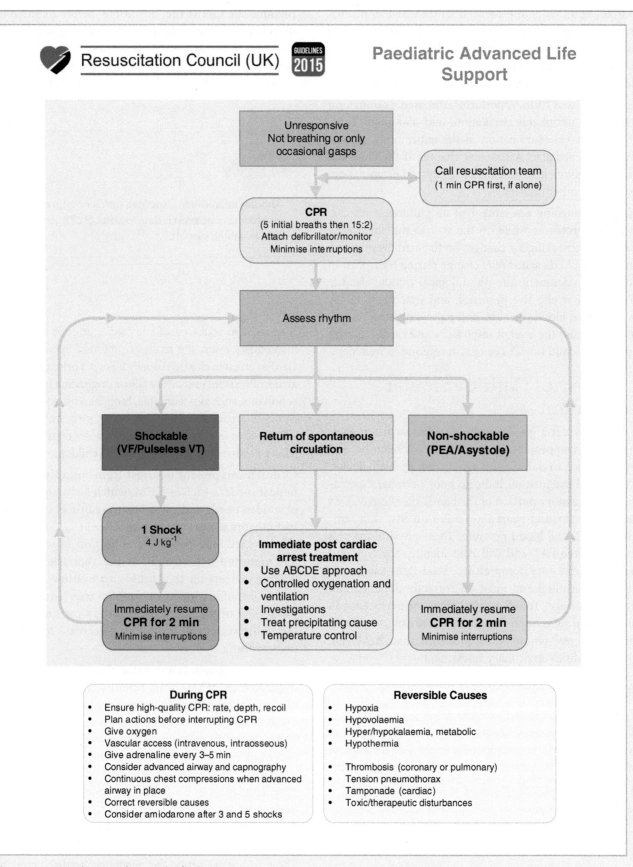

Figure 5-1 Paediatric Advanced Life Support.

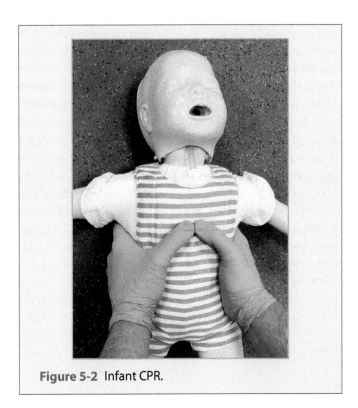

Figure 5-2 Infant CPR.

this older age group, the most likely causes are haemorrhagic shock and blunt trauma from either vehicle-related injuries or falls.

Assessment in Cardiac Arrest

A child in cardiac arrest is unresponsive, apnoeic, and pulseless. The cardiac monitor will show a cardiac arrest rhythm: asystole, PEA, VT, or VF. Asystole is the most frequent rhythm. SVT and VT are rare causes of cardiac arrest.

Asystole reflects profound hypoxia and ischaemia. PEA may represent a variety of ischaemic, hypoxic, hypothermic, and traumatic insults. Some PEA may arise from low-flow states with blood pressures too low to record in the out-of-hospital setting. VF occurs in children usually older than 2 years from a variety of conditions, including myocarditis, congenital anomalies, poisoning, electrocution, or hypoxia.

Chest Compressions

Chest compressions have become the focus of care in a patient in cardiac arrest. Compression techniques differ for a child and infant. For a child, the hand(s) should be placed on the lower half of the sternum, rate should be at least 100–120 per minute, and compression depth should be at least 2 inches (5 cm) with complete recoil (to ensure adequate preload). For an infant, as a single rescuer one places two fingers at the nipple line and compresses at a rate of at least 100 per minute with a depth of at least 1.5 inches (4 cm) with complete recoil. When performing two-rescuer CPR for an infant, the recommended technique is the two fingers encircling the

chest technique (Figure 5-2). For the child and infant, when performing single-rescuer CPR, the ratio is 30:2 and changes to 15:2 for two health care rescuers.

Defibrillators

Cardiac arrest in children is usually the result of profound hypoxia or shock, which leads to asystole, the most frequent rhythm of paediatric cardiac arrest. VF, however, does occur in paediatrics. The typical VF case is a child out of the infant age group who has had a witnessed collapse. Aetiologies for VF arrest in children include myocarditis, an infection of the heart muscle; the "long QT syndrome", a congenital cardiac conduction problem; and hypertrophic cardiomyopathy (HCM), a hypertrophy of the ventricular septum and ventricles. One other special circumstance for VF arrest is commotio cordis, which develops usually in a young athlete who is struck in the chest by a ball, stick, or other blunt object.

Perform rapid assessment for VF on all unresponsive children, begin CPR, and administer defibrillation if VF is present on the cardiac monitor. Be especially vigilant for VF when the child is older and has suffered a witnessed collapse. There is no demonstrated benefit to defibrillation of asystole, and this procedure will only delay the key interventions of oxygenation, ventilation, and chest compressions.

Use of a defibrillator (**Figure 5-3** and **Figure 5-4**) allows early recognition of VF/pVT and rapid defibrillation. The

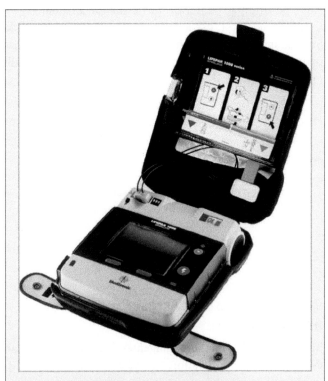

Figure 5-3 An AED.
LIFEPAK 1000 Defibrillator courtesy of Physio-Control. Used with permission of Physio-Control, Inc.

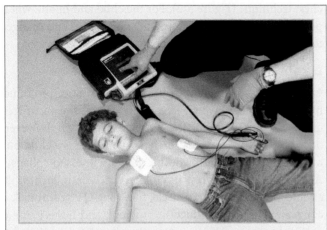

Figure 5-4 Using an AED with CPR in unresponsive children.
© Jones & Bartlett Learning. Courtesy of MIEMSS.

2015 European Resuscitation Council guidelines recommend the use of a defibrillator for treatment of VF/pVT in children of all ages, including infants.

AEDs have been shown to accurately identify VF and VT in young children and are also accurate in identifying paediatric rhythms that do not require defibrillation. When used with a designated paediatric pad-cable system, these AEDs deliver an energy dose that is smaller than that delivered with adult pads. Use a paediatric AED or paediatric AED pads if available; however, an adult AED can be used on a child or an infant (one may consider putting pads anterior–posterior for an infant). For a paediatric arrest, use a defibrillator as soon as possible. Studies show that even school-aged children with no prior experience or education in defibrillation can successfully operate an AED.

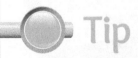 Tip

AEDs can be used on anyone. Preferably use a paediatric specific pads, but adult pads can be used (with anterior-posterior placement). For an unwitnessed arrest, begin CPR, and use an AED as soon as it is available.

Presenting Cardiac Arrest Rhythm and Treatment

The top priority in the management of a patient in cardiac arrest is circulation (emphasis on high-quality compressions); airway and breathing (bag-valve-mask ventilation with an airway adjunct is adequate); and defibrillation (if indicated). The presenting cardiac rhythm is a major determinant of the treatment of cardiac arrest. When the child is pulseless and apnoeic, the treatment of asystole and PEA is the same.

Asystole/PEA. Resuscitation efforts for non-shockable rhythms begin with high-quality CPR with an emphasis on chest compressions without interruption. Management of airway and breathing may be taken care of with bag-valve-mask ventilation (BMV) and airway adjunct as primary intervention as long as chest rise and compliance are noted. If ventilation is unsuccessful with BMV and essential adjuncts (e.g., oropharyngeal airway) then advanced management with a supraglottic device or endotracheal tube MAY be considered. The uncuffed endotracheal tube should be sized with the equation of (age in years divided by 4) + 4. Cuffed endotracheal tubes are sized a half size smaller.

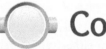 Controversy

Advanced airway management has been shown by Tijssen to worsen outcomes in out-of-hospital paediatric cardiac arrest and should only performed by skilled and competent clinicians in accordance with local policy.

Vascular access can be intravenous (IV) or intraossesous (IO). All medications, fluids, and blood products can be administered through the IO.

Adrenaline (1:10,000) is the drug of choice administered at a dose of 10 mcg/kg IV/IO. High-quality BLS with adequate airway management is continued throughout the resuscitation with the reassessment every 2 minutes and epinephrine administered every 3–5 minutes. Early administration of fluid should also be considered at 20 ml/kg (medical), 10 ml/kg (burns) or 5 ml/kg (trauma).

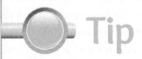 Tip

Vascular access and administration of fluid has been shown to improve outcomes in POHCA by Tijssen.

Table 5-4 Six Hs and Five Ts

Hypovolaemia	Tension pneumothorax
Hypoxia	Tamponade, cardiac
Hypoglycaemia	Toxins
Hydrogen ion (acidosis)	Thrombosis, cardiac
Hypo/ hyperkalaemia	Thrombosis, pulmonary
Hypothermia	

ALS An important component to the treatment of asystole/PEA is rapidly working to identify the cause; therefore, it is imperative the clinician considers the Hs and Ts (**Table 5-4**) while providing care.

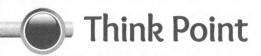 Think Point

When considering toxins, think about cleaning products, medicines, 'grandma's purse' and chemicals from the garage/shed/workshop. Consider this early in your assessment and treat if you are able to do so.

ALS **VF/Pulseless VT.** VF/pVT management should start with quality CPR while attaching the monitor and identifying a shockable rhythm. The initial energy setting for the child should be at 4 J/kg, followed by 2 minutes of excellent CPR. During this time, vascular (IV/IO) access should be gained. Initial airway management should be maintained with a bag-valve-mask device and oropharyngeal airway (OPA) as long as there is adequate chest rise and good compliance (an advanced airway may be considered further down the algorithm). When an airway is not maintainable with a bag-valve-mask ventilation, an endotracheal tube or supraglottic device should be considered as soon as possible.

After 2 minutes of high-quality CPR, the patient is reassessed and a shock is administered at 4 J/kg. CPR is continued, and after the third shock the patient is given 10 mcg/kg of adrenaline (1:10,000) IV/IO, repeated every 3–5 minutes After the third and fifth shock, the patient is given amiodarone at 5 mg/kg. Resume CPR for 2 minutes, then reassess. All subsequent shocks are delivered at 4 J/kg.

Medicine Dosage

Treatment of infants and children in the out-of-hospital setting is difficult because children of different ages require different sizes of equipment, different doses of medications, and different amounts of fluids. JRCALC provides this information in a pocket book version in a 'Page for Age' format, which is easy to locate and determine the dose of each cardiac arrest medicine (**Figure 5-5**).

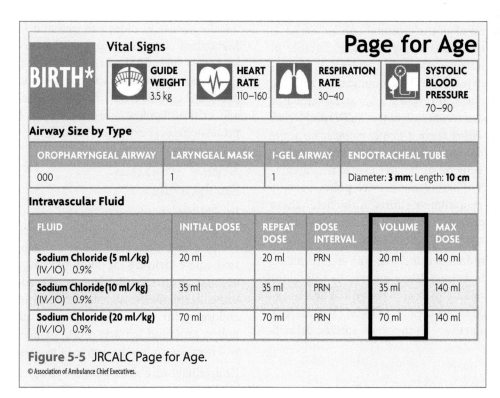

Figure 5-5 JRCALC Page for Age.
© Association of Ambulance Chief Executives.

Length–based tapes are common in the US, but are not regularly used in the UK.

Survival from paediatric cardiac arrest requires good BLS care. IV or IO needle insertion and fluid administration have been shown to increase survival to discharge by Tijssen. Endotracheal tube insertion may offer no benefit to survival and has been shown to worsen survival to discharge.

The Transport Decision: Stay or Go

Deciding which paediatric cardiac arrest patients require hospital transport is another important controversy. Predictors of survival include type of presenting rhythm and early return of spontaneous circulation after BLS on scene. In 2015, Tijssen et al. demonstrated increased survival to hospital discharge with an on scene time of 10–35 minutes. This is the largest study to date looking at the on scene time for children in out-of-hospital cardiac arrest. Importantly, 35 minutes is not a target—if all elements of care are provided within 15 minutes it would not be appropriate to delay on scene. If children in cardiac arrest fail out-of-hospital resuscitation with BLS and ALS, they will not survive unless there is a special circumstance. Patients who have ingested massive amounts of sedative-hypnotic drugs (e.g., barbiturates) may have a greater chance of survival after prolonged resuscitation and deserve extended treatment before death is declared.

In some cases, field resuscitation attempts can be stopped before transport if permitted by local ambulance service recognition of life extinct (ROLE) guidelines. Although survival in unwitnessed out-of-hospital cardiac arrest is rare, prehospital professionals may be uncomfortable in discontinuing resuscitative efforts in children. When resuscitation is terminated, skillful communication with the child's caregivers is critical (**Figure 5-6**), as explained in the *Sudden Unexpected Death in Infancy (SUDI) and Death of a Child* chapter. *Never leave a family member on scene with the deceased child without appropriate supportive personnel.* A system to provide supportive care to the caregivers must be in place if ambulance service policy permits discontinuation of resuscitative efforts in the field. These services might be provided by social services personnel, pastoral care, police, or grief counsellors.

Cardiac arrest in children is associated with high clinician stress. Critical-incident stress debriefing may be helpful for prehospital professionals after such a tragedy. Where available, clinicians should access their local TRiM (Trauma Risk Management representative—as they have specific debriefing skills.

Summary of Cardiac Arrest

Paediatric cardiac arrest is an uncommon event. Survival is unlikely, and asystole has the worst prognosis. VF/pVT

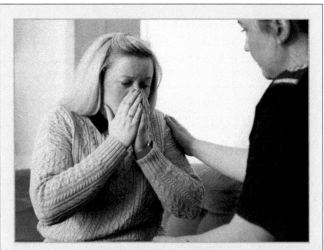

Figure 5-6 Skilled communication with the caregivers and family is imperative after the death of a child.

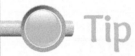

Management of paediatric out-of-hospital cardiac arrest requires clinicians to be confident in their use of the ALS algorithm and for critical interventions to be performed on scene.

usually occurs in older children and has higher survival. Meticulous attention to airway, chest compressions, vascular access (plus fluid when indicated) and early defibrillation, when appropriate, will improve success. In all cases of paediatric cardiac arrest, grief counselling for the caregivers and critical-incident stress debriefing for the prehospital professionals are extremely helpful.

Dysrhythmias
Bradycardia

In children, bradycardia almost always reflects hypoxia, rather than a primary cardiac problem. It is a pre-arrest rhythm, and the prognosis is ominous if left untreated. Immediate delivery of high-flow oxygen and assisted-ventilation are essential. Untreated bradycardia will quickly cause haemodynamic instability and ultimately death. In children with asthma or respiratory distress, bradycardia means profound hypoxia. Pulse oximetry, when available, will help determine the degree of hypoxia in the field.

Congenital heart block is an extremely rare cause of bradycardia in infancy and early childhood. Drug overdose (e.g., β-blockers, calcium channel blockers, digoxin, clonidine) is another possible cause of bradycardia. Bradycardia may also

Case Study 2

You are working at a cross country running event, a 12-year-old patient has collapsed on the course and a bystander has commenced CPR. It will take you 3–4 minutes to get to their location.

1. Working on the assumption this child is in cardiac arrest, what could the presenting rhythm be?

2. What interventions will be important as soon as you arrive on scene?

result from vagal stimulation during medical procedures or gastric tube placement. However, although bradycardia that develops during laryngoscopy or suctioning may be the result of vagal stimulation, hypoxia may be the true cause. If bradycardia does occur in this setting, stop the procedure, administer supplemental oxygen, and reassess the patient.

Bradycardia may also be a normal finding, especially in asymptomatic athletic adolescents. If bradycardia is an isolated finding, without signs of haemodynamic instability in a well-perfused school-aged child or teenager, no treatment is necessary in the field.

Assessment of the Child With Bradycardia

If the child has a heart rate below the normal range for age (see JRCALC), evaluate carefully for signs of respiratory failure or shock. The PAT and <C>ABCDEs, along with a brief history, will establish the likely cause, the severity of the problem, and the need for urgent treatment.

Treatment of Bradycardia

If the child is asymptomatic, consider no treatment, especially if the child is an adolescent, because slow heart rates are common in athletic teenagers. If the child has bradycardia and a primary assessment demonstrates oxygenation, ventilation, or perfusion abnormalities, provide 100% oxygen with bag-valve-mask ventilation and transport. Check effectiveness of ventilation by observing for chest rise and an improvement in the PAT, heart rate, perfusion, and blood pressure.

In rare situations, chest compressions for bradycardia are necessary. If the heart rate is below 60 beats/min and the child shows signs of poor systemic perfusion after oxygenation and assisted ventilation, begin chest compressions.

Drug Therapy for Symptomatic Bradycardia. Oxygenation and ventilation are the primary treatments for bradycardia. If there is increased vagal tone (or poisoning by cholinergic drugs or agents, such as organophosphates) or an atrioventricular heart block, administer atropine, 0.02 mg/kg IV or IO (minimum dose of 0.1 mg, maximum dose of 0.5 mg) or refer JRCALC for doses by age. When the child has a known reason for cholinergic-mediated bradycardia, such as congenital heart block, give atropine and monitor the response as per JRCALC guidelines.

Before administering any medicine, always assess for mechanical problems with oxygen delivery and ventilation. Check for disconnected oxygen tubing, poor mask seal, airway obstruction, inadequate chest rise, endotracheal tube blockage, or malposition. Other causes of bradycardia from hypoxia or ischaemia are pneumothorax, hypovolaemia, cardiomyopathy, poisoning, or increased intracranial pressure.

When oxygenation, ventilation, and drug therapy for bradycardia fail, consider external electrical cardiac pacing of the heart.

Tachycardia

Tachycardia may be a non-specific sign of fear, anxiety, pain, or fever and may not represent serious injury or illness. Tachycardia may also be a sign of a life-threatening problem, such as hypoxia, cardiac abnormality, or hypovolaemia. Sinus tachycardia is the most common dysrhythmia in children, and treatment is generally limited to fluid administration, supplemental oxygen, and transport.

Assessment of the Child With Tachycardia

Tachycardia must be assessed in conjunction with the PAT and <C>ABCDEs. Always ask about a history of congenital heart disease and check for midline chest scars from cardiac surgery.

There are two characteristics in the child's rhythm strip to measure and use as a basis for treatment, along with the perfusion assessment: (1) the heart rate per minute and (2) the width of the QRS complex. First, establish an accurate heart rate electronically from the rhythm strip. As in the assessment of bradycardia, interpret the heart rate based on knowledge of the normal range for age (see JRCALC). Second, establish the width of the QRS from the rhythm strip. If the QRS complex is ≤0.09 seconds (<2¼ standard boxes on the rhythm strip), consider the child to have a narrow complex tachycardia. If the width is >0.09 seconds (>2¼ standard boxes on the rhythm strip), consider the child to have a wide complex tachycardia.

Table 5-5 distinguishes a narrow complex sinus tachycardia from narrow complex supraventricular tachycardia (SVT) and wide complex VT.

Table 5-5 Features of Sinus Tachycardia, SVT, and VT

	History	Heart Rate	Variability	QRS Interval	Assessment	Possible Treatments
Sinus tachycardia	Fever Volume loss Hypoxia Pain Increased activity or exercise	<220 beats/min (infant) <180 beats/min (child)	Yes	Narrow ≤0.09 seconds	Hypovolaemia Hypoxia Painful injury	Fluids Oxygen Splinting Analgesia/ sedation
Supraventricular tachycardia	Congenital heart disease Known SVT Non-specific symptoms (e.g., poor feeding, fussiness)	≥220 beats/min (often 240–300 beats/min) ≥180 beats/min (child)	No	Narrow ≤0.09 seconds	CHF may be present	Vagal manoeuvres (ice to face) Synchronised cardioversion
Ventricular tachycardia	Serious systemic illness	>150 beats/min	Yes	Wide >0.09 seconds	CHF may be present	Synchronised cardioversion Amiodarone

© Jones & Bartlett Learning

Specific Treatment of Tachycardia

If the child presents with tachycardia, determine the appropriate treatment by establishing perfusion status and by assessing the rhythm strip for heart rate and QRS duration.

Narrow Complex Tachycardia. If the child has a narrow QRS tachycardia (≤0.09 seconds), P waves are present, and the heart rate is variable and less than 220 beats/min in an infant or less than 180 beats/min in a child, the cause is usually sinus tachycardia (**Figure 5-7**) from non-cardiac conditions (e.g., hypoxia, hypovolaemia, hypothermia, hypoglycaemia, metabolic abnormalities, toxins, fear, pain, or serious trauma to the chest). No specific cardiac medical management of the sinus tachycardia is needed. Instead, treat with fluids, oxygen, splinting, analgesia, or sedation as indicated by the associated condition. If there is no change in heart rate after treatment, consider other aetiologies, such as SVT.

Specific Treatment of SVT. If the QRS is less than or equal to 0.09 seconds, P waves are absent or abnormal, and the rate is not variable and is ≥220 beats/min in an infant or ≥180 beats/min in a child, consider SVT as the likely aetiology. If the child has no previous history of SVT, and the patient is stable, provide oxygen and transport to the emergency department. Delaying specific treatment for SVT until hospital arrival will permit the hospital staff to confirm SVT, and to run a continuous electrocardiogram while actively managing the dysrhythmia. A patient with a confirmed diagnosis of SVT may need long-term treatment with cardiac medications.

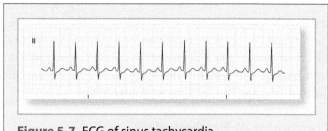

Figure 5-7 ECG of sinus tachycardia.
From 12-Lead ECG: The Art of Interpretation, courtesy of Tomas B. Garcia, MD.

If the patient has a prior history of SVT, and is stable, consider a vagal manoeuvre first. Ice to the face (if available) evokes the "diving reflex" and is an effective management tool for SVT in infants and toddlers. Place crushed ice in a plastic bag, glove, or washcloth and apply firmly over the mid-face (cheeks and bridge of nose) for approximately 15 seconds, until the rhythm changes or the patient's condition dictates immediate cessation of the procedure (**Figure 5-8**). Do not occlude the nose (to allow breathing), and provide constant reassurance to the parent and child. Avoid ocular pressure (pressure on the eyeballs) as a method of vagal stimulation in a child. **Only attempt a vagal manoeuvre once.**

If a child with suspected SVT has signs of poor perfusion and haemodynamic compromise (abnormal PAT, poor pulse quality, abnormal CRT and skin temperature, hypotension), is in shock, or is unconscious, immediately administer

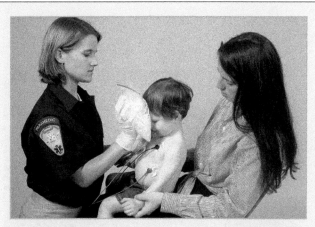

Figure 5-8 Placing a bag of ice on a child's face elicits the "diving reflex" and may convert SVT to sinus rhythm.
© Jones and Bartlett Publishers. Courtesy of MIEMSS.

Wide Complex Tachycardia. If the patient is conscious and has adequate perfusion, a heart rate of greater than 150 beats/min, and a QRS interval of greater than 0.09 seconds, he or she is probably in stable VT. Sinus tachycardia with a conduction abnormality (bundle branch block) may look like VT, but usually occurs in a child with a history of heart disease or cardiac surgery. Likewise, SVT with aberrant conduction can result in a wide complex rhythm. In all such stable cases with wide complex tachycardia's, provide oxygen and transport the patient to an appropriate emergency department, with close cardiac monitoring and equipment for synchronised cardioversion immediately available.

If the child has VT, is stable, and the rhythm is monomorphic and regular, transport to the nearest appropriate emergency department. If the child has VT and shows signs of poor perfusion, treat with synchronised cardioversion (0.5 to 1 J/kg). If a second shock (1–2 J/kg) is unsuccessful, or if the tachycardia recurs quickly, transport rapidly to the nearest appropriate emergency department or seek help from advanced practitioners.

If the child has VT and shock, without pulses, treat as pulseless VT/VF.

synchronised cardioversion at 0.5–1 J/kg as a starting electrical dose. If the initial shock is ineffective, double to 1-2 J/kg. If the child is in shock but still conscious and has vascular access, administer sedation if possible before delivering synchronised cardioversion. Do not delay electrical therapy for sedation. If electrical therapy fails to convert the child to sinus rhythm undertake rapid removal to the nearest appropriate emergency department or seek help from advanced practitioners.

 Controversy

Ice to the face for SVT is a controversial field procedure. It has not been evaluated for efficacy or safety in the prehospital setting, especially in children. If in doubt, prioritise early removal to an appropriate hospital and monitor en route.

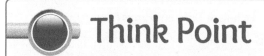 **Think Point**

Most tachycardia in children is a response to non-cardiac stimuli (fever, fear, pain) and does not require dysrhythmia treatment. Treat the cause and monitor for improvement.

Summary of Dysrhythmias

Unlike adults, primary cardiac rhythm disturbances are rare in children. Bradycardia, a pre-arrest rhythm, almost always reflects profound hypoxia and bag-valve-mask ventilation

Case Study 3

You are dispatched to the location of an unresponsive 2-year-old boy recently removed from a swimming pool. Estimated downtime is unknown, but the parents are on scene and state that the child had been missing for more than 30 minutes. The parents initiated CPR immediately. Upon arrival you find the child to be cool, blue, apnoeic, and pulseless.

1. What is the most important intervention for this patient to improve his chances of survival?

2. Should the child be actively rewarmed?

should be initiated rapidly. Tachycardia is most commonly a sinus rhythm, but may represent SVT or VT. Although children can develop sinus tachycardia greater than 200 beats/min, do a careful evaluation for hypovolaemia and hypoxia and other treatable causes, and then treat the identified causes. Assume all rates over 220 beats/min in infants or over 180 beats/min in children and all wide complex (QRS >0.09 seconds) tachycardias are primary cardiac dysrhythmias. The stable patient may need only general supportive care, regardless of cardiac rhythm. <u>Symptomatic ventricular dysrhythmias</u> may require drug therapy and cardioversion or defibrillation.

Congenital Heart Disease

Children with congenital heart disease are at increased risk for the types of cardiovascular emergencies more commonly seen in the adult population, including dysrhythmias and CHF. These complications may present in infancy or as late as the teenage years (**Table 5-6**). Advances in cardiovascular surgery have allowed the medical community to prolong the lives of children who just decades ago would have died in infancy. Many of these children are now living productive

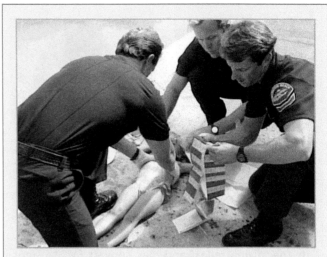

Figure 5-9 Drowning is the third leading cause of death due to unintentional injury in children younger than 14 years.
© Jones & Bartlett Learning

lives at home. Prehospital professionals must be prepared to treat "adult problems" in this younger population.

The primary assessment and management of any child experiencing a cardiovascular emergency are the same: airway, breathing, and circulation. However, in any child with a possible cardiac pathology, include a "quick look" at the cardiac rhythm. These children may have treatable cardiac dysrhythmias.

Drowning

Drowning is suffocation after submersion in water. Globally, the highest drowning rates are among children 1–4 years, followed by children 5–9 years. In the WHO Western Pacific Region children aged 5–14 years die more frequently from drowning than any other cause (**Figure 5-9**). Unfortunately, drowning is not limited to the summer months. In warmer climates it occurs year-round, and in cooler climates it may occur due to submersion in lakes, buckets, hot tubs, and bathtubs.

Prevention

The best management for near-drowning is prevention. The installation of four-sided fencing prevents up to 90% of childhood residential swimming pool drownings and near-drownings. Eighty-five percent of boating-related drownings are preventable by wearing personal flotation devices.

Table 5-6 Congenital Heart Disease Causing Congestive Heart Failure at Different Times During Infancy

Age	Type of Congenital Heart Disease
Newborn	Hypoplastic left heart Severe pulmonic insufficiency Tetralogy of Fallot Severe tricuspid insufficiency Third-degree atrioventricular block SVT Total anomalous pulmonary venous return Transposition of the great vessels
First month	Aortic coarctation with patent ductus arteriosus Ventricular septal defect Tricuspid atresia Truncus arteriosus
First 6 months	Ventricular septal defect Patent ductus arteriosus
6–12 months	Ventricular septal defect Endocardial fibroelastosis

© Jones & Bartlett Learning

Treatment

Early recognition of cardiac arrest and immediate bystander CPR has an important association with survival from severe submersion injuries. ALS care has an unproven benefit.

First remove the patient from the water and begin CPR. If the child is pulseless, begin chest compressions, then open the airway and provide two ventilations. Protect the cervical spine if there is potential head or neck trauma. Perform chest compressions, airway management, oxygenation, and ventilation, and follow protocols for drug therapy and defibrillation/cardioversion depending upon presenting cardiac rhythm.

If the child has a pulse, open the airway and ensure appropriate oxygenation and ventilation, usually with a bag-valve-mask device. Obtain IV or IO access and transport. Provide drug therapy, and rarely defibrillation, as indicated for shock or dysrhythmias.

CASE STUDY ANSWERS

Case Study 1 — page 90

The most likely cause of deterioration is sepsis, resulting in this presentation of septic shock and peri-arrest state. The important observations to recognise sepsis/septic shock in this child are the delayed central CRT and cold peripheries. The working diagnosis is supported by tachypnoea and tachycardia and history of illness for 5 days.

Airway and breathing need to be managed as a priority. Another important intervention to try and prevent cardio-respiratory arrest is vascular access (IV or IO) and a fluid bolus of 20 ml/kg. This should occur on scene, before moving the child and may be repeated if necessary.

Case Study 2 — page 99

The collapse during a sporting event and age of the child may mean a previously undiagnosed cardiac disorder and as such an increased likelihood of finding a shockable rhythm.

You should begin 30 chest compressions to 2 ventilations and apply the defibrillator. Analyse the rhythm and if indicated, deliver a shock. Then resume CPR for 2 minutes, then re-analyse the rhythm. If shockable, deliver a shock, and resume CPR.

This child was in VF due to a previously undiagnosed disorder known as "prolonged QT syndrome". Survivors from this disease often give a history of "blackouts" associated with exercise and stress. Other family members may also be affected by the same disorder. A look back at the family history can uncover unexplained deaths of relatives at young ages.

The initial treatment for children in VF, as in adults, is rapid defibrillation. With the increasing availability of AEDs, many of these children will receive rapid recognition and defibrillation by bystanders.

Case Study 3 — page 101

After removal from the water, begin CPR, starting with chest compressions, then provide bag-valve-mask ventilation with 100% oxygen. Rushing to intubate this child, before providing effective bag-valve-mask ventilation with 100% oxygen, may result in worsened hypoxia and hypercarbia. Most drownings cause airway spasm with little or no water entering the lungs, so bag-valve-mask may be effective. The best anatomical location for palpating a pulse in a 2-year-old child is over the brachial artery, which is located just proximal to the elbow and medially to the biceps muscle.

Although there have been promising results in adult studies of hypothermia after cardiac arrest, paediatric studies have found no benefit. The hypothermic state may be protective of brain function, and rapid rewarming can introduce dysrhythmias. Therefore, remove wet clothing and provide rapid transport.

SUGGESTED READINGS

References

Association of Ambulance Chief Executives. *UK Ambulance Services Clinical Practice Guidelines 2016. JRCALC.* Bridgwater: Class Professional Publishing; 2016.

deCaen AR, Maconochie IK, Aickin R, et al. Part 6: Pediatric basic life support and pediatric advanced life support: 2015 International consensus on Cardiopulmonary Resuscitation and Emergency Cardiovascular Care Science with Treatment Recommendations. *Circulation.* 2015;132 (suppl 1): S177–S203.

Dieckmann RA, et al. *Pediatric Education for Prehospital Professionals.* 2nd ed. Burlington, MA: Jones and Bartlett Learning; 2006:76–103.

Gausche M, Lewis R J, Stratton SJ, et al. Effect of out-of-hospital pediatric endotracheal intubation on survival and neurological outcome: a controlled clinical trial *JAMA.* 2000; *283*(6):783–90. Retrieved from http://www.ncbi.nlm.nih.gov/pubmed/10683058

Hauda WE II. Resuscitation of Children. In: Tintinalli J, Stapczynski J, John Ma O, Cline D, Cydulka R, Meckler G, eds. *Tintinalli's Emergency Medicine*, 7th ed. New York, NY: McGraw-Hill; 2010:80–90.

Kleinman ME, Chameides L, Schexnayder SM, et al. *Pediatric Advanced Life Support.* Part 14. 2010 American Heart Association Guidelines for Cardiopulmonary Resuscitation and Emergency Cardiovascular Care. *Circulation.* 2010;122(suppl 3):S876-S908.

London Ambulance Service. *Cardiac Arrest Annual Report 2016/17.* London: London Ambulance Service; 2017.

Maconochie I, Bingham R, Eich C, et al. European Resuscitation Council Guidelines for Resuscitation 2015. Section 6. Paediatric life support. *Resuscitation,* 2015. 95: 233–248.

Moler FW, Silverstein FS, Holubkov R, et al. Therapeutic Hypothermia after Out-of-Hospital Cardiac Arrest in Children. *N Engl J Med.* 2015;372:1898–1908.

Perondi M, Reis A, Paiva E. A comparison of high-dose and standard-dose epinephrine in children with cardiac arrest. *N Engl J Med.* 2004;350(17):1722–1730.

Raghavan SS. *Pediatric long QT syndrome.* Available at http://emedicine.medscape.com/article/891571-overview. Accessed September 12, 2012.

Shah SN. *Hypertrophic cardiomyopathy.* emedicine. http://emedicine.medscape.com/article/152913-overview. Accessed September 13, 2010.

Tijssen J A, Prince D K, Morrison L J, et al. Time on the scene and interventions are associated with improved survival in pediatric out-of-hospital cardiac arrest. *Resuscitation.* 2015; 94;1–7.

Yabek SM. *Commotio cordis.* Available at http://emedicine.medscape.com/article/902504-overview. Accessed September 12, 2012.

Yee LL, Meckler GD. Pediatric Heart Disease: Acquired Heart Disease. In: Tintinalli J, Stapczynski J, John Ma O, Cline D, Cydulka R, Meckler G, eds. *Tintinalli's Emergency Medicine*, 7th ed. New York, NY: McGraw-Hill; 2010:827–830.

Young K, Gausche-Hill M, McClung C, et al. A prospective population-based study of the epidemiology and outcome of out-of-hospital pediatric cardiopulmonary arrest. *Pediatrics.* 2004;114(1):157–164.

WHO (2018). *Drowning.* http://www.who.int/news-room/fact-sheets/detail/drowning. Accessed 11 July, 2018.

Zevitz ME. Hypertrophic cardiomyopathy. emedicine. 2012. http://emedicine.medscape.com/article/152913-overview. Accessed September 13, 2010.

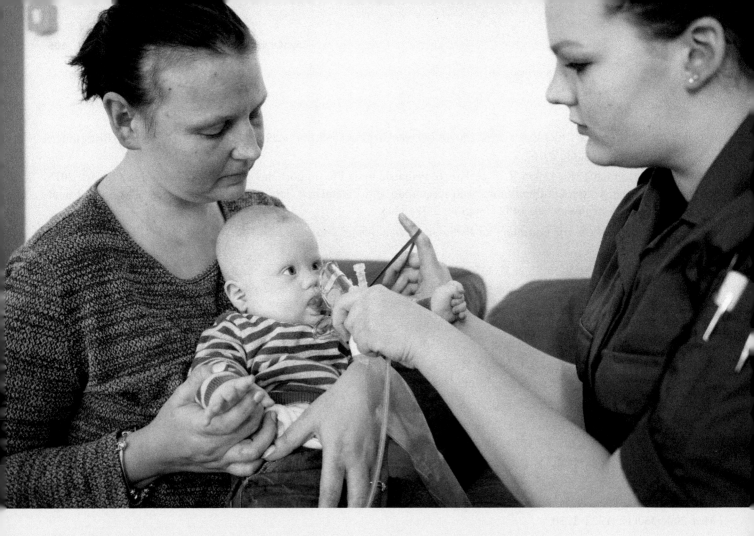

Learning Objectives

1. Describe the major types of seizures and the management priorities for each.
2. Compare the advantages and disadvantages of various benzodiazepines and their routes of administration in status epilepticus.
3. Distinguish the common causes of altered mental status in infants and children, and outline management priorities.
4. Describe signs and symptoms of hypoglycaemia and outline management priorities.
5. Discuss the association of fever and serious illness.
6. Outline the assessment and management of common environmental emergencies, including temperature emergencies, bites, and stings.

Medical Emergencies

Chapter

6

Introduction

Approximately 5–10% of all 999 calls in the UK relate to a child and only a small proportion of these will require urgent intervention. However, calls involving children with paediatric medical complaints tend to be viewed as more serious as a whole, and the varied nature of these complaints makes this patient group especially challenging to assess and treat. This chapter reviews common out-of-hospital paediatric medical emergencies: seizures, altered mental status (AMS), fever, endocrine disorders, gastrointestinal (GI) illness, and environmental emergencies.

Respiratory illness (see the *Respiratory Emergencies* chapter) and seizures are two of the more common out-of-hospital paediatric medical emergencies. Fever is a common medical complaint, but is rarely an emergency in isolation. Fever is usually a symptom of an underlying illness. Although most children with fever have relatively benign, self-limited conditions (e.g., ear infection, croup, viral syndrome), it is important to identify those febrile children with potentially more serious conditions (e.g., meningitis, sepsis) who require immediate pre-hospital management. Fevers may be associated with seizures in infants and nursery-aged children. AMS is a less common characteristic of paediatric 999 patients, but the presence of an AMS usually means the child has a serious or life-threatening medical emergency. Endocrine emergencies in childhood frequently involve AMS and altered blood glucose levels.

Environmental emergencies occurring during childhood include heat and cold-related emergencies and stings and bites. The young child is at increased risk for these environmental emergencies because of physiological, behavioural, and developmental characteristics.

Accurately assessing a child with a medical illness requires an age-based approach to history taking and physical examination, as discussed in the *Paediatric Assessment* and *Using a Developmental Approach* chapters. Communicating with the child and family is essential. Effective communication is fundamental to good clinical care, establishment of trust, and development of comfortable interactions with the child.

The National Institute for Health and Care Excellence offers a traffic light system to help identify the risk of serious illness in children. It is based on the elements of the paediatric assessment triangle and offers guidance on how to identify and stratify the risk of serious illness. The NICE traffic light table should be used in conjunction with the recommendations in the NICE guideline on feverish illness in children.

Red, high risk factors are:
- Skin: Pale/mottled/ashen/blue
- Activity: No response to social cues; Appears ill to a healthcare professional; Does not wake or if roused does not stay awake; Weak, high-pitched or continuous cry

107

Case Study 1

A 2-year-old boy playing on a floor mat at nursery develops jerking of his arms and legs for 1–2 minutes. The nursery teacher calls 999. On arrival at the scene, you find a child who appears drowsy, opens his eyes but does not answer questions, and cries when touched. There are no abnormal airway sounds, work of breathing is not increased, and skin colour is normal. Respiratory rate is 30 breaths/min, heart rate is 100 beats/min, blood pressure is 110/58 mm Hg, and the oxygen saturation is 95%. There are no focal neurological findings. The child's temperature is 38.6°C. He becomes more responsive during your assessment and begins to ask for his father.

1. How should you manage this patient?

2. Should the child be transported?

- Respiratory: Grunting; Tachypnoea: respiratory rate >60 breaths/minute; Moderate or severe chest indrawing

- Circulation and hydration: Reduced skin turgor

- Other: Age <3 months, temperature ≥38°C* (some vaccinations have been found to induce fever in children aged under 3 months); Non-blanching rash; Bulging fontanelle; Neck stiffness; Status epilepticus; Focal neurological signs; Focal seizures

Amber, intermediate risk factors are:

- Colour: Pallor reported by parent/caregiver

- Activity: Not responding normally to social cues; No smile; Wakes only with prolonged stimulation; Decreased activity

- Respiratory:
  ∘ Nasal flaring
  ∘ Tachypnoea
    ▪ RR >50 breaths/minute, age 6–12 months
    ▪ RR >40 breaths/ minute, age >12 months
  ∘ Oxygen saturation ≤95% in air
  ∘ Crackles in the chest

- Circulation and hydration:
  ∘ Tachycardia:
    ▪ >160 beats/minute, age <12 months
    ▪ >150 beats/minute, age 12–24 months
    ▪ >140 beats/minute, age 2–5 years
  ∘ CRT ≥3 seconds
  ∘ Dry mucous membranes
  ∘ Poor feeding in infants
  ∘ Reduced urine output

- Other: Age 3–6 months, temperature ≥39°C; Fever for ≥5 days; Rigors; Swelling of a limb or joint; Non-weight bearing limb/not using an extremity

Green, low risk factors are:

- Colour: Normal colour

- Activity: Responds normally to social cues; Content/smiles; Stays awake or awakens quickly; Strong normal cry/not crying

- Circulation and hydration: Normal skin and eyes; Moist mucous membranes

- Other: None of the amber or red symptoms or signs

Seizures

Seizures are caused by abnormal, sustained electrical discharges from a cluster of cerebral neurons. Seizures have varied physical manifestations, depending on the location of the abnormal electrical seizure activity in the brain and the age of the child. Seizures in the infant, whose central nervous system (CNS) is immature, can be very subtle, consisting only of abnormal gaze, horizontal nystagmus, sustained muscle contractions, sucking motions, or "bicycling" (pedalling movements of the legs). In the older child, who has a more mature CNS, seizures are usually more obvious, and typically manifest as repetitive muscular contractions (tonic-clonic activity) and unresponsiveness. Sustained or repetitive muscular contractions may be associated with upper airway obstruction, resulting in poor air exchange, hypercarbia, and hypoxia. As a result, cyanosis is common.

"Generalised" seizures are the most common type in children. These seizures are divided into convulsive (with motor activity, such as tonic-clonic movements) and non-convulsive (no motor activity, such as an absence seizure). "Partial" seizures are classified based on whether consciousness is maintained. Partial seizures with no loss of consciousness are known as "simple partial seizures"; those associated with a loss of consciousness, are known as "complex partial seizures". Partial seizures are further subdivided based on signs and symptoms, such as motor activity (can be focal and then spread), sensory (paraesthesias, vertigo, visual, or auditory symptoms), or autonomic changes (sweating, pupillary changes). During a complex partial seizure, the child may have motor automatisms, such as chewing or bicycling movements of the legs. There are also epilepsy syndromes, and these infants and children may demonstrate a variety of seizure types. The term epilepsy refers to a chronic disorder that causes recurrent seizures over time, with or without a known underlying cause. Although caregivers of children with epilepsy may be very calm at the scene of a 999 call, those who are witnessing a first-time seizure are usually very frightened, may fear that the child is dying, and may have initiated cardiopulmonary resuscitation efforts.

Febrile Seizures

The most frequent type of seizure in childhood is the febrile seizure. About 5% of all children have at least one seizure by 6 years of age. More than half of these children never have another seizure. By definition, a simple febrile seizure is a generalised, tonic-clonic seizure of less than 15 minutes duration that occurs in a febrile child between 6 months and 5 years of age with no underlying neurological abnormalities. "Simple" febrile seizures do not cause brain injury, even if the child has repeated febrile seizures. Most simple febrile seizures stop spontaneously before the arrival of prehospital clinicians. Risk factors for recurrence include age less than 18 months at the time of the first febrile seizure, a family history of febrile seizure, and complex nature of seizure. There is a 15 to 70% recurrence risk in the first two years after an initial febrile seizure.

Complex febrile seizures consist of any of the following: duration longer than 15 minutes; focal rather than generalised; more than one seizure in a 24-hour period. This type of seizure has a higher association with serious illness and requires evaluation in the hospital. Most children with febrile seizures have relatively benign aetiology of the fever (e.g., otitis media, viral syndrome). Although there may be a brief postictal period, these children generally have improving level of conscious and appear to be well. Children with more serious aetiologies (e.g., meningitis) usually appear ill after the seizure resolves or may have associated symptoms (e.g., petechiae, neck stiffness). A child who has a seizure and a fever may not necessarily have had a febrile seizure and may require a doctor's evaluation to exclude a serious disease. *A prehospital professional cannot make a definitive diagnosis of a febrile seizure.*

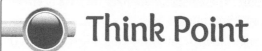

Think Point

A prehospital professional cannot make a definitive diagnosis of a febrile seizure.

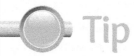

Tip

If the child begins to have another seizure, ensure ABCs. If the seizure does not stop in 5 minutes, begin medication administration as per JRCALC guidance.

Afebrile Seizures

Although childhood seizures are frequently associated with fever, there are many other possible causes of seizures. These include trauma, especially head injury (including child abuse), hypoxia, hypoglycaemia, infection, toxic ingestion, CNS bleeding, metabolic disorders, and congenital neurological problems. A common group of children with afebrile seizures are those with known epilepsy who have not received therapeutic doses of their anti-convulsant medication and experience "breakthrough" seizures. There is a significant group of children who have breakthrough seizures despite medication compliance. In this group, parents call when normal methods of controlling seizure activity are unsuccessful.

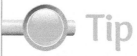

Tip

A seizure with a fever is not the same as a febrile seizure.

Status Epilepticus

The classic definition of status epilepticus is either a series of two or more seizures without recovery of consciousness, or a continuous seizure more than 20 minutes long. An "operational" definition of status epilepticus was developed in the late 1990s by a group of neurologists specialising in seizure management. Based on data indicating that most seizures stop spontaneously in less than 5 minutes, they redefined the term "status epilepticus" and set a threshold for initiating pharmacological treatment as a seizure lasting longer than 5 minutes. Accordingly, consider any child who is actively seizing on arrival of the prehospital professional to be in status epilepticus, and treat with drug therapy to stop the seizure. These patients are likely to have been seizing for at least 15 minutes.

Status epilepticus may occur as the child's first seizure. The age of the child in status epilepticus helps forecast the likely cause of the seizure. Children younger than 3 years of age tend to have acute, sometimes progressive causes of status epilepticus, such as hypoxia, infection, or toxic ingestion. Children older than 3 years of age who present with status epilepticus tend to have chronic, static causes (e.g., epilepsy, neurological disorder, an inborn metabolic disorder, or inadequate anticonvulsant treatment). Therefore, be especially vigilant in care of infants and young children with status epilepticus, especially if they do not have a history of fever or epilepsy.

Status epilepticus is a medical emergency. Early treatment in the field is critical because prolonged seizure activity is difficult to control pharmacologically. Stopping the seizure also facilitates airway management and support of oxygenation and ventilation, and transport. However, the risk of long-term neurological injury is most closely associated with the underlying *cause* and associated complications (hypercarbia, hypoxia) rather than with the *duration* of the seizure. For example, a child who has a 20-minute febrile seizure is unlikely to sustain brain injury, whereas a child with meningitis who has a seizure of the same duration is at high risk for long-term neurological problems.

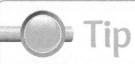

Tip

During status epilepticus, the risk of brain injury is most closely related to the cause of the seizure, not the length of the seizure.

Controversy

When to treat a seizure is a matter of debate. Although most seizures stop spontaneously and do not need any treatment, some untreated children go on to the dangerous condition of status epilepticus. The best practical approach is to offer treatment if the child is seizing on arrival.

Classification of Seizures

The type of abnormal motor activity and the age of the child are factors important to classify seizures, as shown in **Table 6-1**. The main distinction is whether the seizure involves the entire body (generalised seizures affect both hemispheres of the brain) or only one part of the body (focal seizures affect only one hemisphere of the brain).

Table 6-1 Classification of Seizures

Type	Description
Generalised	
Tonic-clonic	• Trunk rigidity and loss of consciousness, with sudden jerking of both arms and/or both legs; may be only tonic (muscle contraction, rigidity), or clonic (muscle relaxation, jerking)
Absence	• Brief loss of awareness without any abnormal body movements; the child may appear to be staring or may be blinking his or her eyes repetitively
Partial	
Simple	• Focal motor jerking, without loss of consciousness; may be sensory, autonomic, or psychic; may progress to complex seizure activity
Complex	• Focal motor jerking, with loss of consciousness; sometimes there is secondary generalisation to a tonic-clonic seizure
Tonic	• Rigid posturing of trunk and extremities, may have fixed eye deviation
Clonic	• Rhythmic twitching of muscle groups, particularly the extremities and face
Multifocal	• Similar to clonic with multiple muscle groups involved
Myoclonic	• Brief focal or generalised jerks of extremities or parts of the body with distal muscle groups, may occur as a single jerk or series of repetitive jerks
Neonatal	
Subtle	• Chewing motions, excessive salivation, blinking, eye deviation, swallowing, swimming arms, pedalling legs, apnoea, or colour change

A generalised seizure usually involves abnormal muscle jerking (tonic-clonic seizure), but may be non-convulsive with only a loss of attention or eye blinking (absence seizure). When the child has had a partial seizure, establish whether consciousness and verbal interaction are preserved (simple partial seizure) or impaired (complex partial seizure). Simple partial seizures can progress to complex partial seizures or to generalised seizures. When a partial seizure evolves to a generalised seizure, it is called "secondary generalisation". Neonatal seizures tend to be more subtle, because tonic-clonic activity may not occur during the first month of life. Deviated gaze or horizontal nystagmus and myoclonic seizures (a sudden, single muscle jerk) may be the only evidence of seizures in infants.

Complications

Seizures may cause hypoxia from airway obstruction, aspiration, or inadequate respiratory drive. Good clinical management minimises these complications. A second concern is brain injury from prolonged seizure activity in a child with a serious underlying condition, such as infection, intoxication (including toxic exposures), haemorrhage, or congenital neurological problems. Children have fewer energy reserves than adults and active seizures use those reserves. Hypoglycaemia can cause and prolong seizure activity. Blood glucose should be checked in all children with seizures, and hypoglycaemia should be rapidly corrected.

Support of airway and breathing, control of seizure activity, checking and treating for hypoglycaemia, and rapid transport to a facility with paediatric intensive care capability are the best strategies for minimising morbidity in this population of critically ill children.

Assessment and Treatment of the Actively Seizing Child

If a child is actively seizing when the prehospital professional arrives, there are several essential steps:

1. *Open the airway.*

   Managing the airway is the most important initial action (**Table 6-2**).

   Positioning is the easiest method to maintain a clear airway in a young child. For an infant, toddler, or nursery-aged child, perform the chin lift or jaw thrust. Be mindful of the child's anatomy (size of occiput) and whether some padding under their body may allow for better airway positioning. If there are a lot of secretions, open the airway while placing the child in the recovery position. The insertion of a nasopharyngeal airway is the most useful tool in stepwise airway management after doing chin lift or jaw thrust. It provides an open airway around clenched teeth. Although an oropharyngeal airway can also be used, it is more difficult to insert if the teeth are clenched, and may cause vomiting if the

Table 6-2 Initial Airway Management in Seizing Children

Position the head to open the airway.
Clear the mouth with suction.
Consider the recovery (lateral decubitus) position if the child is actively vomiting and suction is inadequate to control the airway (**Figure 6-1**).
Provide 100% oxygen by non-rebreathing mask or blow-by.
Consider a nasopharyngeal airway.

© Jones & Bartlett Learning.

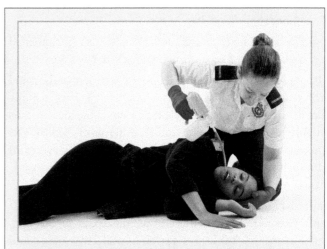

Figure 6-1 Position the head to open the airway, place the child in the recovery position, and clear the mouth of vomitus with suction.
© Jones & Bartlett Learning.

patient has a gag reflex. Suction the mouth of secretions, if possible.

Without the use of neuromuscular blockade agents, successful endotracheal intubation during a seizure is extremely difficult, and complication rates are high. *Do not attempt to intubate a seizing child.* If the airway is not maintainable, attempt to stop the seizure through the administration of anti-convulsant medications as per JRCALC guidelines. After the seizure is stopped, perform airway management as needed.

Consider spinal stabilisation as part of airway management in a post-traumatic seizure, although it is not very effective until the seizure activity has stopped.

2. *Ensure adequate breathing.*

   Seizures are associated with some degree of hypoventilation. Attempt to assist ventilation if the child is cyanotic, or has an oxygen saturation less than 90% on supplemental oxygen. Be aware, however, that it is difficult to obtain an accurate pulse oximetry reading in a child who is having a seizure, secondary to poor perfusion. Again, stopping the seizure is the key to successful ventilation. Opening the airway, co-ordinating positive-pressure ventilations with the patient's spontaneous respiratory effort, and expanding a rigid chest wall are technically difficult procedures during a generalised seizure. Often the result of <u>assisted ventilation</u> is stomach inflation with air. Trained advanced life support (ALS) providers should consider a nasogastric tube to decompress the stomach if bag-valve-mask ventilation visibly distends the abdomen.

3. *Safeguard circulation.*

   Unless a child has seizures associated with sepsis or trauma, fluid resuscitation on scene or in transport is not necessary. Signs of poor perfusion are most likely associated with prolonged seizure activity, hypoxia, and metabolic acidosis. Once again, treating the seizure addresses these problems.

4. *Manage any disability.*

   Check the bedside glucose level and treat documented hypoglycaemia, as described in **Table 6-3**.

Although most seizures stop before the arrival of prehospital professionals, the child who is still actively seizing usually benefits from pharmacological treatment. Consider options for anti-convulsant administration, in terms of medications approved in the ambulance service and available routes of administration. The goal is to stop the seizure, while minimising medication side effects.

<u>Benzodiazepine</u> drugs are excellent first-line anticonvulsants. Common drugs in this class are diazepam, midazolam, and lorazepam. **Table 6-4** provides indicative doses and

routes of administration, but these should be checked against the JRCALC guidelines where appropriate.

Although each of the benzodiazepines has the same mechanism of action, differences in specific agent and route of administration lead to significant clinical differences in the time to peak effect and the duration of action.

Diazepam. Diazepam is a long-established drug for status epilepticus. IV diazepam is an effective treatment for status epilepticus or prolonged seizures, but rapid IV administration may cause <u>respiratory depression</u>. Do not give diazepam intramuscularly (IM), because it is not well absorbed and is irritating to muscle tissue. Sublingual and intranasal administrations have been described, although there is little out-of-hospital experience.

The requirement for cannulating a peripheral vein in a seizing child often slows down delivery of essential ALS drugs, especially in infants and toddlers. *The rectum is an effective alternative route for emergency diazepam administration.* PR diazepam is effective, causes less respiratory depression, and is easy to administer. Rates of respiratory depression associated with PR diazepam are lower than for IV diazepam. However, onset of action is longer, with time to clinical effect in the range of 5 minutes. IV administration is considered to be the route of first choice but if cannulation proves difficult or too time consuming, then PR should be used. For a step-by-step explanation of the rectal diazepam administration procedure, see **Rectal Administration of Benzodiazepines, Procedure 17**.

Diazepam begins to work quickly but its anticonvulsant action does not last long, which is a serious limitation in protracted on-scene or transport times. Another dose of diazepam should not be given. It is possible to follow up a PR dose with an IV dose if the PR medication has not been effective. If the child is on phenobarbital or has received other benzodiazepines in the previous few hours, seek further advice before administration of diazepam due to the risk of respiratory depression.

Midazolam. Buccal midazolam is another benzodiazepine that can be given to a patient without IV access if they have their own medication and treatment plan. Follow the patient's

---

Table 6-3 Dextrose Administration Guidelines During Seizures

Indications
- Glucose level <4 mmol/Litre

Treatment
Consider whether to offer glucose gel (minding the airway), IV 10% glucose or IM Glucagon. The dosages of these options vary with age, check against the JRCALC guidelines.

© Jones & Bartlett Learning.

Table 6-4 Benzodiazepine Administration During Seizures. Refer to the JRCALC guidelines for dosages

Generic Name	Route	Pros	Cons
Diazepam	IV, IO	Rapid onset Inexpensive No refrigeration	Sedating Respiratory depression Short duration of action for seizure control (15 min)
Diazepam	PR	Rapid onset No IV required	Sedating Respiratory depression
Midazolam	IV, IM, IO	Rapid onset	Medium duration of action for seizure control (30–120 min)

© Jones & Bartlett Learning.

specific treatment plan or Epilepsy Passport for administration. When administering any benzodiazepine by any route, watch closely for respiratory depression, a common side effect of this class of drugs, and be prepared to provide bag-valve-mask ventilatory support. Even in the case of <u>apnoea</u> after benzodiazepine administration, a bag-valve-mask device usually suffices, because the respiratory depressant effects of the drugs are transitory. Endotracheal intubation is rarely necessary.

If the seizure does not stop after two doses of a benzodiazepine, seek further medical advice. If unsure about the use of midazolam, then ambulance clinicians should use IV or PR diazepam.

Lorazepam. Of the benzodiazepines, lorazepam probably has the best pharmacological profile for prehospital seizure management. It has a rapid onset of action, can be given intravenously (IV) or intraosseously (IO), and has a long half-life. Lorazepam is used to stop a seizure and can help to prevent further seizure activity for up to 8 hours, depending on dose. There is little experience with out-of-hospital PR lorazepam administration in children, and drug doses are not well established. In general, this drug has not been widely used by prehospital professionals because of the manufacturer's recommendation regarding refrigeration. Lorazepam may be stocked unrefrigerated in an ambulance service vehicle if it is replaced every 30 days.

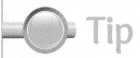

Tip

Always administer oxygen to a child who is having a seizure or who is postictal.

Transport

After providing airway and breathing support and administering a benzodiazepine, transport should be initiated. Perform history taking and physical examination and the detailed physical examination (trauma patients), if possible, on the way to the hospital. During transport, ongoing assessments should be performed using continuous cardiac monitoring and pulse oximetry. If a patient has not stopped seizing after administration of a benzodiazepine the risk for a prolonged seizure is high. Consider options in terms of transport destination because this subset of children is likely to require intensive care.

Assessment of the Postictal Child

Usually the child's seizure is already over when the prehospital professional arrives. This "postictal" state is characterised by abnormal appearance with sleepiness, confusion, irritability and decreased interactivity that may last from minutes to hours.

If the child is physiologically stable, perform a complete assessment in the field, including history taking and physical examination, observing particularly for any rash or discolouration of the skin, and the detailed physical examination (trauma patients). Check blood glucose levels and correct hypoglycaemia if present.

An example of a stable postictal patient is the child with a previous diagnosis of epilepsy who experiences a brief tonic-clonic seizure or the child younger than 6 years of age with fever and a possible febrile seizure. Most children who have had a brief seizure show steady improvement in level of alertness, muscle tone, and interactivity within 15–30 minutes. Failure to reach normal mental status over a 30- to 60-minute period after the seizure may reflect a serious underlying problem and trigger early transport with completion of the assessment en route to the hospital. **Table 6-5** lists some of the conditions that might lead to a prolonged postictal state that requires urgent treatment in the emergency department (ED). If the child has a seizure after closed head injury, always stabilise the <u>cervical</u> spine, as discussed in the *Trauma* chapter.

If the postictal patient has a previous diagnosis of epilepsy, include the name and dosage of anticonvulsant medications and when the last dose was given in the history. Enquire when the last blood levels were obtained and whether the levels were adequate. Determine the duration of the seizure and ask for a description of the motor activity, including where it started, how it progressed, and how long the child was unconscious. From this information, determine the type of seizure (e.g., generalised or partial, or partial with secondary generalisation). Ask carefully about head trauma. Consider the possibility of ingestion or overdose especially in toddlers and adolescents. Keep in mind that overdose of many non-prescription medications (e.g., antihistamines) can cause seizures.

Table 6-5 Worrisome Circumstances With the Postictal Child

Post-traumatic seizure
Post-ingestion seizure
Seizure and sustained hypoxia
Seizure in a neonate (<4 weeks of age)
First seizure in a child >6 years
More than one seizure
Seizure time >5 minutes
Low glucose level

© Jones & Bartlett Learning.

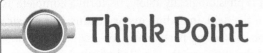

Think Point

Calm caregivers' fears about the seizure, but do not diagnose or provide them uncertain information about the cause of the seizure or chance of recurrence.

Attempt to allay the caregiver's fears. If this was the child's first seizure, the caregiver may be extremely frightened.

Summary of Seizures

Seizures are common in children, and frightened caregivers frequently call 999 to assist in managing this problem. Usually the seizure has stopped before ambulance arrival, in which case the tasks include only assessment of the postictal child and transport to the hospital with supportive care. Support of the frightened caregiver is also important because their demeanour can further upset the child.

Sometimes the child is seizing on arrival and requires medical management. The treatment includes opening and clearing the airway; providing oxygen; and then administering a benzodiazepine medication. The benzodiazepine medications may cause temporary respiratory depression, which requires bag-valve-mask ventilation support without endotracheal intubation in most cases. Transport to the hospital should not be delayed.

Altered Mental Status

AMS is an abnormal neurological state in which the child is less alert and interactive than is age-appropriate. The term AMS refers to a range of abnormal appearances, from irritability to total unresponsiveness. Sometimes the concern of the caretaker is vague, and the complaint is simply that the child is "not acting right". Understanding normal developmental or age-related changes in behaviour and listening carefully to the caregiver's opinion about alterations from an individual's normal state are key features in the assessment. A mnemonic recalls many of the severe causes of AMS (**Table 6-6**). The mnemonic is the five vowels in the alphabet (AEIOU), followed by tips (TIPPS), and reflects the major causes of AMS.

Assessment

Use the Paediatric Assessment Triangle (PAT) and the disability component of the hands-on <C>ABCDEs to quickly assess neurological status. These two parts of the primary assessment work in concert to evaluate both cortical and brainstem functions; see the *Paediatric Assessment* chapter. There is a difference between "abnormal appearance" and AMS. Abnormal appearance is a more subtle measure of brain function and is evaluated using the TICLS mnemonic (Table 1-1). AMS is a more severe signal of mental status alteration and is evaluated with the alert-verbal-painful-unresponsive (AVPU) scale. Although AMS is always associated with an abnormal appearance, some children with more subtle abnormalities in appearance would not have AMS using the AVPU. For example, a child who is irritable or listless and has abnormal appearance on the PAT

Table 6-6 AEIOU TIPPS: Possible Causes of AMS

Alcohol
Epilepsy, endocrine, electrolytes
Insulin
Opiates and other drugs
Uraemia
Trauma, temperature
Infection, intussusception
Psychogenic
Poison
Shock, stroke, space-occupying lesion, subarachnoid haemorrhage

© Jones & Bartlett Learning.

Case Study 2

You respond to a call about an unresponsive child. The caregiver states that the 3-year-old boy could not be awakened from his nap. The child is "sleeping" on your arrival, with no abnormal airway sounds or retractions. He is pale. Respiratory rate is 20 breaths/min, cardiac monitor shows a narrow complex with a rate of 160 beats/min, and blood pressure is 80/50 mm Hg. Pupils are small and slow to constrict to light, and the child withdraws to pain. There is no sign of trauma. The caregiver states that the child was playful and appeared healthy before his nap.

1. What are the immediate treatment priorities for this child?

2. What additional history may be helpful?

may be "alert" on the AVPU scale of disability during the <C>ABCDE hands-on evaluation.

The AVPU system is a quick way to determine level of consciousness and to assess major changes in mental status during transport. A child with sepsis or brain haemorrhage from inflicted injury, for example, has a serious degree of brain dysfunction and may score "verbal" or lower on the AVPU.

Finally, observe motor activity and check the pupils. In the assessment of motor activity, watch for purposeful and symmetric movement of extremities, ataxia, seizures, posturing (decorticate or decerebrate), or flaccidity (hypotonia). In the assessment of pupils, check size (small or large), equality, and response to light. Pupils may have abnormal size or reactivity in the presence of drugs, ongoing seizures, hypoxia, or impending brainstem herniation. The presence of a deviated gaze is abnormal and should be noted and reported.

Look for a Medical Alert Bracelet, and ask about important medical history that may account for the child's AMS, such as diabetes or a seizure disorder (**Figure 6-2**).

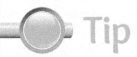

> **Tip**
>
> There are many causes of AMS, but management must focus on the ABCs.

Management

Regardless of the cause of AMS, focus on the ABCs.

1. *Open the airway.*

   In the poorly responsive patient with compromised airway reflexes, suction the mouth to relieve potential obstruction

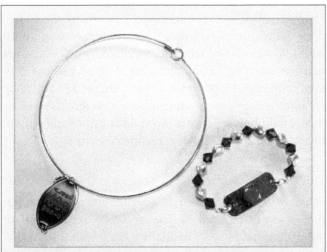

Figure 6-2 In a child with AMS, look for a bracelet with his or her medical history.
Courtesy of Rhonda Beck.

from secretions or vomitus. If there is no gag reflex or if the patient is totally unresponsive, position the head and insert an oropharyngeal or nasopharyngeal airway. Keep the spine stabilised if there is suspicion of head or neck injury.

2. *Ensure adequate breathing.*

   Patients with AMS may have inadequate breathing despite spontaneous respiratory effort, based on inadequate respiratory rate or inadequate tidal volume. Administer 100% oxygen by non-rebreathing mask. Start bag-valve-mask ventilation with 100% oxygen if the patient is cyanotic, has oxygen saturation less than 90% on 100% oxygen by non-rebreathing mask, is breathing at a rate too slow for age, or has shallow or irregular respiratory effort.

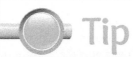

> **Tip**
>
> There is a difference between abnormal appearance and AMS. Abnormal appearance is a more subtle measure of brain function and is evaluated using the TICLS mnemonic. AMS is a more severe signal of mental status alteration and is evaluated with the AVPU.

Consider the airway cascade from basic manoeuvres to advanced airway management to protect the airway and to avoid aspiration. This may mean the introduction of a supra-glottic airway device or intubation. The choice of whether to intubate will be made considering service policy and the clinician's decision based on competence and confidence. Ventilate the patient with suspected brain injury, but do not hyperventilate (see the *Respiratory Emergencies* chapter). Use end-tidal CO_2 ($EtCO_2$) or capnography to guide ventilations. Place the patient on a cardiac monitor and a pulse oximeter.

3. *Safeguard circulation.*

   Establish vascular access and obtain blood for serum glucose measurement. If IV cannulation is required for drug or fluid administration then this should be attempted. If this fails then intraosseous (IO) access should be used. Reassess the child's level of consciousness.

4. *Perform a bedside blood glucose test* (**Figure 6-3**).

   Administer glucose only to children with hypoglycaemia. Neurological outcome in patients with diffuse brain injury is worse when the child also has hyperglycaemia. If a bedside glucose test shows hypoglycaemia (<4 mmol/l), give an IV glucose bolus, or IM glucagon as outlined in Table 6-3. Administer oral glucose to a child with diabetes and hypoglycaemia who is conscious and has a gag reflex.

5. *In the child with AMS and depressed respirations, consider naloxone administration.*

   The naloxone dose should be given IV as per JRCALC guidelines. As outlined in the *Emergency Delivery and*

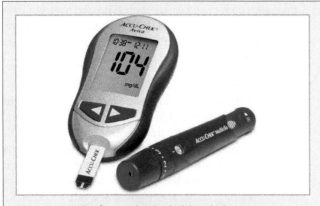

Figure 6-3 Perform a bedside blood glucose test.
Accu-Chek® Aviva used with permission of Roche Diagnostics.

Newborn Stabilisation chapter, naloxone should not be administered to the newly born. Outside of the newly born, narcotic overdose is a less likely cause of AMS in children but should be considered. It is an important consideration in teenagers. Constricted pupils are a universal finding in pure opiate overdoses. This is not necessarily the case with *synthetic* narcotics, such as oxycodone.

Endocrine Disorders

In children, endocrine disorders include diabetes, congenital adrenal hyperplasia (CAH), panhypopituitarism, and cortisol deficiency. Of these disorders, diabetes is the most common.

Diabetes Mellitus

Diabetes is a disorder of the hormone insulin. Insulin, produced by the pancreas, helps regulate blood glucose levels. Glucose is needed in the production of energy by cells in the body. Without adequate amounts of insulin, muscle cells cannot access circulating glucose and thus cannot create energy. The disease called diabetes mellitus is a result of a lack of functioning insulin.

Diabetes mellitus is a disease of children and adults. Of the two types, Type 1 (insulin-dependent diabetes mellitus, IDDM) and Type 2 (non–insulin-dependent diabetes mellitus, NIDDM), younger children are more likely to have type 1 diabetes, which is insulin-dependent. These children are more prone to develop antibodies to the cells in the pancreas that produce insulin. The underlying cause is unknown.

There is an increasing prevalence of type 2 diabetes (NIDDM) in childhood. Such children are usually adolescents, often with associated obesity. The child may be on oral hypoglycaemic agents, rather than insulin.

Regardless of the type of diabetes, the onset of symptoms is relatively slow, over days (as in type 1 diabetes) to weeks (as in type 2 diabetes). The disease process begins as insulin production is diminished. Diminished amounts of insulin

increasingly impair the availability of glucose to the muscle cells. The diminished amounts of glucose available for energy production stimulate the release of fat stores. As fat stores are mobilised, they are converted to ketones and other metabolic acids. Together the accumulation of glucose and metabolic acids cause the symptoms of diabetic ketoacidosis (DKA).

If the blood glucose level exceeds the renal threshold for reabsorption, osmotic diuresis occurs. This results in frequent urination (polyuria) with corresponding loss of body water. As blood glucose levels rise, increasing amounts of body water are lost in the urine. Loss of body water causes intense thirst (polydipsia). Fat breakdown leads to increased hunger (polyphagia) in the presence of abdominal pain along with the hallmark symptom of Kussmaul respirations. These respirations are rapid and deep, and have the odour of ketones or rotten fruit. These children may fall asleep in school, begin wetting the bed, and have abnormal thirst. The odour of ketones is often prevalent.

Ambulance services may be called for a child with AMS with a history of abdominal pain, vomiting, and excessive thirst. The child is often severely dehydrated. In the presence of abdominal pain, nausea, and vomiting, sepsis may be suspected. The presence of a blood glucose level higher than 30 mmol/l or hyperglycaemia may lead one to suspect the presence of DKA.

Assessment

Signs and symptoms of hyperglycaemia can be difficult to detect, especially because the onset is relatively slow. The primary sign of hyperglycaemia is dehydration. Depending on the blood sugar level, signs and symptoms may range from mild to severe hypoperfusion. Tachycardia, rapid/deep respirations, and dry skin are all signs of volume depletion. In general, the higher the blood glucose level, the more extreme the dehydration.

Management

After general treatment measures are implemented, initiate an IV and administer fluid as advised by JRCALC. Care must be taken when administering IV fluid because children with high blood glucose levels are prone to develop cerebral oedema in the presence of excess fluid. Therefore, repeat fluid boluses only if the child is hypotensive. If not hypotensive, keep IV fluids at maintenance rate.

Hypoglycaemia

Hypoglycaemia is defined as a serum glucose concentration of less than 4 mmol/l. The most frequent scenario for out-of-hospital hypoglycaemia is a child with known diabetes who uses too much insulin; exerts himself or herself excessively; or delays a meal (transient hypoglycaemia) after taking insulin. Hypoglycaemia may also occur in children with a history of almost any endocrine problem.

In non-diabetic infants, hypoglycaemia may occur when increased metabolic demands deplete glycogen stores (e.g., when compensating for a cardiac defect or for an extreme respiratory rate). This is more common in infants and toddlers.

Hypoglycaemia may also occur in children with sepsis. Check a bedside glucose level in any acutely ill appearing child, especially in the presence of abnormal appearance or AMS. Other causes of hypoglycaemia in children are poor food intake in the face of an acute illness, such as gastroenteritis, especially in infants and toddlers with limited glycogen reserves.

Assessment

Signs and symptoms of hypoglycaemia may be difficult to detect, especially in younger infants who have mild hypoglycaemia. The changing signs and symptoms are noted in **Table 6-7**. Depending on the blood glucose level, signs and symptoms may range from mild to severe. Tachycardia, tachypnoea, sweating, agitation, and tremor all reflect increased catecholamine release as the body responds to inadequate sugar supplies to support cellular metabolism. When blood sugar is dangerously low, seizures, coma, and death can occur.

Management of Hypoglycaemia in Diabetes Mellitus

Children with type 1 IDDM are often well aware of the signs and symptoms of hypoglycaemia, based on past experiences with insulin. If a patient with diabetes is at least physiologically stable and cooperative but is hypoglycaemic by blood sugar testing, allow him or her to attempt oral glucose replacement. Give 0.5–1.0 g/kg of sugar. There are 20 g glucose in one glass (230 ml) of a regular (not dietetic) fizzy drink, as well as orange or apple juice. Milk may be the preferred replacement with a balance of 12 g glucose, 8 g protein, and 8 g fat in 230 ml of whole milk.

Children taking oral hypoglycaemic agents (type 2 diabetes) are also prone to hypoglycaemia, although not as frequently. When present in the child with type 2 diabetes, hypoglycaemia can be more difficult to stabilise. Give the child oral glucose replacement if signs and symptoms of hypoglycaemia

occur and the child is physiologically stable and cooperative, or treat with IV glucose or IM glucagon if the child has AMS. Administration values are outlined in JRCALC.

Treatment of Hypoglycaemia

Treat hypoglycaemia if the child has AMS and measured serum glucose of less than 4 mmol/l, as outlined in Table 6-3. Children have different tolerances to hypoglycaemia, so a child may be alert and cooperative with a blood sugar level between 4 and 5 mmol/l. A child in this condition can take oral glucose or an infant can breastfeed.

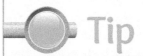

Tip

Signs and symptoms of hypoglycaemia can be non-specific.

For the physiologically unstable patient with hypoglycaemia and AMS, IV or IO glucose should be administered immediately. Recheck the serum glucose if scene time or transport is prolonged and repeat glucose doses as needed. It is important to avoid infiltration because the solution even when diluted, is quite irritating to skin tissues.

If there is no IV access, glucagon should be administered (as per JRCALC guidelines). Glucagon stimulates a transient increase of the blood glucose level as long as there are liver stores of glycogen (long chains of stored glucose molecules). It is important to note that the incidence of vomiting is increased in children when glucagon is administered. Take care to position the child to ensure airway patency within the first 15–20 minutes after administration.

Congenital Adrenal Hyperplasia

Congenital adrenal hyperplasia (CAH) is another endocrine disorder. This disorder involves the hormones of the adrenal glands. The adrenal glands help keep the body in balance by making the right amounts of cortisol, aldosterone, and androgens. Although there are many different types of CAH, the most common type (95%) results in a deficiency of cortisol and sometimes aldosterone. As a result, the body cannot adjust to illness or injury. Hypotension, hypoglycaemia, and dehydration may be severe and a threat to life.

Most children with this disorder carry emergency medication with them at all times. Usually, the medication includes dexamethasone or hydrocortisone. Parents should be asked if they have given the needed medication, such as hydrocortisone. If not, have them administer the medication if possible. Because the body is unable to adjust to a stress, checking blood glucose level and administering dextrose as needed, monitoring blood pressure and replacing fluids as necessary are all part of assessment and treatment.

Table 6-7 Signs and Symptoms of Hypoglycaemia		
Mild	**Moderate**	**Severe**
Hunger, irritability, weakness, agitation, tachypnoea, tachycardia	Anxiety, blurred vision, stomach ache, headache, dizziness, sweating, pallor, tremors, confusion	Seizure, coma

© Jones & Bartlett Learning.

Cortisol Deficiency

This deficiency occurs when the adrenal glands do not produce enough cortisol. This may occur for a variety of reasons, including CAH, pituitary gland malfunction, and failure of the adrenal gland itself or when steroids are already present. When children are prescribed steroids for a period of time, they must be gradually withdrawn to give the adrenal glands sufficient time to resume function. Normal management includes oral hydrocortisone or IM injections. In certain circumstances, the amount of hydrocortisone should be increased quickly. This is done by administering either oral or IM hydrocortisone.

In any case, when a child with cortisol deficiency becomes sick, many body systems are affected, including the ability to balance blood glucose and regulate body water. These children should always have a blood glucose check. Asking the parent or caregiver if the child's normal medication has been administered is important. If the medication has not been administered, calling the receiving facility or following the care plan (found with the rescue medication) is also encouraged.

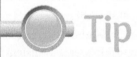

Tip

In a child with impaired adrenal gland function, administration of steroids (dexamethasone or hydrocortisone) can be life-saving.

Panhypopituitarism

This condition affects the pituitary gland, particularly the anterior pituitary where thyroid-stimulating hormone (TSH), adrenocorticotropic hormone (ACTH), growth hormone (GH), and others are produced. As a result, many other glands of the child's endocrine system are also affected. These children are usually diagnosed in infancy, or can develop the condition after removal of certain brain tumours, and parents or other caregivers are well educated in their child's condition. When a child suffering this condition becomes ill, hypoglycaemia is common and dehydration may also be present.

Transport

With any child having an endocrine issue, transport is important. If the child is suffering from hyperglycaemia, do not delay transport for administration of fluid. The child needs to be transported, so IV/IO starts en route are appropriate.

However, if a low blood glucose level is present, treatment should be initiated immediately. After giving IV or IO glucose or IM glucagon, reassess. Watch for a return to normal appearance and behaviour. If the child with AMS does not return to normal in a few minutes after IV or IO administration or 15–20 minutes after IM glucagon, transport immediately and conduct additional assessment on the way to the ED. If the child returns to normal, consider doing additional assessment on scene. If the child has no history of diabetes or other endocrine problems, and has either hyperglycaemia or hypoglycaemia, transport is indicated.

Additional Assessment

Perform history taking when possible. Ask key questions, such as:

- How quickly did the symptoms progress?
- Does the patient have diabetes or any other known illness?
- If the patient is a diabetic, or has another endocrine problem, has there been a recent change in medication or meals?
- Is the child on insulin, an oral hypoglycaemia drug, or any other replacement medication?
- Is this the first episode? If not, how often does this happen?
- Is it possible that the child was exposed to drugs or alcohol?
- If the patient is a newborn, has the mother received prenatal care?
- Has the mother had any medical problems with the pregnancy?
- Is the mother a diabetic?
- What is the newborn being fed and how often?
- When was the last time the child had medication?
- How many caregivers are giving medications? Are they doubling up doses?

After the history, a physical examination should be performed. It is important to continually reassess the patient. If the child has diabetes and received too much insulin, and there are no physiological or anatomical abnormalities on reassessment, or if the child has another endocrine problem, consider requesting additional clinical advice. In some services, the child with type 1 diabetes, who is not in DKA, may be left at the scene with management directed by the general practitioner (GP) in consultation with the caregiver. However, the circumstances with type 2 diabetes are somewhat different, because the oral drugs that are taken for this condition have a longer duration of action than most insulin and the child may need ongoing administration of glucose to maintain blood sugar. *Patients with type 2 diabetes on oral agents, who have experienced hypoglycaemia, should not be left on the scene.* If the child has an emergency medication that needs to be administered, or if the child is a type 2 diabetic with an episode of hypoglycaemia, transport the child to the ED.

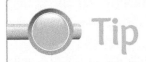

Do not leave patients with type 2 diabetes on oral agents, who have experienced hypoglycaemia, on the scene.

Summary of Altered Mental Status and Endocrine Disorders

There are many causes of AMS in children. The caregiver may be the best judge of AMS, especially in the infant or toddler where developmental assessment is more challenging. Appearance and the AVPU scale work in concert to help assess AMS. Address the ABCs first and especially consider causes of dehydration, such as hyperglycaemia, and reversible causes, such as hypoglycaemia. Transport the child with hyperglycaemia immediately.

Fever

Fever is a sign of infection or inflammation, rather than a problem itself, and is often misunderstood. Most infections in childhood are systemic and result in fevers. Children can run high fevers in response to either bacterial or viral infections. High fever (>40°C) can be caused by minor illnesses, such as a cold, or serious problems, such as pneumonia, meningitis, or sepsis. Fever of any cause leads to an increase in basal metabolic rate, causing a more rapid respiratory rate, increased cardiac output, higher oxygen consumption, and a greater need for fluids and calories. The ill child frequently is not interested in eating or drinking and, with the increased metabolic demands of fever, may be at risk for volume depletion and hypoglycaemia. A body temperature less than 41.1°C is not itself harmful. However, body temperatures greater than 41.1°C may have the potential to be harmful, and the child should be carefully evaluated. In general, fevers are a common cause of concern for most parents, and high temperatures are a cause of concern to caregivers who fear brain damage as a result of a high fever despite the fact that there is no evidence to support that concern.

Determine the presence of fever by history and field evaluation. Knowing the temperature, however, usually does not change field management.

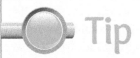

Fever less than 41.1°C by itself does not cause brain damage.

Assessment

The primary assessment helps determine the severity of the child's illness and the urgency for treatment. If the primary assessment is normal, take a history and perform a physical examination. Ask about important signs and symptoms of infection, such as chills, malaise, poor feeding, lethargy, pulling of ears, vomiting, diarrhoea, abdominal pain, presence of a rash or skin discolouration, stiff neck, headache, and irritability.

Ask about exposure to known childhood communicable diseases. Many childhood illnesses begin with a fever before any other symptoms are present. Determine if the child has any significant medical history, because febrile children who may be immune deficient (e.g., patients with sickle cell disease, cancer, human immunodeficiency virus (HIV), or post-organ transplantation) are at higher risk for serious infection as the cause of fever.

Febrile respiratory infections are very common in children and are characterised by fever, tachycardia, tachypnoea, nasal congestion, cough, and respiratory distress. Fever may make a child with a minor illness appear sicker than he or she really is, and parents often report a marked improvement in symptoms after administration of antipyretics, such as paracetamol or ibuprofen. After the history, if the child has no physiological abnormalities, a physical examination should be performed to look for possible sources of infection.

Although the height of fever is not reflective of the degree of illness, certain findings suggest a serious underlying illness and must prompt rapid transport. These include a bulging fontanelle (if <12 months of age, palpate with the child sitting up), photophobia (sensitivity to light), nuchal rigidity (stiff neck), paradoxical irritability (an infant who is crankier when picked up and held than when left alone) (**Figure 6-4**), seizures, prolonged capillary refill time, or a petechial or purpuric rash (**Figure 6-5**).

Age and Fever

In addition to signs and symptoms, the age of a child is important in assessing the significance of fever. A fever in an infant less than 6 months old may be the only indication of serious infection, but the degree of temperature may be lower in comparison to the severity of illness or in comparison to older children with the same problem. The symptoms of serious bacterial infection in a young infant may be non-specific, such as fussiness, poor feeding, and sleepiness. Because these very young infants have an immature immune system and are difficult to assess because of their limited range of behaviours and activities, any infant less than 4 weeks old with fever greater than or equal to 38°C requires blood, urine, and spinal fluid cultures and empiric antibiotics in the ED. In the first few days of life, jaundice may be a sign of serious bacterial infection. Infants 28 days to 2 months of age usually require a similar evaluation but may be discharged from the ED if the physical examination

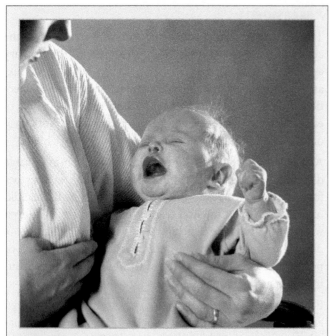

Figure 6-4 An infant suffering from paradoxical irritability.
© Stock Connection Distribution/Alamy Images.

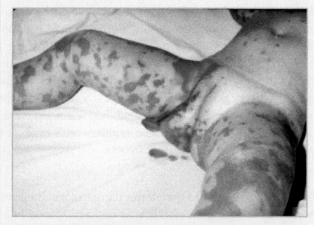

Figure 6-5 Purpuric rash in a child with meningococcemia.
Courtesy of Ron Deickmann, MD.

and laboratory evaluation are normal. A seizure in the presence of a fever in a child less than 6 months of age also warrants transport.

Management

Management of fever in the child who has a normal primary assessment includes the following:

1. *Prevent transmission of disease to the prehospital professional.*

   Use standard precautions for infection control.

2. *In a febrile child who is older than 6 months, consider administration of antipyretics if none have been administered in the past 4 hours.*

   Give paracetamol at a dose indicated in JRCALC guidelines. Another option for the alert paediatric patient is ibuprofen at a dose suggested by JRCALC guidelines if awake. Ibuprofen is not recommended by JRCALC for infants less than 3 months of age. A paediatric patient's level of consciousness or history of recent vomiting should be considered before administering anything by mouth. Aspirin should be avoided in a febrile infant or child because prior studies suggest that there is an increased incidence of Reye's syndrome in children who receive aspirin for a viral illness. Parents may need explanation that overdressing a febrile child retains heat and may increase fever.

3. *Cool the feverish child by undressing him or her, but avoid hypothermia.*

   Do not use cold water, fans, ice, or alcohol baths to lower temperature.

4. *Transport with ongoing reassessment for deterioration.*

5. *Explain to the caregiver that fever alone is not dangerous to the child.*

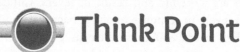

Think Point

Never use ice, cold water, fans, or alcohol baths to cool a feverish child.

Summary of Fever

Fever is usually a response to any type of infection. It is rarely a problem in and of itself. However, the longer the child has sustained a fever the more likely the child has become dehydrated. The age of the child and other associated signs and symptoms are important in determining probability of serious illness. The presence of a petechial or purpuric rash, stiff neck, light sensitivity, and/or AMS in a child with a fever is highly suspicious for a more serious problem. In most cases, simple cooling measures and transport are the primary actions for the prehospital professional.

Communicable Diseases

Many communicable diseases are common during childhood. Although most are viral in origin, and mild in terms of severity, infectious diseases on occasion cause significant compromise in the paediatric patient, resulting in the need for prehospital transport. Many childhood diseases have a respiratory component, a GI component, or both. Respiratory diseases are addressed in the *Respiratory Emergencies* chapter. This chapter concentrates on the GI signs and symptoms of nausea, vomiting, and diarrhoea.

Nausea, Vomiting, and Diarrhoea (Gastroenteritis)

Collectively, nausea, vomiting, and diarrhoea are termed gastroenteritis. Gastroenteritis is an inflammation of the GI tract that presents as vomiting and diarrhoea in the paediatric patient. There are numerous causes of gastroenteritis ranging from food and waterborne diseases, viruses, bacteria, side effect of antibiotics, and parasites, many carried by animals, especially pets. Of all the causes, viral agents are most common, with the Norwalk virus being especially contagious. No matter the cause, this infectious illness can result in volume depletion, particularly in younger children. Beware that signs and symptoms most commonly associated with gastroenteritis, such as fever, abdominal pain, or vomiting, can also herald more serious abdominal emergencies, such as appendicitis and bowel obstruction.

It is important to determine the presence and sequence of nausea, vomiting, diarrhoea, and/or fever. Conditions of malrotation of the gut (in newborns) and pyloric stenosis (vomiting shortly after nursing but no diarrhoea or fever) are conditions more common in young infants. Food poisoning, such as salmonella, usually occurs after eating (sometimes as much as 6–8 hours) and causes vomiting and diarrhoea in that order, followed by a fever. The diagnosis of gastroenteritis requires exclusion of more serious causes, and this determination is not possible in the field.

Assessment

Focus the assessment of a child with presumed gastroenteritis on the child's state of hydration.

The history should include questions regarding:

- The onset, sequence of events, and frequency of vomiting or diarrhoea
- Relationship to eating
- Amount of oral intake
- Number of wet nappies or times of urination in the past 8 hours
- Character of stool including the presence of blood
- Last urination or wet nappy

The physical examination should include attention to:

- Presence or absence of fever
- Level of consciousness
- Hydration of mucous membranes (moist or dry)
- Presence or absence of tears
- Extremity warmth and pulse quality
- Abdominal tenderness or distention

Always check a bedside glucose level in a child with a history of vomiting, diarrhoea, and poor oral intake.

Management

Management of the paediatric patient with presumed gastroenteritis depends on the degree of dehydration. Prevention of disease transmission to the prehospital professional is an additional component of care.

1. *Use standard precautions to reduce the likelihood of disease transmission.*

   Gastroenteritis, whether bacterial, viral, or parasitic in origin, is transmitted by the faecal-oral route. Ingestion of even a few pathogenic organisms can lead to disease in some cases. Some organisms can survive on examination instruments and surfaces for hours, so special care of clothes and instruments and careful hand washing are essential.

2. *Provide supplemental oxygen and airway management for the unstable paediatric patient.*

3. *Provide fluid replacement for severe clinical dehydration.*

   Establish vascular access, IV or IO, and initiate fluid replacement using crystalloid fluid at 20 ml/kg initial bolus if the child has severe clinical dehydration as evidenced by elevated heart rate, poor pulses, delayed capillary refill time, cool extremities, and abnormal colouration. Repeat the bolus until perfusion is stabilised or up to the maximum dose recommended by JRCALC.

4. *Treat documented hypoglycaemia.*

5. *Reassess vital signs.*

6. *Transport.*

   Transport decisions depend on the degree of dehydration and local resources. A child with mild to moderate dehydration and ongoing vomiting and diarrhoea may require transport alone without treatment. Provide oral fluids in the field to children with dehydration, if permitted by the ambulance service guidelines. The child with signs of severe dehydration or shock benefits from immediate fluid replacement before hospital transport.

Sepsis and Meningitis

Sepsis implies an overwhelming, life-threatening bacterial bloodstream infection. Some children with sepsis also have meningitis, resulting from infection and inflammation of the meninges, the membranes that cover the brain and spinal cord. Other children present with sepsis or meningitis alone. The causative agent of meningitis may be aseptic (non-bacterial) or bacterial. Although children with viral or aseptic meningitis may appear quite ill, the infection is not often life-threatening. However, bacterial meningitis is rapidly progressive, with death sometimes following the onset of symptoms within hours to days. Although fever is usually present, except occasionally in the neonatal period, other symptoms may vary from stiff neck and headache to impending brainstem herniation. **Table 6-8** outlines the JRCALC criteria for suspecting sepsis.

Infants in the first year of life are at highest risk for sepsis and bacterial meningitis, and the organisms vary with age. Since the introduction of the *Haemophilus influenzae* type B vaccine in the late 1980s, this previously common cause of childhood illness has almost disappeared.

Table 6-8 JRCALC guideline on suspecting sepsis in children.

High risk criteria suspect 'Red flag' sepsis:	
Colour	• Pale/mottled/ashen/blue.
Activity	• No response to social cues. • Appears very ill to a healthcare professional. • Does not wake or, if roused, does not stay awake. • Weak, high-pitched or continuous cry.
Respiratory	• Grunting. • Severe tachypnoea. • Moderate or severe chest indrawing. • Oxygen saturations ≤90% on air.
Hydration	• Reduced skin turgor. • Severe tachycardia (see below). • Bradycardia <60. • Not passed urine/no wet nappies in last 18 hours.
Other	• Temperature <36°C. • Non-blanching rash. • Bulging fontanelle. • Neck stiffness. • Status epilepticus. • Focal neurological signs. • Focal seizures.
Sepsis likely/intermediate risk for sepsis (if history suggestive of infection)	
Colour	• Pallor reported by parent/caregiver.
Activity	• Not responding normally to social cues/not wanting to play. • Wakes only with prolonged stimulation. • Significantly decreased activity. • No smile.
Respiratory	• Nasal flaring. • Moderate tachypnoea (see below). • Oxygen saturations ≤ 92% on air. • Crackles.
Hydration	• Dry mucous membranes. • Moderate tachycardia (see below). • Poor feeding in infants. • CRT ≥3 seconds. • Reduced urine output. • Cold feet or hands.
Other	• Age 0–3 months ≥38°C. • Age 3–6 months ≥39°C. • Fever for ≥5 days. • Rigors. • Swelling of a limb or joint. • Leg pain. • Non-weight bearing/not using an extremity.

Republished with kind permission of the Association of Ambulance Chief Executives.

Bacterial sepsis and meningitis in the first month of age is most commonly caused by bacteria acquired from the maternal vaginal area during delivery. These include *Escherichia coli*, group B streptococcus, and *Listeria monocytogenes*.

Outside of the youngest age group, community-acquired infection is the source of sepsis and meningitis, with common bacterial causes in immune-competent children including *Streptococcus pneumoniae* (also the most common cause of bacterial ear infections, sinusitis, and pneumonia in children) and *Neisseria meningitidis* (meningococcus). *H. influenzae* type B meningitis has also decreased significantly because of widespread vaccine use. The enteroviruses are also common causes of viral meningitis, especially during summer and autumn months.

Another group of children who are at risk for sepsis are those who are immunodeficient (e.g., cancer, post-organ transplantation), especially if they have an indwelling central line.

Meningococcal sepsis or meningitis is a life-threatening emergency that presents acutely with high fever, AMS, and a characteristic petechial rash or purpura. The presence of such a rash should always trigger rapid transport by the highest level of provider to the highest level of care available, because these children can deteriorate very quickly, requiring aggressive life support.

Assessment

In a physiologically unstable child with presumed sepsis or meningitis, limit the scene assessment. Perform the focused history and physical examination during transport, if possible. The focused history should include:

- Known exposure to illness
- Perinatal history for infants <1 month of age
- Onset of symptoms and rapidity of progression
- Presence or absence of fever
- Associated symptoms and signs, such as irritability, vomiting, stiff neck, rash (petechiae or purpura)
- Immunisation history

The physical examination should include attention to:

- Fever
- Level of consciousness
- Adequacy of perfusion
- Stiff neck (nuchal rigidity)
- Presence of a rash (petechiae or purpura)
- Photophobia

Because children with sepsis and meningitis are in a hypermetabolic state, they can develop hypoglycaemia and dehydration. Check a bedside glucose level on any patient with presumed sepsis or meningitis.

Management

Management of the paediatric patient with sepsis or meningitis must include infection control precautions. Interventions vary based on the patient's clinical presentation.

1. *Prevent disease transmission.*

   The prehospital professional should use standard and respiratory precautions, including gowns, gloves, and masks to avoid contact with patient secretions.

2. *Provide supplemental oxygen.*

   Unstable patients may need assisted ventilation or airway management.

3. *Establish vascular access.*

4. *For inadequate perfusion, initiate fluid replacement.*

   For the paediatric patient with inadequate perfusion, initiate fluid replacement using crystalloid fluid at 20 ml/kg initial bolus as fast as possible. Because of the effects of fever, dehydration may be present. Because of the effects of bacterial toxins on the blood vessels, children with sepsis may develop distributive shock requiring aggressive fluid resuscitation. Therefore, repeat fluid boluses of 20 ml/kg of crystalloid fluid may be required.

5. *Consider antibiotic treatment.*

   In a patient with suspected meningococcal septicaemia, a repeatable dose of benzyl penicillin may be given either IV, IO, or IM as per JRCALC guidance. Refer to **Figure 6-6**.

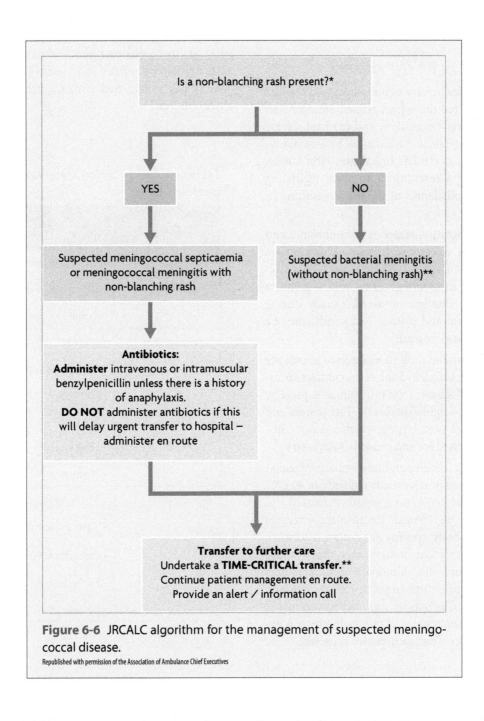

Figure 6-6 JRCALC algorithm for the management of suspected meningococcal disease.

Republished with permission of the Association of Ambulance Chief Executives

6. *Treat hypoglycaemia.*

7. *Reassess vital signs frequently.*

   Use continuous cardiorespiratory monitoring and pulse oximetry, if available. Anticipate deterioration in transport.

8. *Transport.*

   Because these children are at risk for rapid deterioration and may need ALS intervention, transport by the highest level of service available. Children with sepsis or meningitis generally require intensive care. Consider this when determining a transport destination.

Environmental Emergencies

Common paediatric environmental emergencies include temperature-related problems and stings. Each of these emergencies can range from mild to severe. Match the intensity of the intervention to the severity of the illness or injury.

Heat-Related Emergencies

Heat-related emergencies involve two separate and distinct processes leading to three main heat-related emergencies: (1) heat cramps, (2) heat exhaustion, and (3) heat stroke. Heat cramps and heat exhaustion are caused by a combination of fluid deficit and electrolyte imbalance. Heat stroke, however, is a result of a resetting of the heat-regulating mechanism in the hypothalamus of the brain, resulting in hyperthermia.

Heat cramps are a combination of electrolyte imbalance and dehydration where the electrolyte imbalance precipitates spasms of the muscle, typically of the long bones. These children complain of pain in their legs, arms, and sometimes the abdomen. Because this has occurred, usually during activity, the skin is warm and sweaty. Tachycardia may be present and may be caused by pain.

Heat exhaustion is a combination of electrolyte imbalance and dehydration where the dehydration precipitates dizziness and/or syncope. Because a volume deficit is present, the skin is often pale, cool, and diaphoretic. Tachycardia and tachypnoea are also common. Hypoglycaemia is not common but should be assessed for and treated as necessary.

Heat stroke occurs when the temperature-regulating mechanism is reset to a higher set point, usually higher than 40.6°C. As a result, the basal metabolic rate is greatly increased and every body organ can be affected. Because the enzymes within the organs and body systems are designed to work between a relatively narrow temperature range, organ failure occurs. AMS, heart failure with pulmonary oedema, kidney and liver failure, and profound hypotension are evident. Because of the increased metabolic rate, hypoglycaemia is common. The skin is usually dry and red; tachycardia is extreme (usually >150 bpm); and tachypnoea is present.

Heat-related emergencies, however, are rarely as clear-cut as they are described. The child with heat exhaustion may have AMS, or the child with heat stroke may be sweating. Regardless of the type of heat-related emergency, it is very important that a heat-related emergency is recognised and treatment implemented. In the paediatric population, heat-related emergencies occur most commonly when young children are left in a closed car or older children who are not heat-acclimated participate in sports during periods of high environmental temperatures and do not hydrate adequately. Because of the difficulty of obtaining temperature readings in the field, the assessment of such patients often occurs without the benefit of an objective temperature.

Physiological considerations in infants and toddlers with heat-related emergencies include immature thermoregulatory systems, greater body surface area-to-mass ratio, and a lesser ability to dissipate heat (**Table 6-9**). These characteristics predispose infants and toddlers to heat-related emergencies, particularly heat stroke, much more quickly than in older children.

Table 6-9 Typical Clinical Presentation of Heat-Related Emergencies

Clinical Presentation	Signs and Symptoms
Heat cramps	• Normal level of consciousness • Slightly elevated body temperature • Painful muscle spasms
Heat exhaustion	• Mild AMS • Tachycardia, tachypnoea, hypotension • Core temperature 38°–40°C • Fatigue • Headache • Diaphoresis
Heat stroke	• Severe AMS; confusion to coma • Tachycardia, hypotension • Core temperature >40.6°C • Flushed, dry skin • Nausea and vomiting

© Jones & Bartlett Learning.

Assessment

The history should include:

- Environmental temperature
- Duration of environmental exposure
- Activities and events before symptom development
- Pre-existing medical conditions

Management

The management of heat-related illness depends on the severity of symptoms, especially the patient's level of consciousness and cardiovascular status. Because the mechanism is different, use of antipyretics is not effective.

Heat Cramps

- Cool environment
- Remove excess clothing
- Oral rehydration with an electrolyte-containing solution
- Establish vascular access with normal saline at TKO rate

Heat Exhaustion

- Cool environment
- Cool mist or light sponging with tepid water and allow moisture to evaporate
- Establish vascular access and initiate fluid replacement with crystalloid fluid at 20 ml/kg for treatment of shock

Heat Stroke

- Airway management, assist ventilations, intubate if indicated
- Establish vascular access and fluid replacement with crystalloid fluid at 20 ml/kg
- Cool mist or light sponging with tepid water and allow moisture to evaporate
- Aggressive cooling measures: wet sheets, ice bags to axilla, groin, and neck
- Frequent re-measurement of core temperature
- Treat hypoglycaemia
- Avoid shivering
- Treat for shock

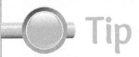

Tip

Early recognition and frequent reassessment of a heat-related emergency is important, because the patient's temperature may continue to rise despite initial management techniques.

Summary of Heat-Related Emergencies

Rapid recognition of heat-related emergencies is essential to effective management. Reassess vital signs frequently to evaluate the patient's response to treatment. Aggressive cooling measures are required for heat stroke.

Cold-Related Emergencies

Hypothermia is a core temperature of less than 35°C. Infants and toddlers are at especially high risk for hypothermia because of their greater body surface area-to-mass ratio, decreased body fat, increased permeability of thin skin, and limited ability to shiver and produce heat. Extended exposure to a cold environment and immersion in cold water are the two most common causes of hypothermia in young children. Children with severe illness or injury may also develop hypothermia. Finally, infants and young children may become hypothermic while being exposed for medical evaluation, especially in cold environments. The presence of hypothermia may precipitate or extend shock and complicate resuscitation, regardless of the underlying condition.

Assessment

History taking should include recent illness or injury and circumstances of exposure. The physical examination should include special attention to airway and breathing. Because hypothermia leads to a slowing of metabolism, the child may hypoventilate, with slow or shallow respirations.

Circulation

Bradycardia and hypotension may be present because of hypothermia itself or because of a concurrent hypoxic insult. Hypothermia may also lead to cardiac dysrhythmias. The skin is often pale and cool.

Disability

Mental status may range from confusion to coma, depending on the degree of hypothermia. Again, hypoxia may be the underlying cause of AMS, especially in submersion victims, so ensure the adequacy of oxygenation and ventilation. Depending on the circumstances, hypoglycaemia may also be present.

Core Body Temperature

Obtain core body temperature, when possible, with a thermometer that registers less than 34°C.

Determine degree of hypothermia:

- Mild: 35°–36°C
- Moderate: 30°–34°C
- Severe: less than 30°C

Loss of the compensatory mechanism of shivering to generate heat is characteristic of moderate to severe hypothermia.

Management

Management of the patient with hypothermia depends on the core temperature.

1. *Support airway, breathing, and circulation as indicated.*

2. *Prevent heat loss.*

   It is crucial to prevent further heat loss. Remove wet clothing, dry the skin, and cover the patient after the examination is completed (**Figure 6-7**). Apply a hat or head wrap because a high proportion of heat is lost through the head.

3. *Rewarm.*

   External, passive rewarming is appropriate for mild to moderate hypothermia. In the case of severe hypothermia, external rewarming may shunt cold blood to the core, leading to further complications. Core rewarming in the ED is the appropriate therapy for these patients.

   a. Mild hypothermia: apply warm blankets, increase ambient temperature of the ambulance. Prehospital professionals should be uncomfortably warm!

   b. Moderate hypothermia: warm blankets, heat packs to axilla and groin.

   c. Severe hypothermia: cautious movement with gentle handling; warmed, humidified oxygen if available; warmed IV solution; treat hypoglycaemia if present; rapid transport to a definitive care facility for core rewarming.

Summary of Cold-Related Emergencies

Paediatric patients' physiological and developmental characteristics place them at risk for the development of cold-related emergencies. Accurate assessment of the degree

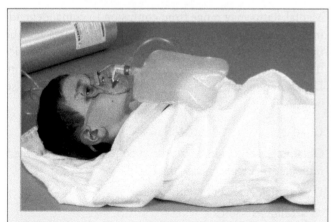

Figure 6-7 Cover patient after examination.
© Jones & Bartlett Learning.

of hypothermia is essential to effective management of children in the prehospital environment.

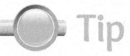

Tip

Use caution when rewarming the severely hypothermic paediatric patient in the prehospital environment, because cold acidemic blood from the periphery could lead to further deterioration. Focus instead on preventing further heat loss and supporting the ABCs.

Bites and Stings

Bites and stings typically result in a puncture-type wound or laceration and sometimes significant injury. Some stings, such as from a bumblebee or wasp, may produce a severe allergic or anaphylactic reaction. Some bites, such as from a snake or exotic pets such as certain spiders, or scorpions, can cause life-threatening envenomation or bleeding problems. Bites and stings may pose a greater risk to the paediatric patient because of his or her smaller body weight and higher metabolic rate. In the case of dog bites, consider reporting any dangerous dog to the police.

Assessment

History taking should include:

- Time and type of bite or sting
- Identification of causal creature
- Activities since the injury
- Known allergies to bites or stings
- Immunisation history

The physical examination should include special attention to:

- Clinical presentation varies depending on the type of bite, the presence or absence of envenomation, and the time since the bite occurred.
- Assess airway, breathing, and circulation; respiratory distress and anaphylaxis may be the initial signs of a bite envenomation.
- Inspect for type, anatomical location, and number of punctures or wounds.
- Assess for swelling, discolouration, and pain at or around the site.
- Note whether bites appear to be human.

Management: Bites

Management depends on the type of insect or animal involved in the incident.

General Management

- Ensure rescuer safety.
- Support airway, breathing, and circulation; establish vascular access.
- Treat anaphylaxis if present (see the *Shock* chapter).

Local Management

- Stop bleeding and perform wound care.
- If an envenomation is suspected, rinse area with water and consider cool compresses to the affected area to reduce spread of venom.
- Minimise the activity level of the paediatric patient. Most venom is transported through the lymphatic-system, and increased physical activity increases the rate spread throughout the body.
- Immobilise an affected extremity at or below the level of the heart.
- Transport rapidly with a detailed pre-alert to evaluate for possible antivenin administration and for definitive care.
- Remove any clothing or jewellery on the affected area or limb.
- Consider any safeguarding issues that may be present especially if bites appear to be from a human.

Management: Stings

General Management

- Support airway, breathing, and circulation; establish vascular access.
- Treat anaphylaxis if present (see the *Shock* chapter).

Local Management

- Apply cold compresses.
- Consider medications based on clinical presentation: epinephrine in the case of anaphylaxis, salbutamol in the case of wheezing, or chlorphenamine in the case of hives, itching, or swelling.

Tip

Abnormal behaviour may be the first clue that the paediatric patient has been bitten or stung. A thorough inspection of the patient's skin, particularly around the waist, distal extremities, axillae, and neck, may reveal the location of the bite or sting.

Summary of Bites and Stings

Insect bites are common in children and may result in complications ranging from mild local reaction to life-threatening anaphylaxis. Other types of envenomation, such as snake bites are unusual in the UK. Early recognition of the nature of the injury is important. On-scene treatment of anaphylaxis may be life-saving. Consider whether the bite could be a non-accidental injury and report appropriately. Report any dangerous dog to the police.

Case Study 3

A 6-year-old boy with a known allergy to bee stings has been playing outside in the garden. The caregiver calls 999 when the child develops noisy breathing. On arrival at the scene, the PAT reveals a pale, irritable child, with audible wheezing, and supraclavicular and subcostal retractions. Respiratory rate is 32 breaths/min, heart rate is 140 beats/min, and blood pressure is 90 mm Hg by palpation. His skin is covered in pink welts.

1. What are the possible causes of respiratory distress in this child?

2. What are the immediate management priorities?

CASE STUDY ANSWERS

Case Study 1 — page 108

The child is physiologically stable and can be further assessed on the scene. As you manage the child, allay the caregiver's fears. Use the opportunity to provide the caregiver with education regarding seizures and fever. Take a history, which suggests a possible febrile seizure.

All children with a history of seizure activity should be transported to the hospital because it is impossible to diagnose a febrile seizure in the field. There are many causes of seizures, including serious infections, such as meningitis.

Field treatment should be limited to simple cooling methods, such as a cool towel to the forehead if the child is still febrile. There is no need to apply ice packs to the body, unless the child has heat stroke. Reassess the patient frequently and be prepared for repeat seizures.

ALS If multiple seizures occur or a seizure lasts longer than 5 minutes, treat with a benzodiazepine: rectal or IV diazepam. Although brief seizures do not require pharmacological treatment, prompt treatment of seizures lasting longer than 5 minutes have the greatest success in terms of seizure cessation. Continuous, careful monitoring during transport is especially important if drug therapy has been given, because administration of benzodiazepines can result in apnoea or respiratory depression.

Case Study 2 — page 114

The aetiology of the child's AMS is wide and includes head trauma, toxin, hypoglycaemia, or postictal period after a seizure, yet the initial treatment is the same. Open and manage the airway with positioning. Consider 100% oxygen by non-rebreathing mask. If there is no trauma, place the patient in the sniffing position and use the jaw-thrust manoeuvre to maintain the airway. If respirations are shallow or irregular, or if oxygen saturation is less than 90% on supplemental oxygen, assist ventilation with the appropriate-sized bag-valve-mask device. Insert an oropharyngeal or nasopharyngeal airway as needed to maintain a patent airway.

ALS Use a length-based resuscitation tape or computer software program to determine drug doses.

Rapidly assess the serum glucose. If the glucose level is less than 4 mmol, establish an IV and give 10% glucose by IV bolus. If there is no IV access, give glucagon IM. If bedside glucose determination is normal, consider other causes of AMS and consider administering naloxone as per JRCALC guidelines.

Case Study 3 — page 127

A previously healthy child playing outdoors with an acute onset of respiratory distress should be assessed for bites and stings. This child's prior history of hymenoptera (bumblebee) allergy, the presence of hives in addition to respiratory distress, and the sudden onset of symptoms all suggest anaphylaxis.

Supplemental oxygen and inhaled bronchodilators for wheezing should be provided. In addition, IM adrenaline could be administered.

ALS Establish vascular access and give IV chlorphenamine.

Even if the child shows marked improvement with these treatments, transport urgently, because symptoms may recur as the medication effect wears off. Monitor carefully during transport.

SUGGESTED READINGS

Textbooks

Advanced Life Support Group. *Advance Paediatric Life Support: A Practical Approach to Emergencies*. 6th ed. Chichester: Wiley-Blackwell; 2016.

Association of Ambulance Chief Executives, Joint Royal Colleges Ambulance Liaison Committee JRCALC *Clinical Practice Supplementary Guidelines 2017*. Bridgwater: Class Professional Publishing.

Baram T, Shinnar S. *Febrile Seizures*. San Diego: Academic Press; 2002.

Greaves I, Porter K. *Oxford Handbook of Pre-hospital Care*. Oxford: Oxford University Press; 2012.

Paediatric Formulary Committee. *The British National Formulary, British National Formulary for Children*. London: Pharmaceutical Press; 2017.

Roper TA. *Clinical Skills*. 2nd ed. Oxford: Oxford University Press; 2014.

Articles

Holsti M, Sill BL, Firth SD, et al. Prehospital intranasal midazolam for the treatment of pediatric seizures. *Pediatr Emerg Care*. 2007;23:148–153.

Patel N. Febrile seizures. *British Medical Journal*. 2015;351:h4240.

Warden CR. Evaluation and management of febrile seizures in the out-of-hospital and emergency department settings. *Ann Emerg Med*. 2003;41(2):215–222.

Websites

National Institute for Health and Clinical Excellence. *Sepsis: Recognition, Diagnosis and Early Management* (NG51). London: NICE, 2017. https://www.nice.org.uk/guidance/ng51. Accessed March 3, 2018.

National Institute for Health and Clinical Excellence. *Fever in Under 5s* (CG160). London: NICE, 2013. https://www.nice.org.uk/guidance/cg160. Accessed March 3, 2018.

Royal College of Paediatric and Child Health. *Standards for Children and Young People in Emergency Care Settings*. 2012. https://www.rcpch.ac.uk/emergencycare. Accessed March 3, 2018.

Royal College of Physicians. *National Early Warning Score (NEWS)*. London: The Royal College of Physicians, 2012. https://www.rcplondon.ac.uk/projects/outputs/national-early-warning-score-news. Accessed March 3, 2018.

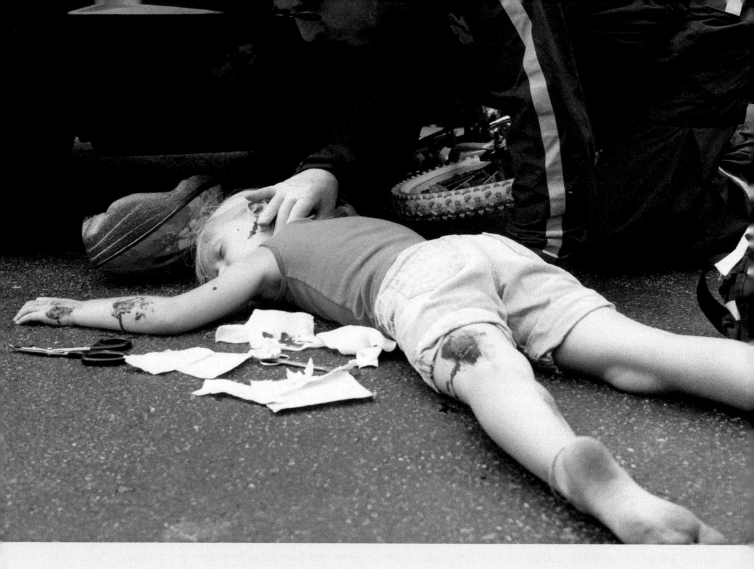

Learning Objectives

1. Explain the unique anatomical features of children that predispose them to injuries.
2. Sequence the primary assessment of the injured child.
3. Integrate the essential trauma interventions into the hands-on <C>ABCDEs.
4. Distinguish different approaches in airway management of injured children.
5. Discuss assessment and treatment of paediatric burn patients.

Trauma

Introduction

Injury is still the leading cause of death and disability in children according to the Trauma and Audit Research Network. Fortunately, the most common injuries are minor problems, such as lacerations, minor or superficial burns, mild closed head injuries, and extremity fractures. In minor trauma, the role of the prehospital professional is straightforward: Perform a scene assessment, assess for physiological or anatomical problems, pre-alert and transport to the emergency department (ED). Treatment depends on the presentation and injury of the child.

Multisystem trauma, in contrast, provides the prehospital professional with a great challenge, and demands a rigorous assessment and a child-specific approach to treatment. Most principles of adult trauma management can be effectively and safely applied to children. Important modifications in assessment are related to differences in mechanisms of injury, anatomy, and physiological responses. Modifications in treatment are related to differences in equipment sizes and emergency procedures.

From infancy through to adulthood, injuries are the most common cause of death. Severe traumatic brain injury is the most common injury type to cause death with the highest mortality from asphyxia and drowning.

Most injuries are preventable. Correctly sized child car seats and seatbelts, bicycle helmets, swimming pool fences, and window barriers have significantly reduced the incidence of blunt injuries and drowning. There are reduced incidence of fires, but in the UK 110 children per day are seen in emergency departments with burn injuries—46 as a result of a hot cup of tea or coffee spill. Paediatric trauma challenges the prehospital professional to manage not just the injury and related physiological abnormalities, but also to treat the child's pain and communicate with and support the injured child and their family or care givers.

Death or serious injury of a child from trauma causes tremendous emotional stress on prehospital professionals. Experience and education in the care of ill and injured children helps the prehospital professional have a greater sense of confidence, competency, and control in these stressful situations. Critical incident stress management or staff wellbeing support programmes may be valuable to the prehospital professional after treating a seriously injured child.

Case Study 1

Your ambulance is dispatched to a residential neighbourhood where a child has had a fall. You are greeted in the street by a teenage girl who leads you to a 7-year-old boy who is lying supine on the grass next to a tall tree. The teenager indicates that she observed the child fall about 20 feet out of the tree. No one has moved him. Your primary assessment reveals a child who is only responsive to painful stimuli. His breathing is shallow, with audible snoring sounds. His colour is pale with slight cyanosis. Respiratory rate is 12 breaths/min, heart rate is 130 beats/min, and blood pressure is 80 mm Hg/palp. His skin is cool, the radial pulse is weak, and capillary refill time is greater than 3 seconds. Pupils are equal and reactive, lung sounds are absent on the right and decreased on the left. The oxygen saturation is 82%. He has a haematoma on the right side of his head. His abdomen feels rigid. His right upper leg is swollen, with an obvious deformity of the right femur.

1. Based on the primary assessment and mechanism of injury, what are the child's most likely injuries?

2. Discuss the initial stabilisation and prehospital management of this child.

Severe Injury Mechanisms

Analysis of injury mechanism data shows a high incidence of road traffic collisions and falls of less than 2 m (**Table 7-1**). 10.1% of the patients are aged under 2 and were injured intentionally, recorded as Non-Accidental Trauma (NAT).

Unique Anatomical Features of Children: Effect on Injury Patterns

Head

Head injury is the most common cause of serious trauma in children. Even in multisystem trauma, the severity of traumatic brain injury (TBI) usually defines the patient's medical and functional outcome. Many of the essential interventions in managing paediatric trauma are directed at preserving brain function.

Until early school age (5–6 years old), the child's head is disproportionately large in relationship to overall body mass and surface area compared to adults. Because of this anatomical feature, in a fall or in an acceleration deceleration event, such as a road traffic collision, the head may be the site of initial impact and because it is large and heavy, will absorb a higher percentage of forces applied (**Figure 7-1**).

Table 7-1 Serious Injury Mechanism Number (%)

This report concentrates on the 737 children in 2012 who sustained the most serious injuries—an Injury Severity Score (ISS) greater than 15.	
Road Traffic Collision	284 (38.5%)
Fall < 2m	164 (22.3%)
Fall > 2m	110 (14.9%)
NAI under 2 years	74 (10%)
Penetrating	10 (1.4%)
Blows	46 (6.2%)
Other (e.g., sport/drowning)	49 (6.6%)

Source: Trauma Audit and Research Network (2012) Severe Injury in Children 2012, England & Wales. Available at: https://www.tarn.ac.uk/Content/ChildrensReport/files/assets/common/downloads/TARN%20document.pdf

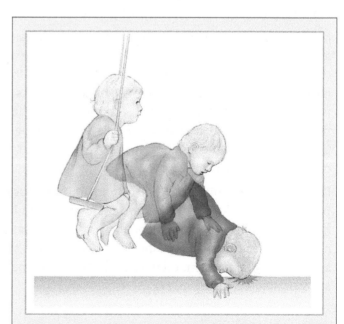

Figure 7-1 A disproportionately large head size in children explains their tendency to fall "head first", leading to a high rate of TBI.

© Jones & Bartlett Learning

Consequently, the head and brain of a child are more commonly injured in blunt trauma compared to adults.

Spinal Column

As a group, children do not suffer many vertebral fractures or dislocations. When vertebral fractures do occur, the event typically involves a high-energy mechanism (e.g., road traffic collision or diving incident) with axial loading of the spine or extreme flexion or extension. Traumatic spinal cord injury, or disruption of the central nerve pathways, is also uncommon in children.

The most common cervical spine injuries in children occur at the level of the high cervical spine. Weaker neck muscles and spinal ligaments, in conjunction with a "heavy" head, create greater vulnerability to acceleration-deceleration forces common in road traffic collisions and falls.

The most common lower spine injuries occur in the mid to lower thoracic spine. Mechanisms include direct blows, falls, or spinal compression during a road traffic collisions from improper seat belt use. The use of booster seats in vehicles may reduce these types of injuries by allowing proper fitting of the lap and shoulder belt.

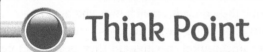

Think Point

It is difficult to find a cervical collar that really fits an infant or toddler. When a properly sized collar is not available, stabilise the child's spine on a scoop stretcher or vacuum mattress to prevent movement.

Chest

The ribs of the child are more pliable and compressible than those of the adult because they are comprised mainly of cartilage. For this reason, rib fractures and flail chest are uncommon in younger children, even with high-energy transfers. However, this bony compressibility in conjunction with a chest wall that is poorly protected by fat or muscle leads to direct transfer of energy to the lungs and heart on impact (**Figure 7-2**). Serious injuries of the thoracic organs can be present with or without external signs of injury, such as abrasions, bruises, or tenderness.

Pulmonary contusion, or bruising of the lung tissue itself, is a form of serious lung injury in children. You may suspect this condition in a child who sustains blunt chest trauma and has hypoxia or respiratory distress; however, pulmonary contusions may take time to fully develop and can only be diagnosed by X-ray, which makes the distinction between pulmonary contusion and pneumothorax difficult in the field.

If a child has a blunt injury mechanism, be careful when differentiating between a contusion and tension pneumothorax

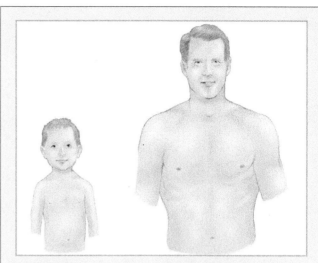

Figure 7-2 The child's chest wall is not well muscularised, so it lacks the soft-tissue protection from injury that is present in adolescents and adults.
© Jones & Bartlett Learning

as a contusion is more likely than a tension pneumothorax. In contrast, a child with progressive hypoxia and respiratory distress after a penetrating injury probably does have a tension pneumothorax, and needle decompression is indicated.

Penetrating chest trauma may cause serious problems in oxygenation and ventilation. When the chest wall, back, or high abdomen is penetrated, look for tension pneumothorax and sucking chest wounds. These injuries are unusual in children but, if present, require specific immediate life-saving treatment in the field. Needle decompression may save the life of a child with a tension pneumothorax. The procedure is the same for a child and adult. Needle decompression is a skillset undertaken by paramedics who have completed the training and are competent with the task. Advanced paramedics can perform finger thoracostomy plus and minus the chest range if trained in this skill set. This is usually a procedure paramedics with advanced skill sets can initiate.

The diaphragm of a child can rise as high as the nipple line during full expiration. When there is blunt or penetrating trauma to the chest below the nipple line or below the scapula, internal injury may include chest and abdominal organs (**Figure 7-3**).

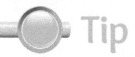

Because the child's chest wall is smaller, thinner, and less muscular than an adult's, lung sounds may be transmitted throughout the chest cavity, making it difficult to appreciate asymmetric breath sounds. Listening along the lateral sides of the chest wall under the axilla's (armpits) may improve the ability to distinguish sound variability between the right and left lungs.

A.

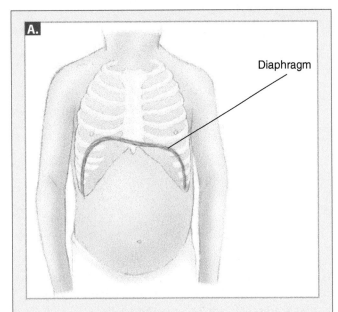

Diaphragm

B.

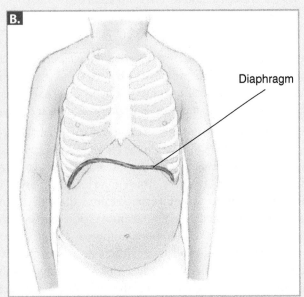

Diaphragm

Figure 7-3 The diaphragm can rise as high as the nipple line during full expiration **A.** and can flatten to the level of the lowest ribs during full inspiration **B.** Therefore, injuries to the abdominal organs may occur after chest trauma.

© Jones & Bartlett Learning

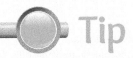 **Tip**

If there is penetration of the chest wall below the nipple, or below the scapula, anticipate abdominal injury as well as tension pneumothorax.

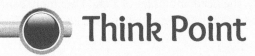 **Think Point**

Remember that young children rely heavily on their diaphragm to breathe. Do not restrict the abdomen when immobilising the patient's spine.

Abdomen

The abdomen can often be a site of serious blood loss in paediatric patients and is a common site of injury causing shock. The solid organs of the upper abdominal cavity are the liver, spleen, and kidneys. These organs are disproportionately larger and more exposed than in adults and are poorly protected by the child's softer ribs and relatively undeveloped abdominal muscles (**Figure 7-4**). The liver is the largest abdominal organ, located in the right upper quadrant of the abdomen, and extends below the rib cage in infants, toddlers, and preschool-aged children. The spleen, located in the left upper quadrant, is also commonly injured. The spleen and liver are the organs most commonly affected in blunt abdominal trauma. Injuries to the hollow organs of the abdomen—the stomach, small bowel, and bladder—are less common than solid organ injuries. Although pelvic fractures are uncommon in children, they become more frequent in adolescents, who have adult anatomy.

Assume that every child with a serious trauma has a life-threatening abdominal injury. Many children with abdominal injury have no localizing signs and may not complain

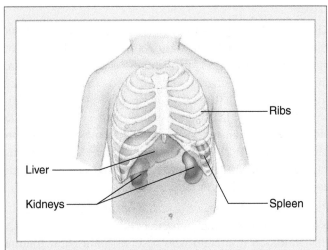

Ribs

Liver

Kidneys

Spleen

Figure 7-4 The solid organs of the upper abdominal cavity are disproportionately large and more exposed in children than in adults. They are poorly protected by the thin chest wall and undeveloped abdominal muscles.

© Jones & Bartlett Learning

of pain. Fear, young age, or other distracting injuries may hide signs and symptoms. When present, signs include abdominal wall contusions or abrasions, progressive abdominal distension, tenderness, rigidity, and haemodynamic instability. Ongoing assessment may improve the accuracy of abdominal assessment.

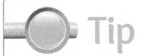

Tip

The abdomen is often a site of injury causing shock. Ongoing assessment can greatly improve the accuracy of assessment of abdominal injury.

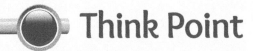

Think Point

Never overlook the possibility of solid organ injury when there has been blunt injury, because fear, young age, or other distracting injuries may mask signs and symptoms.

Extremities

Children's bones are more flexible, and their muscles are not as well developed as those of adults. They are especially vulnerable to fractures at the weak, cartilaginous growth plates near the ends of the bones (**Figure 7-5**). Fractures that disrupt the <u>periosteum</u> on only one side of the bone (often called <u>greenstick fractures</u>) are common, as are "<u>buckle fractures</u>" (also known as torus fractures) in which the pliant bone is compressed with <u>axial loading</u>. These fractures may be present in the absence of significant swelling, bruising, or

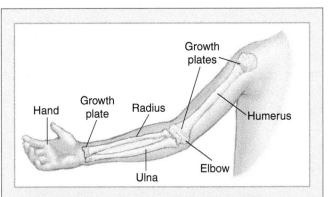

Figure 7-5 The physeal (growth) plates at the ends of children's bones are easily fractured.

© Jones & Bartlett Learning

deformity. *Suspect a fracture whenever there is point tenderness or limited range of motion, especially around a joint.*

The most serious complications of extremity injuries are <u>neurovascular</u> problems and blood loss into the soft tissues at the fracture site. Blood loss may be severe in long-bone fractures (e.g., fractures of the femur) or in pelvic fractures. The symptom usually associated with serious extremity injuries is pain.

Pain is frequently underestimated and undertreated in children. Analgesia should normally be introduced in a step-by-step manner, titrating to effect. A variety of analgesia's and non-pharmacological methods are available to clinicians. Consider the most appropriate analgesia for pain management in children depending on the severity of their injury. Pain management protocols vary across ambulance services so it is important that you know the protocols and clinical guidelines for your own area.

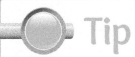

Tip

Suspect an extremity fracture whenever findings include point tenderness or limited range of motion.

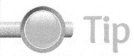

Tip

Injuries to the <u>physeal plate</u> or growth plate of a long bone can be permanently damaging to the limb.

Skin

The skin provides temperature regulation. Children's skin is thinner and has a greater surface area in relation to their overall size and weight than does the skin of adults. Because of this, heat transfer (loss or gain) from the skin can be rapid. Even without injuries that damage the skin, such as burns, injured children are at increased risk for hypothermia, which can in turn compromise core organ function. The signs and symptoms of hypothermia can mimic those of hypovolaemia and shock. In infants, hypothermia may deplete vital glucose stores. To avoid hypothermia, especially in an infant and toddler, prevent heat loss by ensuring that the child is dry and covered, and limiting time that the undressed child is exposed for assessment and procedures, recognising the importance of full exposure for assessment of injuries balanced against heat loss. Turn up the heat in the ambulance! In extremely hot environments, beware of

Table 7-2 Common Mechanisms and Associated Patterns of Paediatric Injury*

Mechanism of Injury	Associated Patterns of Injury	
Motor vehicle crash (child is passenger)	• Unrestrained • Air bag • Restrained	Multiple trauma, head and neck injuries, scalp and facial lacerations Head and neck, facial and eye injuries Chest and abdominal injuries, cervical and lower-spine fractures
Motor vehicle crash (child is pedestrian)	• Low speed • High speed	Lower-extremity fractures Chest and abdominal injuries, head and neck injuries, lower-extremity fractures
Fall from a height	• Low • Medium • High	Upper-extremity fractures Head and neck injuries, upper- and lower-extremity fractures Chest and abdominal injuries, head and neck injuries, upper- and lower-extremity fractures
Fall from a bicycle	• Without helmet • With helmet • Hitting handlebar	Head and neck injuries, scalp and facial lacerations, upper-extremity fractures Upper-extremity fractures Internal abdominal injuries

*Adapted from *Teaching Resource for Instructors in Prehospital Pediatrics (TRIPP)*. Version 2.0. New York, NY: Center for Pediatric Emergency Medicine; 1998.

© Jones & Bartlett Learning

hyperthermia. Regular monitoring of temperature is part of managing paediatric patients.

Mechanism of Injury: Effect on Injury Patterns

The different mechanisms of injury in children in combination with their unique anatomical features lead to predictable patterns of injury (**Table 7-2**). Head injury caused by blunt trauma is very common in children. Although there are many cases of minor closed head injuries associated with play that do not have neurological consequences, high-energy impacts are often associated with traumatic brain injury (TBI). Because of a child's small size, high-energy blunt impacts can lead to multisystem trauma, including the head, chest, abdomen, and long bones.

Figure 7-6 illustrates several typical injury sequences in children.

Assessment of the Injured Child

The initial steps in assessing the injured child follow the generic approach for all children outlined in the *Paediatric Assessment* and *Using a Developmental Approach* chapters. This includes pre-arrival mental preparation based on dispatch information and a scene assessment on arrival. Always use personal protective equipment to prevent potentially harmful or infectious exposures to bodily fluids.

The on-scene trauma evaluation includes (1) general assessment using the Paediatric Assessment Triangle (PAT); (2) the primary assessment with the hands-on <C>ABCDEs; and then (3) additional assessment consisting of a focused

history and physical examination and a detailed physical examination (trauma). A child with multisystem injuries needs a prioritised, efficient on-scene approach to assessment and treatment, and rapid transport to the nearest major trauma centre.

The General Assessment
The PAT

The PAT is the first part of the primary assessment of trauma as well as medical patients, and allows rapid determination of the type of physiological disturbance, severity of injury, and urgency of treatment.

Appearance

Appearance reflects brain function, which may be abnormal in injured children because of primary brain injury (caused by direct trauma to the brain tissue itself) or secondary brain injury (caused by an indirect insult to the brain tissue by hypoxia or ischaemia). The most likely causes of abnormal appearance in a paediatric trauma patient are closed head injury, hypoxia, haemorrhage, and pain from fractures, burns, and soft-tissue injuries.

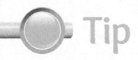

Tip

There are many potential causes of abnormal appearance in a paediatric trauma patient, including closed head injury, hypoxia, haemorrhage, and pain from fractures, burns, and soft-tissue injuries.

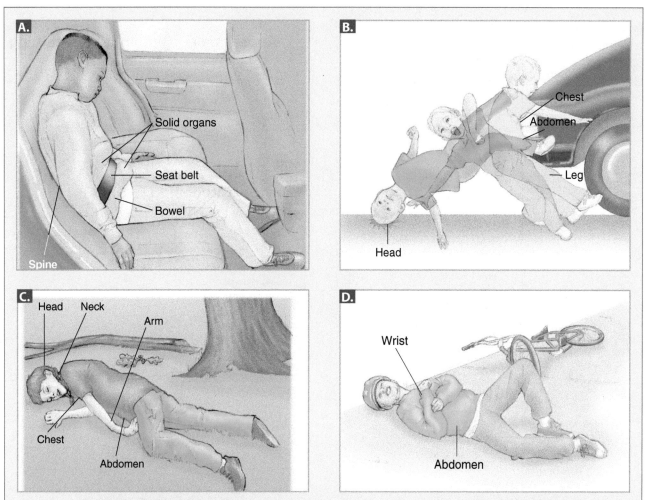

Figure 7-6 A. A restrained child in a motor vehicle crash may have a lap belt injury involving solid organs, bowel, and spine. **B.** Children frequently sustain multisystem injuries involving the head, chest, abdomen, and long bones. **C.** A fall from height frequently involves injuries to the head and neck, chest, abdomen, and the extremities. **D.** A fall over the handlebars of a bike may result in injuries to the abdomen and extremities.

© Jones & Bartlett Learning

Toxins may also cause an abnormal appearance, but are uncommon causes of poor responsiveness in the pre-school and school-aged trauma patient. However, toxins (most often alcohol or recreational drugs) are an important contributor to trauma in the adolescent, who may incur injuries caused by high-risk behaviours while "under the influence". **Table 7-3** lists common causes of abnormal appearance in injured children.

Work of Breathing

Work of breathing is increased by injuries that affect the airway, lungs, pleura, or chest wall. **Table 7-4** summarises the causes of increased work of breathing in paediatric trauma patients. Effortless tachypnoea, or a rapid respiratory rate in the absence of increased work of breathing, may be seen in a child with traumatic shock. This is a reflexive mechanism to compensate for metabolic acidosis caused by hypoperfusion by "blowing-off" carbon dioxide.

Listen for abnormal airway sounds, such as stridor or change of speech, which may reflect tracheal injury or obstruction. Wheezing reflects lower airway irritation and bronchospasm. This may occur from inhalation of vaporised toxins. When children are confined in a house fire, this type of inhalation should always be suspected.

Grunting, an infant's method of positive end-expiratory pressure (PEEP), indicates decreased gas exchange at the level of the alveoli, and may be seen with pulmonary contusion. After listening, look for retractions and nasal flaring to further assess for hypoxia.

Circulation to Skin

Circulation to skin reflects the blood flow to the skin and mucous membranes. If skin colour and skin temperature are abnormal in an injured child who is not in a cold environment, it suggests hypovolaemia and poor perfusion. Haemorrhage

Table 7-3 Common Causes of Abnormal Appearance in Injured Children

Category of Injury	Examples
Primary brain injuries	• Closed head injury • Concussion • Contusion • Intracranial haematoma • Intracranial haemorrhage • Penetrating brain injuries

Secondary brain injuries	• Brain oedema
	• Haemorrhage with hypoperfusion/ shock due to:
	  - Solid organ abdominal injury
	  - Haemothorax
	  - Pelvic fracture
	• Hypoxia due to:
	  - Aspiration of gastric contents
	  - Failure of central respiratory drive
	  - Pulmonary contusion
	  - Smoke inhalation
	  - Tension pneumothorax

Pain	• Burns • Fractures • Soft-tissue injuries
Toxins	• Alcohol • Recreational drugs • Carbon monoxide

© Jones & Bartlett Learning

Table 7-4 Injury Causes of Increased Work of Breathing in Injured Children

Cause	Examples
Airway injuries	• Haematomas or lacerations of the tongue, mouth, or neck • Smoke and gas inhalation · • Penetrations into the upper airway
Chest injuries	• Pulmonary contusion • Sucking chest wound • Tension pneumothorax/haemothorax
Abdominal injuries	• Diaphragmatic injury • Solid or hollow viscus injury with pain and "splinting"

© Jones & Bartlett Learning

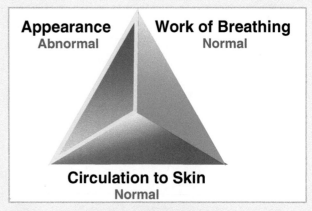

Figure 7-7 A patient with closed head injury has an abnormal appearance, but normal work of breathing and normal circulation to skin.
© Jones & Bartlett Learning

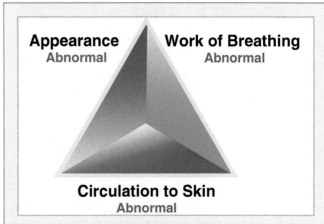

Figure 7-8 A patient with multiple system injury has an abnormal appearance, abnormal work of breathing, and abnormal circulation to skin.
© Jones & Bartlett Learning

to account for signs of hypoperfusion or hypovolemic shock in children outside of infancy, because the closed space of the skull cannot accommodate a significant volume of blood. However, infants can lose large volumes of blood based on intracranial bleeding, because the plates of their skull (sutures) are not yet fused, and the skull can expand under pressure.

Figure 7-7 and **Figure 7-8** show the PAT findings for the two most common patterns of major paediatric trauma: closed head injury and multisystem injury.

The Primary Assessment
Hands-on <C>ABCDEs

The <C>ABCDEs are the hands-on primary assessment. The trauma <C>ABCDEs have a special focus on spinal precautions and control of blood loss.

from abdominal solid organ injury is the most common cause of hypoperfusion and shock in paediatric trauma patients. The use of tourniquets in children with exsanguinating haemorrhage from an extremity to prevent blood loss should be based on local protocols. An isolated closed head injury is unlikely

Table 7-5 Paediatric Trauma <C>ABCDEs

Element of Assessment	Special Interventions
Catastrophic haemorrhage	Apply tourniquet on the limb over a single bone as close to the joint as practical
Airway	Chin lift or jaw-thrust manoeuvre while maintaining manual cervical spine immobilisation High concentration oxygen Consider airway adjunct
Breathing	Needle thoracostomy Dressing to sucking chest wound
Circulation	External haemorrhage control Splinting of fractured extremity Where possible, vascular access can be gained en route to hospital (5 ml/kg fluid boluses are used and repeated as needed)
Disability	Record AVPU (GCS en route) Stepwise disability management Measure blood glucose levels
Exposure	Prevent heat loss
Secondary survey	Systematic and careful review of each part of the injured child and reassess analgesia Pre-alert hospital (for example, with ATMIST tool)

The paediatric assessment, including the PAT and ABCDEs, does not require any specialised equipment. Potentially life-threatening problems should be treated as they are identified in the <C>ABCDE sequence. **Table 7-5** lists the key features of the paediatric trauma <C>ABCDEs and interventions specific to the trauma patient.

Catastrophic Haemorrhage

Identify and manage the site of any catastrophic haemorrhage. Consider the use of pressure, trauma bandages, tourniquets, and other agents to stop the bleeding.

Airway

Airway is the next priority. Trauma victims are at risk for airway obstruction from bleeding, emesis, oedema, or foreign objects. TBI may cause loss of protective airway reflexes or impair central respiratory drive.

Consider spinal injury in an unconscious child with any of the following:

- A mechanism of injury involving high-velocity forces transmitted to the head or spine (e.g., fall from a height, ejection from a vehicle)

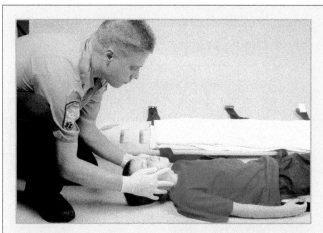

Figure 7-9 If airway obstruction is suspected in a child with possible spine injuries, use the modified jaw-thrust manoeuvre combined with manual immobilisation.
© Jones & Bartlett Learning. Courtesy of MIEMSS.

- Physical evidence of trauma to the head or spine (e.g., scalp haematoma, tenderness to palpation of the cervical spine); altered mental status (AMS)
- Neck or back pain
- Weakness or numbness

If the child has any of these findings, manually in-line stabilise the C spine while managing the airway. Although great care must be taken to prevent further injury in the unlikely event of an unstable spine injury, these concerns must not take precedence over appropriate management of the child's airway. *An injured child is far more likely to die from untreated hypoxia or shock than spinal trauma.*

Actions. If airway obstruction is present, use a modified jaw-thrust manoeuvre combined with manual in line stabilisation (**Figure 7-9**) to establish and maintain airway patency. Insert an airway adjunct if unable to maintain an open airway and the child has no gag reflex. Consider postural drainage if no indications of spinal injury and/or use suction to clear any fluid from the mouth, nose, or upper airway, or Magill forceps to remove foreign bodies. Quickly but carefully logroll the patient if vomiting occurs before he or she is secured to a spine board or stretcher. After the spine is fully immobilised, the entire backboard can be turned if necessary to protect the child from aspiration.

Immobilisation. The spinal column is made of 33 articulating bones, the vertebrae, and its structure changes significantly during childhood growth. The incidence and type of spinal injuries depend on the age of the child and the mechanism of injury, and in turn are influenced by the child's developmental level and activity. Cervical spine trauma can lead to quadriplegia, the most devastating type of spinal injury. If cervical spine injury is suspected, an appropriately-sized cervical collar should be applied. The use of a spinal board for extraction only should follow

Case Study 2

You are dispatched to a local cricket field where a 4-year-old boy was struck in the head by a cricket ball that was hit into the stands. The child has a large haematoma on his forehead and is crying inconsolably in his father's arms. The child did not lose consciousness but is not making eye contact with you or his dad. Other than his altered appearance, the PAT is normal and the hands-on <C>ABCDEs reveal normal vital signs and no other apparent injuries. The child becomes increasingly drowsy during your assessment, and is difficult to arouse.

1. What is the child's greatest threat to life?

2. What interventions are required?

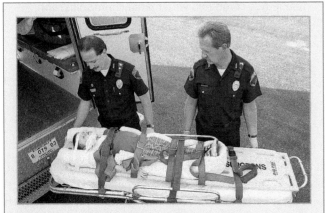

Figure 7-10 Immobilisation
© Jones & Bartlett Learning

local trust guidelines (**Figure 7-10**). Spinal cord injuries and lifelong paralysis may follow thoracic or lumbar trauma. For a step-by-step explanation of this procedure, see **Spinal Immobilisation, Procedure 18.**

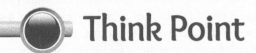

Think Point

Never let concern for spinal injury compromise appropriate management of the child's airway.

Breathing

Breathing is an important priority in the <C>ABCDEs (**Table 7-6**). Injuries to the airway, chest wall, lungs, or abdomen as well as gastric distention caused by air swallowing may compromise oxygenation and ventilation. Head and cervical spine injuries sometimes depress central respiratory drive mechanisms or diminish protective airway reflexes. Pulmonary aspiration of gastric contents is a common and potentially serious complication of head injuries that results in hypoxia and increased work of breathing.

Table 7-6 Normal Respiratory Rates

<1 year	30–40 breaths per minute
1–2 years	25–35 breaths per minute
2–5 years	25–30 breaths per minute
5–11 years	20–25 breaths per minute
>12 years	15–20 breaths per minute

Source: JRCALC, 2016.

Look for soft-tissue or penetrating injuries of the chest or back. Watch for the adequacy and symmetry of chest rise, and then auscultate to assess air entry and equality of breath sounds. Feel the chest wall for crepitus, pain, or instability. Apply a pulse oximeter to assess for hypoxia, because pallor and cyanosis can be late findings. A normal pulse oximetry reading does not, however, rule out respiratory distress. A child with profound tachypnoea or increased work of breathing may need assisted ventilation regardless of the reading on the oximeter, before he or she exhausts compensatory mechanisms.

Actions. If breathing is inadequate, position the child and assist with bag-valve-mask ventilation and high flow oxygen. Lift the jaw into the mask. Pushing the mask onto the face to make a seal may cause cervical spine movement. The C-E grip (**Figure 7-11**) helps with proper hand placement for good mask-to-face seal. Consider inserting an airway adjunct to help maintain an open airway, although an oral airway is not tolerated by a child with an intact gag reflex.

Give 100% oxygen with bag-valve-mask ventilation. Use a properly fitted oxygen mask. Provide assisted ventilation with a bag-valve-mask device if the child's respiratory effort is inadequate or if he or she has deteriorating cardiopulmonary or mental status. Use the "squeeze-release-release" timing technique, because the tendency is to bag too fast. Allow a brief pause between each breath to minimise the

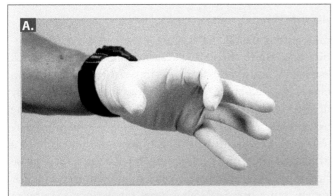

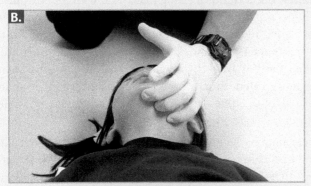

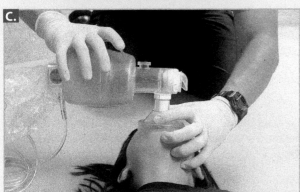

Figure 7-11 The C-E grip technique facilitates proper hand placement for good mask-to-face seal. **A.** Hand displaying C-E shape. **B.** Fingers resting on bony ridge of jaw. **C.** Bag-valve-mask ventilation in place.

© Jones & Bartlett Learning

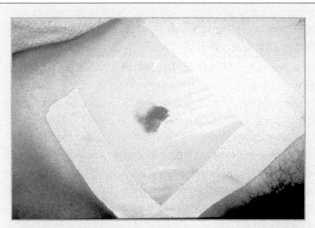

Figure 7–12 Management of a sucking chest wound. Cover sucking chest wounds with an occlusive dressing.

Courtesy of the State of North Carolin EMSC.

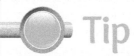 Tip

Pulmonary aspiration of gastric contents is a common and potentially serious complication of head injuries.

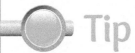 Tip

If a patient with penetrating chest trauma also has respiratory distress, hypoxia, and hypoperfusion, consider needle decompression to treat possible tension pneumothorax. Needle decompression is a skillset undertaken by paramedics who have completed the training and are competent with the task. Advanced paramedics can perform finger thoracostomy plus and minus the chest range if trained in this skill set.

chance of gastric distention. The best gauge is by using wave form capnography with an aim to keep the ETCO$_2$ 35–44 mm Hg (4.6–6.0 kPa). In each breath, provide only enough tidal volume to just achieve chest rise.

Treating penetrating chest injuries, sucking chest wounds, impaled objects, and tension pneumothorax in paediatrics is the same as in adults. Cover sucking chest wounds with an occlusive dressing, such as gauze, taped on three sides (**Figure 7-12**) or a specially designed bandage/seal for sucking chest wounds. This technique allows trapped air to escape while helping to prevent the entrance of air and development of tension pneumothorax. Do not remove impaled objects. Instead, stabilise them in place.

Management of Tension Pneumothorax. If a patient with penetrating chest trauma has increasing respiratory distress, hypoxia, and hypoperfusion, consider a needle decompression (needle thoracentesis) to treat possible tension pneumothorax.

Needle decompression may also be necessary in the child with blunt chest injury if the child has serious blunt chest-wall injury and respiratory distress, especially if he or she worsens with assisted ventilation. In this situation, when there is a closed pneumothorax, positive pressure ventilation quickly increases the air pressure in the pleural space, creating a dangerous level of "tension". Tension pneumothorax not only compromises ventilation of the affected lung, but impairs venous return to the heart. This can lead to shock unresponsive to fluid resuscitation. Needle decompression of the tension pneumothorax improves oxygenation, ventilation, and perfusion.

Management of Gastric Distention With a Nasogastric Tube.

This is a procedure not done routinely by frontline ambulance crews, however, paramedics with enhanced skills such as critical care paramedics may consider this intervention, depending on their local trust protocols. Assisted ventilation or prolonged crying can cause air swallowing and gastric distention. Nasogastric (NG) tube placement may improve ventilation by decreasing the upward pressure on the diaphragm caused by the distended stomach, and reduce the risk of vomiting.

Fluid Management.

Where possible gain vascular access en route to hospital. In paediatric trauma, use 5 ml/kg fluid boluses and repeat as necessary to improve clinical signs which include respiratory rate, heart rate, capillary refill and conscious levels. Hypotensive resuscitation should not be used in children. Following IV fluid resuscitation, in a paediatric major trauma with catastrophic haemorrhage, a bolus of tranexamic acid should be given (Clinical Practice Guidelines, JRCALC, 2016).

Circulation

Multisystem paediatric trauma more often involves respiratory failure than shock. Sometimes, however, shock develops because of external or internal bleeding, tension pneumothorax, spinal injury, or pump failure caused by cardiac contusion or tamponade. The combination of the PAT and the hands-on <C>ABCDEs allows ongoing perfusion evaluation. Measure heart rate continuously with a cardiac monitor, or with frequent brachial or carotid pulse checks. Tachycardia may be caused by pain, fear, cold, or anxiety, but a trend of rising heart rate with a poor pulse volume suggests shock. Blood pressure measurement is not a good indicator of hypovolaemia, because a child can be in compensated shock with a normal blood pressure. When there is frank hypotension, assume the child is in decompensated shock. If it is significantly higher than normal in a child with possible TBI, consider possible intracranial hypertension.

There may be technical challenges of obtaining a reliable blood pressure (mainly because of having the proper cuff size) therefore consider additional signs such as capillary refill time and pulse quality when considering perfusion (**Table 7-7**).

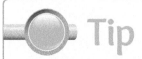

Frequently monitor and reassess heart rate. Tachycardia may be a response to pain, fear, cold, or anxiety, but a trend of rising heart rate suggests ongoing blood loss.

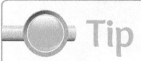

Consider pelvic and long bones fractures—and the indications for early splinting, traction, and full immobilisation, which can reduce blood loss and pain.

Table 7-7 Normal Blood Pressure by Age Group (mm Hg)

Age	Systolic Pressure	Diastolic Pressure	Systolic Hypotension
Birth (12 h, <1000 g)	39–59	16–36	<40–50
Birth (12 h, 3 kg)	60–76	31–45	<50
Neonate (96 h)	67–84	35–53	<60
Infant (1–12 mo)	72–104	37–56	<70
Toddler (1–2 y)	86–106	42–63	<70 + (age in years × 2)
Preschooler (3–5 y)	89–112	46–72	<70 + (age in years × 2)
School-age (6–9 y)	97–115	57–76	<70 + (age in years × 2)
Preadolescent (10–11 y)	102–120	61–80	<90
Adolescent (12–15 y)	110–131	64–83	<90

Source: Novak C, and Gill P (2016).

Actions. Stop any visible external bleeding with an appropriate dressing and apply direct pressure on the wound. Where possible, elevate the bleeding point above the level of the heart. Don't forget your personal protective equipment. Splint any extremities with obvious deformity. Apply high flow oxygen and place the child in a supine position for transport.

Begin transport when the airway is properly secured, ventilation is adequate, and the child's spine is appropriately stabilised.

Volume Resuscitation. If the child has signs of shock or significant ongoing blood loss, where possible obtain vascular access and start volume resuscitation on the way to the ED/A&E. Look first for peripheral intravenous (IV) sites in the upper extremities. Insert an intraosseous (IO) needle if IV access is problematic and the child has signs of decompensated shock. Use 5 ml/kg fluid boluses and repeat as needed until clinical signs such as respiratory rate, heart rate, capillary refill and conscious level are within normal ranges, using a three-way tap approach as seen in **Figure 7-13**.

Due to the physiological reserves, children maintain their systolic blood pressures during major blood loss, with hypotension only occurring at a very late stage. Cardiac arrest or significant cardiovascular compromise may occur if volume resuscitation were to be delayed until a child reached such an advanced stage of hypovolaemia. Following fluid resuscitation, in paediatric cases with catastrophic haemorrhage, a bolus of tranexamic acid should be given according to age per page guidelines (Clinical Practice Guidelines, JRCALC, 2016).

Disability

Confusion or agitation in an injured child may be due to a significant head injury, but equally may also be secondary to hypoxia from an impaired airway or compromised breathing, or due to hypoperfusion from blood loss and shock. Children may have primary or secondary brain injuries, or both. Primary brain injury is the direct result of the traumatic insult and may include brain haemorrhage, cerebral oedema (brain swelling), or diffuse axonal shearing. Increased intracranial pressure may develop quickly after primary brain injury. Untreated, the downward spiral of increased intracranial pressure can lead to brainstem herniation, cardiopulmonary arrest, and brain death. By the time the prehospital professional reaches the scene, any damage incurred from the primary brain injury is complete.

Secondary brain injury results from central nervous system hypoxia or ischaemia and disorders of blood glucose. The prehospital professional has a key role in preventing secondary brain injury. Hypoxia may be the result of airway or chest injury, or of compromised central respiratory drive

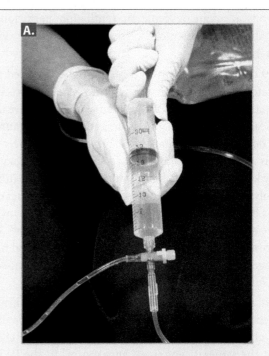

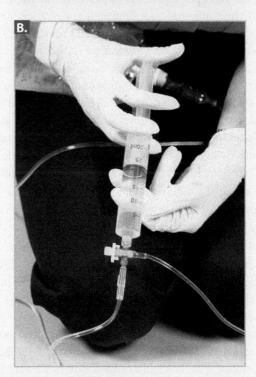

Figure 7–13 Infuse boluses using a a three-way tap system with a large syringe. **A.** Pull fluid bolus into syringe after turning off the three-way tap to patient. **B.** Push fluid bolus into patient after turning off the three-way tap to IV bag.
© Jones & Bartlett Learning

caused by the primary brain injury. Brain ischaemia may result from haemorrhage, usually in the abdomen or chest. Central nervous system (CNS) cells cannot survive without sufficient blood glucose levels.

Ensuring adequate oxygenation, ventilation, perfusion, and normal blood glucose are the keys to preventing secondary brain injury.

A 999 call sometimes involves an infant with altered mental status, apnoea, or seizures with no report of preceding trauma. Assessment of these infants may not reveal any physical examination findings suggestive of head trauma or TBI, despite the fact that they have sustained severe TBI. This is a typical scenario in non-accidental head injury (formerly known as shaken baby syndrome), where the infant is forcibly shaken by a caregiver, sometimes with impact of the baby's head against a fixed object. This mechanism involves severe acceleration–deceleration forces to the infant's brain and consequent diffuse axonal injury or intracranial haemorrhage. Non-accidental head injury is further discussed in the *Child Maltreatment* chapter.

Assess the injured child's degree of neurological disability with the AVPU scale (see Table 1-7 in the *Paediatric Assessment* chapter). Disability, as categorised in the AVPU scale, is not the same as "abnormal appearance" in the PAT. An injured child may have an abnormal appearance for many reasons other than brain or spinal cord injury, such as pain, fear, shock, hypoxia, or intoxication. Appearance may be quite abnormal in a child who is "alert" on the AVPU scale. Appearance is a more subtle indicator of overall physiological function in children than AVPU. The AVPU scale is more helpful in categorising children with severe neurological insults, including critical primary or secondary brain injuries. A formal Paediatric GCS (**Table 7-8**) en route may be useful to the receiving hospital but should not delay transfer.

When using the GCS, pay special attention to the motor component of the score, which has the highest value in predicting neurological outcome from TBI.

Record the time of the AVPU assessment, pupil size, shape, symmetry, and response to light; whether the child was moving some or all limbs; and any abnormalities of posture. If the child is not alert, they are time critical. After evaluating the level of consciousness with AVPU or the GCS, note abnormal positioning (including posturing) and seizures, and check for pupil size, symmetry, and reactivity. Seizures are common with head injury in children. Beware of persistent horizontal nystagmus, which may indicate persistent seizure activity.

The pupils provide important information about brainstem function, and the pupillary examination helps determine the need for hyperventilation in patients who are comatose. Concussion, a form of mild TBI, can result from rotational and acceleration forces on the brain, or a bump, blow, or jolt to the head. A direct blow to the head is not needed. Frequently sports-related, loss of consciousness is seen in very few concussed patients. Symptoms of confusion, amnesia, loss of co-ordination, slow reaction time, and delayed thought processing put the player at increased risk for further

Table 7-8 Paediatric Glasgow Coma Scale

Score	Child	Infant
Eyes		
4	Opens eyes spontaneously	Opens eyes spontaneously
3	Opens eyes to speech	Opens eyes to speech
2	Opens eyes to pain	Opens eyes to pain
1	No response	No response
_____ = Score (Eyes)		
Motor		
6	Obeys commands	Spontaneous movements
5	Localises	Withdraws to touch
4	Withdraws	Withdraws to pain
3	Flexion	Flexion (decorticate)
2	Extension	Extension (decerebrate)
1	No response	No response
_____ = Score (Motor)		
Verbal		
5	Oriented	Appropriate words or social smiles, fixes on and follows objects
4	Confused	Cries, but is consolable
3	Inappropriate words	Persistently irritable
2	Incomprehensible words	Restless, agitated
1	No response	Silent
_____ = Score (Verbal)		
_____ = **Total Score (Eyes, Motor, Verbal). Scores will range from 3 to 15.**		

Source: James HE, Anas NG, Perkin RM. *Brain Insults in Infants and Children*. Orlando, FL: Grune & Stratton; 1985. Reprinted with permission.
© Jones & Bartlett Learning

injury. Recovery requires physical and cognitive rest and may take weeks to months. A "second impact" during the recovery phase may lead to rapid brain swelling and death.

Actions. In paediatric trauma patients with AVPU scores of P or U, ensure an adequate airway, provide assisted ventilation to maintain good oxygenation and adequate ventilation. Hypoxia is an important cause of secondary brain injury in these children with TBI. Hypoxia may be associated with

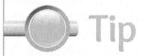

> A child with head trauma has impending brainstem herniation if the AVPU score is P or U, or if the PGCS is less than 9, or there is a fixed dilated pupil, asymmetric pupils, or active posturing.

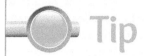

> Use assisted ventilation to maintain oxygenation and continue monitoring with end-tidal CO_2 monitoring to avoid carbon dioxide retention in paediatric trauma patients with AVPU scale scores of P or U.

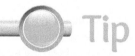

> In the out-of-hospital environment, endotracheal intubation is not always the optimal airway management tool, consider other airway adjuncts such as supra-glottic devices.

increased intracranial pressure, a situation that may occur rapidly and sometimes deceptively in a child with a primary brain injury.

Children with TBI require careful oxygenation and ventilation. Ventilated patients should be adequately paralysed, sedated, and ventilated to maintain a $PaCO_2$ of 4.5 kPa. Ensure you continue monitoring the child with end-tidal CO_2 monitoring. Saturation levels should be above 96%.

Management of Elevated Intracranial Pressure. If the child has AMS (not alert on AVPU or <15 on the GCS), anticipate elevated intracranial pressure. Take a graded approach to intracranial pressure management, always balancing risks and benefits of treatment.

- Support the patient's head in a midline position to facilitate jugular venous return to the heart.
- Consider loosening the cervical collar.
- If the patient is not in shock, elevate the head of the backboard or stretcher to approximately 30 degrees. Ensure adequate paralysis and sedation (according to local protocols), oxygenation and ventilation, maintaining a PaCOs of 4.5 kPa.

Exposure

Exposure is the last step in the primary assessment. Good exposure allows full assessment of the child's entire anatomy, including the extremities. Quickly examine the back during the spinal stabilisation procedure for soft-tissue or penetrating injuries. Assess circulation and neurological function distal to obvious or suspected extremity injuries. Although not usually life-threatening, complicated extremity injuries (e.g., open fractures of the humerus or femur) may cause significant blood loss and pain. Remember to cover the patient after the examination to prevent heat loss and hypothermia. If the child is time critical, pre-alert (for example, using ATMIST) the receiving hospital. Also consider a secondary survey en route if the primary survey is intact.

Summary of Primary Assessment

The assessment of the injured child requires knowledge of anatomical and developmental differences that lead to paediatric-specific patterns of injury. The child's airway is small and easily obstructed, the lungs are vulnerable to contusion, and the solid organs and long bones are poorly protected. The prehospital professional's primary role in multisystem trauma is to ensure an open airway, assist ventilation, control external haemorrhage and minimise secondary brain injury. Treatment goals are to avoid hypoxia and hypotension. Short time on scene and rapid transport to the ED/A&E are overriding priorities for all children who are physiologically unstable or have concerning mechanisms of injury. Vascular access and volume resuscitation are secondary tasks to be considered on the way to the hospital.

Special Airway Considerations in Paediatric Trauma

Children with severe head injuries with neurological disability and impending herniation often require advanced field interventions to:

- Protect the airway and prevent aspiration
- Improve or control ventilation
- Improve or control oxygenation

Optimal airway management balances the potential risks of the procedure against the potential benefits to the patient. Although endotracheal intubation has long been considered the best method for airway management in a critically injured patient, the procedure is not without risk, particularly when performed without drugs in patients who are not in cardiac arrest. These risks may include prolonged scene time, worsened hypoxia, vomiting and aspiration, elevation of intracranial pressure during laryngoscopy, or a misplaced tube.

Following trauma, a child may obstruct their airway either through loss of airway reflexes or the airway may become blocked by blood or vomit. Airway management and ventilatory support should follow an algorithmic approach starting with basic manual manoeuvres and simple adjuncts as the primary management step. There are several factors to consider when balancing the need to escalate airway management intervention and the patient's clinical condition:

- Ability to access the airway
- Actual or impending airway compromise
- Inadequate respiratory drive or ventilatory failure
- Length of on-scene and transport times
- Personnel availability and experience
- Anticipated clinical course

Should a child be unable to be managed using basic manual techniques and adjuncts, then a supraglottic device, such as an iGel or Larygeal Mask Airway (LMA), should be the next step in achieving optimal airway management. However, in the context of a soiled airway, either due to blood or vomit, both of these interventions are but temporising measures. The child requires swift evacuation or rendezvous with personnel capable of performing rapid sequence induction and endotracheal intubation.

Advanced Airway Management of the Paediatric Trauma Patient

Rapid sequence induction of anaesthesia followed by endotracheal intubation is the definitive method of securing an airway in patients who have sustained major trauma and who are unable to maintain their own airway or adequately ventilate. If a severely injured child needs endotracheal intubation, the preferred path is orotracheal, with manual neutral stabilisation of the cervical spine (see **Endotracheal Intubation, Procedure 9**).

RSI for paediatric endotracheal intubation, with sedatives and paralysing drugs, is standard practice in Emergency Departments and, more recently, in ambulance services via critical care teams responding on behalf of the ambulance service. These teams, comprising of doctors, nurses, and paramedics, are educated and skilled in the practice and provision of pre-hospital emergency anaesthetics.

See **Advanced Airway Techniques, Procedure 11**, for a detailed explanation of this procedure.

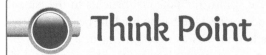

Think Point

Do not attempt blind nasotracheal intubation in children.

The Primary Assessment
The Transport Decision: Stay or Go?

After the primary assessment and initiation of life support, consider the timing for transport. *Immediately transport every paediatric trauma patient who has any abnormal physiological or anatomical findings, severe pain, or a serious mechanism of injury.* Stable trauma patients with apparently minor injuries should be viewed with suspicion. While it may be appropriate to undergo further evaluation and treatment on scene, prehospital providers should retain a low threshold for the conveyance of paediatric patients who have sustained a traumatic injury. If the scene assessment suggests circumstances that could be dangerous to the child or prehospital professional, transport immediately. Potentially dangerous conditions that warrant immediate transport and completion of assessment in the ambulance include proximity to fire or hazardous materials, threatened violence, angry bystanders or caregivers, and suspected non-accidental trauma.

Additional Assessment

The additional assessment consists of the focused history and physical examination, and the detailed physical examination (trauma patient). This part of the assessment is directed at anatomical problems. Perform the focused history and physical examination, and the detailed physical examination in the field only if the patient is physiologically normal and the conditions are safe. Otherwise, address these components of the assessment in the ambulance while on the way to the Emergency Department (ED).

When obtaining the focused history, use the SAMPLE template, as outlined in the *Paediatric Assessment* chapter. Focus only on points likely to affect primary trauma assessment and interventions. **Table 7-9** provides a SAMPLE template oriented to paediatric trauma patients.

The focused physical examination includes a careful look at the anatomy in the suspected areas of injury. This may

Table 7-9 SAMPLE History in Paediatric Trauma

Component	Explanation
Signs/symptoms	Time of event Nature of symptoms or pain Age-appropriate signs of distress
Allergies	Known drug reactions or other allergies
Medications	Chronic medications—timing and dose of last dose Timing and dose of **analgesic**/antipyretic
Past medical problems	Prior surgeries or anaesthetics Immunisations
Last food or liquid	Time of the child's last food or drink, including bottle or breastfeeding
Events leading to the injury	Key events leading to the current incident Mechanism of injury Hazards at the scene

© Jones & Bartlett Learning

involve a conscientious examination by exploration and palpation of the head and scalp for a child with closed head injury, observation and palpation of the back and axillae in a child with a penetrating chest injury, or inspection and palpation of the neck in a child with a strangulation injury.

The detailed physical examination (trauma) is a head-to-toe sequence or (in infants, toddlers, and preschool-aged children) toe-to-head, then front-to-back complete physical examination of the patient. This examination uses the traditional assessment tools of PAT, as outlined in the *Paediatric Assessment* chapter. The clinician should aim to seek out all of the injuries the child has sustained to inform their management plan.

After the child is on the way to the ED, perform on-going reassessments, irrespective of whether the patient has normal or abnormal physiology. This includes serial evaluations of the PAT, <C>ABCDEs, pulse oximetry, vital signs (including heart rate and rhythm on the cardiac monitor), blood pressure, anatomical problems, and response to treatment. Be sure to monitor and treat pain, if possible. When the child arrives in the ED, diagnostic testing with blood tests and imaging studies may assist with continued assessment.

Summary of Additional Assessment

After the primary assessment, determine the timing of transport and the appropriate destination and what other interventions the child is likely to need. Consideration of whether intervention will occur more quickly via rapid transport to hospital or by rendezvous with a critical care team is both an individual patient and geographical consideration. Do a secondary assessment, or on-scene focused history and physical examination, then a detailed physical examination, only on stable patients in safe scene circumstances. All other patients deserve immediate transport with continuation of assessment on the way to the ED. Frequent reassessment is important in all injured patients. Triage to an appropriate Major Trauma Centre or Trauma Unit can be guided by nationally inspired tools to assist decision-making, which are then locally adjusted to suit geographical differences and specialty availability.

Spinal Motion Restriction and Splinting for Transport

Indications for spinal protection for children are the same as for adults and are indicated for any child with a concerning mechanism of injury, signs of significant head injury, or multisystem trauma. Stabilise the neck using a properly sized paediatric extrication collar and immobilise using a scoop stretcher or vacuum mattress. Children should not be conveyed or immobilised on extrication boards.

A child who does not have severe injuries may be frightened and fight the process vigorously. Reassure the child and offer relaxation or distraction techniques to minimise

discomfort. Children who become anxious or who do not want to lie flat should be carried safely in a caregivers arms, and in a position that is comfortable for them.

For a step-by-step description of this procedure, see **Spinal Immobilisation, Procedure 18**.

Pre-school-aged children may not be able to localise or communicate the presence of neck or back pain. Anatomical differences, specifically the large size of an infant's or toddler's head, require modification of spinal stabilisation procedures. For example, placing a thin (1 inch) layer of padding beneath a child's body from shoulders to hips before securing the child to the stretcher (**Figure 7-14**) helps to properly align the airway and spinal column.

The spine does not stop at C-7, and spinal stabilisation is not complete unless the entire body is secured. Secure the patient against all axes of motion on the scoop stretcher. Near vertical positioning may be necessary during extrication. Secure the patient against lateral movement by padding along the sides of the body to eliminate all space between the patient and the straps. Avoid chin straps and other spinal stabilisation aids that might impair ventilation. Leave room for chest expansion during breathing when tightening chest straps. Make sure cervical collars fit properly, or use manual in-line spinal stabilisation until the child can be secured to the stretcher. Ensure that spinal stabilisation equipment does not interfere with assessment and access to the patient.

Splinting deformed or painful extremities is also an important prehospital intervention. Splinting has several important functions: reduction of fracture site crepitus therefore aiding pain control; control of haemorrhage from bone ends; reduction of cytokine release; and preservation of

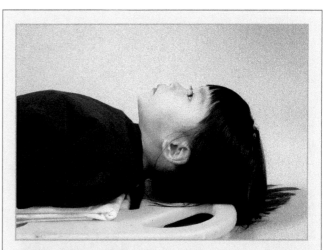

Figure 7-14 Keep the airway and spine in a neutral position by placing a layer of padding beneath the child's body from shoulders to hips before securing the child to the scoop stretcher.
© Jones & Bartlett Learning

neurovascular function. Unless the extremity shows signs of neurovascular compromise or there is severe pain, splint bones that may be fractured or dislocated in an "as is" position (**Figure 7-15**). An open femur fracture should be reduced by traction ONLY if the traction can be maintained. This controls the bleeding at the fracture site and helps to control pain. Otherwise, unless circulation is compromised, leave exposed bone out to avoid introducing further contamination by forcing fractured bone fragments back under the broken skin (**Figure 7-16**). A long box splint is an appropriate management device in this instance.

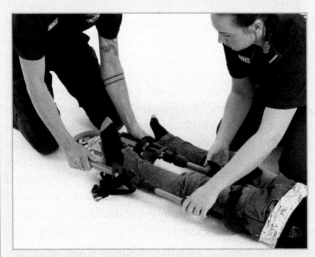

Figure 7-15 Splinting.
© Jones & Bartlett Learning. Courtesy of MIEMSS.

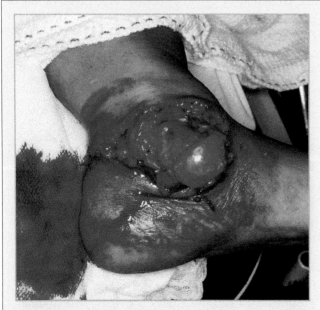

Figure 7-16 Leave exposed bone out. Do not attempt to reduce open fractures, unless circulation is compromised. Do not irrigate open fractures unless grossly contaminated.
© Charles Stewart & Associates

Restraint of Children During Transport

The responsibility for the safe transfer of patients ultimately rests with whomever is driving the ambulance. Make sure all persons riding in an ambulance are appropriately restrained. Secure children with possible spinal injury in a supine position on a scoop stretcher on the ambulance trolley cot. If the child has mild to moderate trauma without suggestion of spinal injury, consult local and national guidelines for age-appropriate restraint. There are well-defined regulations within the Road Safety Act and from the Health and Safety Executive on proper child restraint in a passenger vehicle. The appropriate use of a child restraint seat in an ambulance is dependent upon the model of the child seat and where it is placed in the ambulance. When "car seats" are used for ambulance transport, both the device and the method of securing the seat to the stretcher must conform to industry standards and meet national requirements. If service guidelines permit, have the child's caregiver remain within view or speaking distance of the child, if the caregiver's presence does not compromise the child's treatment or crew safety.

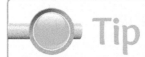 Tip

Although spinal injuries are not common in children, the high frequency of head injury means that spinal stabilisation should be part of the care of many paediatric patients with a significant mechanism of blunt trauma.

Paediatric Burn Patients

The assessment and management priorities for the burn patient are the same as for any other trauma patient. Make sure the scene is safe before approaching the child. Always anticipate exposure to hazardous materials and carbon monoxide, and use protective measures. Get technical help, if needed, from authorities on hazardous materials.

Assessment

Assess the scene for risk factors for airway and breathing. Important considerations in patients with fire and smoke exposures include the following:

- Enclosed space
- Heavy smoke
- Fumes
- Steam
- Hot vapours
- Chemical hazards
- Explosions with blunt or penetrating injury

Assess the patient for signs of smoke or particle inhalation and thermal burns of the airway. Give 100% oxygen for suspected carbon monoxide poisoning in children with

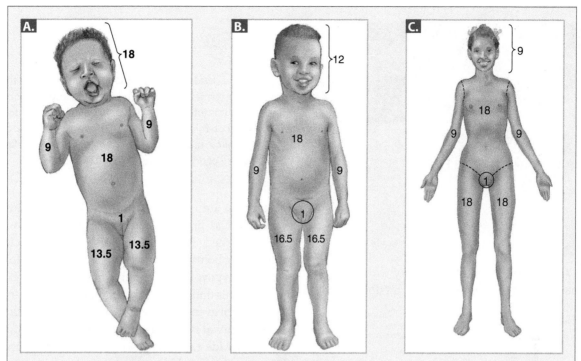

Figure 7-17 Modified anatomical diagrams of children of different ages give an approximation of involved body surface area for calculation of extent of burn in **A.** infant, **B.** child, and **C.** adolescent.

abnormal appearance or altered mental state, or in children exposed to fire or smoke in an enclosed space. Anticipate hidden injuries (especially abdominal) from a fall or a blast injury.

Make a quick estimation of burned body surface area. A modified anatomical diagram of children of different ages gives an approximation of burned body surface area, as shown in **Figure 7-17**. If such a diagram is not available, use the "rule of palms", which states that the patient's palm plus fingers equals 1% of body surface area (**Figure 7-18**). The percentage of burned body surface area is therefore roughly equal to the number of patient palm plus fingers-sized areas burned. This method should be used for small or scattered area burns only.

Although most burns are unintentional, assess all burn patients for risk factors for non-accidental injury. Scald and contact burns are common in children and are frequent findings in non-accidental trauma, as explained in the *Child Maltreatment* chapter. A "pattern" burn (where there is a clear demarcation of an object in the burned skin), "glove" or "stocking" distribution of a scald burn (**Figure 7-19**), or a history that is inconsistent with the injury are suspicious circumstances for intentional injury.

Management

Remove any burnt clothes unless stuck to the wound. Give 100% oxygen to all patients with flame or blast burns. High-flow oxygen therapy is the only field treatment for suspected carbon monoxide poisoning. The risk of hypothermia in the paediatric cohort is high and this risk must

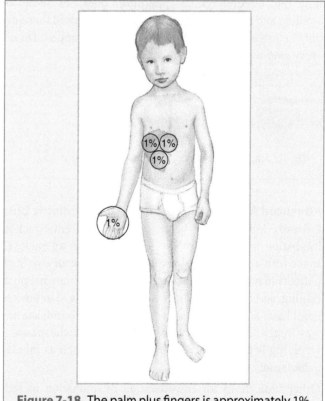

Figure 7-18 The palm plus fingers is approximately 1% of the body surface area.

© Jones & Bartlett Learning

be balanced with stopping the burning process. Evaporative cooling of a burn with water or water-based gel dressings is a simple and effective way to cool a burn and should be performed for a period of 20 minutes. Once cooled, cover

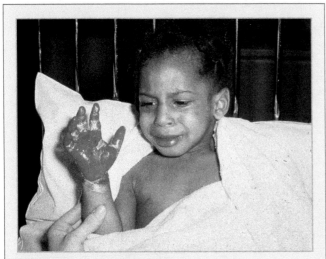

Figure 7-19 Consider intentional injury with a suspicious pattern of the burn, especially a "stocking" or "glove" distribution.
Courtesy of Ron Dieckmann, MD

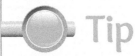

Tip

The Parkland formula (or a modification thereof) is the most common method of determining fluid resuscitation after a burn. It is intended only as a guide for fluid resuscitation. Based on this formula, the patient receives 2 to 4 ml/kg of crystalloid multiplied by the percentage body surface area burned of crystalloid for the first 24 hours.

burned areas with a plastic wrap, such a polyvinylchloride film (Cling Film). Covering helps to reduce pain by minimising exposure to air currents however it is important to note that circumferential application does not allow for swelling and may damage tissues further. It should therefore only be placed onto the skin in sheets, not wrapped. *Do not apply ointments or creams to burn areas.*

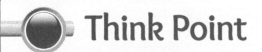

Think Point

Do not apply ointments or creams to burn areas.

Advanced Airway Management of the Paediatric Burn Patient. Consider early (before oedema starts) endotracheal intubation in any patient exposed to a fire in an enclosed space with a suspected inhalation injury to the airway. Such patients may have abnormal airway sounds, abnormal positioning, and respiratory distress or failure. Singed or burned nasal hairs and carbonaceous sputum may also indicate airway injury. Smoke inhalation may cause bronchospasm. If wheezing is present, give a bronchodilator such as inhaled Salbutamol.

Other indications for consideration of intubation include increasing analgesic needs and an altered level of consciousness, which may be attributable to another cause, such as trauma or cyanide poisoning.

Pharmacological Management of the Paediatric Burn Patient. Try to establish at least one IV line in patients with partial or full-thickness burns requiring fluid resuscitation; if necessary, insert IV catheters through a burn site. Fluid

and heat are rapidly lost through disrupted skin, with the rate of loss proportionate to the percentage body surface area burned. If indicated, initiate fluid resuscitation with 10 ml/kg boluses of isotonic crystalloid fluid. However, profound hypovolaemia is not a normal initial response to a burn. This finding should prompt the clinician to review the history of events and assess for occult haemorrhage and the possibility of myocardial dysfunction from cyanide poisoning. Provide early analgesia with oral paracetamol, intravenous opiates and if required, sedation with Ketamine, and titrate to effect.

Pain Management and Sedation. Fear and pain in children are frequently ignored or misinterpreted. Pain management is an important prehospital priority, especially in trauma and burn patients with long transport times. Infants and young children experience the same degree of pain as older children and adults; they just cannot express it in words.

Pain and anxiety are different things and require different treatments. Treat pain with a opiate based analgesic drug, such as morphine or fentanyl. Treating the patient's pain will often alleviate the anxiety the child displays. However, if required, treat anxiety with a sedative drug, such as a benzodiazepine (e.g., diazepam or midazolam). For example, a child with continued pain after stabilisation of an isolated extremity fracture needs morphine or fentanyl to control the principal problem, which is pain. Opiate-based medications, such as morphine or fentanyl, are pain killers but also provide some sedation.

IV/IO opiate analgesics are appropriate in haemodynamically stable trauma patients with burns or with isolated long-bone fractures or dislocations. If serious blood loss or bleeding is suspected, or if assessment suggests hypoperfusion, opiates should be used with caution because of the tendency to contribute to hypotension. The intramuscular (IM) route in patients with major trauma or burns should only be used if the IV/IO routes are not accessible.

If a child has received a prehospital anaesthetic, it is important to ensure that their pain, sedation and paralytics are well managed throughout the transfer to hospital. Signs of increased anaesthetic awareness are tachycardia, hypertension, and lacrimation.

Table 7-10 lists common medications to treat pain or anxiety in a haemodynamically stable child as per local ambulance service guidelines.

All IV sedatives and opiates cause respiratory depression. Give by slow IV push over 3–5 minutes. Some advanced care teams are able to administer stronger opiates such as Fentanyl or Diamorphine. In paediatrics this is commonly given via the intra-nasal route due to its quick onset of action following absorption through the mucous membranes. These drugs may potentially sedate the child due to the anxiolytic and CNS depressant effects. In this case, the clinician should give consideration to the application of supplemental oxygen to all children receiving these medications. Place the child on a cardiac monitor and use pulse oximetry and end-tidal CO_2 when available. Be ready to begin positive pressure ventilation with a bag-valve-mask device if the child develops respiratory depression. Naloxone may temporarily reverse respiratory depression caused by opiate administration; however, dosing should be checked prior to administration against local and national guidance. Keep in mind that use of naloxone also negates any analgesic effect and prevents further positive effects of opiates until the naloxone has been metabolised by the child's body.

Circulatory compromise should be managed with IV fluid boluses, volumes of which are dependent upon both the weight of the child, and the condition for which fluid is being administered.

Table 7-10 ALS: Pharmacological Management of Pain and Anxiety

Pain	
Morphine sulphate	• *Neonates:* 0.05 mg/kg IM, IV, IO, or SQ • *Infants and children:* 0.05–0.1 mg/kg IM, IV, IO, or SQ • *Adolescents:* 3–4 mg IV, IM, or IO
Fentanyl	• 1–2 mcg/kg/IV, IO, IM, or IN every 30–60 minutes
Anxiety	
Midazolam	• 0.05–0.1 mg/kg IV, IM, or IO or 0.2 mg/kg IN • Dosing should be checked prior to administration against local and national guidance.

Tip

Pain and anxiety are different things and require different treatments.

Think Point

Opiate-based analgesics may contribute to hypotension. Consider giving smaller doses in the patient who has sustained multiple trauma.

Summary of Burns

Burns are common paediatric injuries, but are usually small and require only first aid. Burns involving the airway, or more than 5% of body surface area, or of full thickness require important field interventions, including possible airway protection and fluid administration. Closed-space burns raise the possibility of both inhalational injury and carbon monoxide poisoning. Pain is a universal feature of burns, and analgesia using non-pharmacological and pharmacological methods is usually a primary intervention.

Case Study 3

You are dispatched to a child who has been run over by a vehicle. On your arrival you notice a car parked in the middle of the road, and a 6-year-old girl, conscious and alert with a small laceration on her chin, being held in her father's arms. She has no abnormal airway sounds; however, her work of breathing is increased and her skin is pale. You notice the odour of alcohol on the man's breath. According to bystanders, the child was walking behind the car when her dad backed up. The patient is cool and clammy to the touch. Respiratory rate is 40 breaths/min, heart rate is 146 beats/min, and you are unable to obtain a blood pressure. Lung sounds are decreased in lower fields. While exposing the child, you notice a tire track impression across the abdomen and sternum area. Pulse oximetry is 90% on room air.

1. What critical injuries do you suspect?

2. What are your treatment and transport priorities?

CASE STUDY ANSWERS

Case Study 1 — page 132

This patient requires immediate treatment and transport. The patient has sustained multisystem trauma to the head, chest, abdomen, and right lower extremity, and the primary assessment confirms respiratory failure and shock. Snoring respirations are likely caused by airway obstruction by soft tissues or blood. Positioning the airway and suctioning may alleviate the problem. Perform rapid spinal stabilisation.

The patient is hypoxic with abnormal breath sounds from either pulmonary contusion or tension pneumothorax.

ALS If the child does not respond to oxygen at 100% by positive pressure ventilation, consider needle decompression on the right side.

Stabilise the femur with a splint. Start IVs en route to the hospital and initiate fluid resuscitation. Transport rapidly to a trauma centre with paediatric expertise.

Case Study 2 — page 140

This child appears to have an isolated head injury and TBI. The child's rapid deterioration suggests an expanding intracranial haematoma, which may be life-threatening. As with any serious head injury, consider the risk of associated spinal injury. Stabilise and protect the child's spine and be prepared for vomiting. Apply 100% oxygen. Rapidly transport.

ALS Establish an IV en route for the administration of medications and leave at TKO.

Transport to a facility with paediatric neurosurgical capability, or consider rendezvous with an air ambulance service if such care is not available in your community. This is a surgical emergency and immediate access to operative care may make the difference between the life and death of this child.

Case Study 3 — page 151

The injuries to this child are life-threatening and she appears to be in shock. Administer 100% oxygen, transport immediately in the position most comfortable and consistent with safe transport of the child.

ALS Do not prolong scene time with IV attempts as the child is conscious and alert and therefore perfusing her brain. Give fluid resuscitation during transport if required.

This child is at risk for massive internal injury, including abdominal solid organ haemorrhage (liver, spleen, and kidneys); viscous rupture of the stomach, small bowel, and large bowel; haemothorax; pneumothorax; pulmonary contusion; and pelvic fracture. The recognition and treatment of compensated shock is critical. While intra-abdominal haemorrhage cannot be directly controlled in the field, if there is suspicion of a pelvic fracture, a pelvic binder is a life-saving intervention and should be applied as soon as possible.

Transport to the highest level of trauma care available in your community, based on local trauma triage protocol. This child requires rapid radiological assessment of the extent of injury and possibly early operative or endovascular intervention.

SUGGESTED READINGS

Textbooks

American Academy of Orthopaedic Surgeons. *Emergency Care and Transportation of the Sick and Injured*. 10th ed. Burlington, MA: Jones & Bartlett Learning; 2011.

American Academy of Pediatrics and the American College of Emergency Physicians. *APLS: The Pediatric Emergency Medicine Resource*. 5th ed. Burlington, MA: Jones & Bartlett Learning; 2012.

Barss P, Smith G, Baker S, et al. *Injury Prevention: An International Perspective*. Oxford University Press; 1998.

Bledsoe B, Porter R, Cherry R. *Essentials of Paramedic Care*. Upper Saddle River, NJ: Prentice Hall; 2003.

Campbell J. *BTLS for Paramedics and Other Advanced Providers*. 5th ed. Upper Saddle River, NJ: Pearson-Prentice Hall; 2004.

Articles

British Orthopaedic Association and British Association of Plastic, Reconstructive and Aesthetic Surgeons Standard For Trauma (2009) The Management Of Severe Open Lower Limb Fractures. Available at: https://www.boa.ac.uk/wp-content/uploads/2014/05/BOAST-4-The-Management-of-Sever-Open-Lower-Limb-Fractures.pdf

Adelson PD. Guidelines for the acute medical management of severe traumatic brain injury in infants, children, and adolescents. Chapter 4. Resuscitation of blood pressure and oxygenation and prehospital brain-specific therapies for the severe pediatric traumatic brain injury patient. *Pediatr Crit Care Med*. 2003;4(suppl 3):S12–S18.

Gausche-Hill M, Brown KM, Oliver ZJ, Sassoon C, Dayan PS, et al. (2014). An evidence-based guideline for prehospital analgesia in trauma. *Prehosp Emerg Care*. 2014;18(suppl 1):25–34.

Morrison W. Pediatric trauma systems. *Crit Care Med*. 2002;30(suppl 11):S448–S456.

Sadow KB. Prehospital intravenous fluid therapy in the pediatric trauma patient. *CPEM*. 2001;2(1):23–27.

Stafford PW. Practical points in evaluation and resuscitation of the injured child. *Surg Clin North Am*. 2002;82(2):273–301.

Stallion A. Initial assessment and management of pediatric trauma patient. *Respir Care Clin N Am*. Mar 2001;7(1):1–11.

Teasdale G, Maas A, Lecky F, Manley G, Stocchetti N, Murray G. The Glasgow Coma Scale at 40 years: standing the test of time. *The Lancet Neurology* 2014; 13: 844–54.

White IV CC, Domeier RM, Millin MG, and the Standards and Clinical Practice Committee, National Association of EMS Physicians. EMS spinal precautions and the use of the long backboard-resource document to the position statement of the National Association of EMS Physicians and the American College of Surgeons Committee on Trauma. *Prehosp Emerg Care*. 2014;18:306–14.

Resources

Children's Burn Trust. Burns Database. Available at: http://www.cbtrust.org.uk/burn-prevention/database/

Joint Royal Colleges Ambulance Liaison Committee. *UK Ambulance Services Clinical Practice Guidelines 2016*. Bridgwater: Class Professional Publishing; 2016.

Novak C, Gill P. Pediatric Vital Signs Reference Chart. Available at: http://www.pedscases.com/sites/default/files/Vital%20Signs%20Reference%20Chart%201.2_1.pdf. Accessed August 21, 2018.

Trauma Audit and Research Network, Severe Injury in Children 2012, England & Wales, 2012. Available: https://www.tarn.ac.uk/Content/ChildrensReport/files/assets/common/downloads/TARN%20document.pdf. Accessed 19 June, 2018.

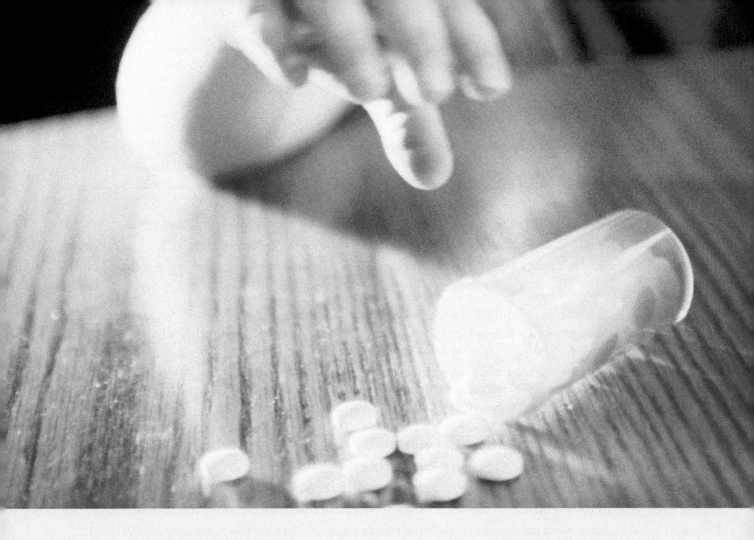

Learning Objectives

1. Identify the age groups at risk for toxic exposures, and the substance and management issues unique to each group.

2. Describe the physical assessment of the child with a suspected toxic exposure.

3. Discuss the risk assessment of the child with a suspected toxic exposure.

4. Explain the risks and the benefits of different forms of gastric decontamination.

5. Identify situations where online contact with the regional poison centre might influence the assessment and treatment of toxic exposures.

Toxic Emergencies

8

Introduction

A toxic exposure is an ingestion, inhalation, injection, absorption, or application of any substance that causes illness or injury. There are a myriad of reasons that children experience such exposures, including unintentional ingestions of poisons, environmental misadventures, and deliberate intoxications. An example of an unintentional exposure is a toddler who ingests a caregiver's medicine. An environmental misadventure might be a child who inhales carbon monoxide during a house fire, or a child with a systemic reaction to a skin contact with an insecticide. Deliberate intoxications include recreational exposures and attempted suicides. The top 10 Toxbase® pages accessed in 2016/17 by ambulance personnel searching for information on poisoning for all age groups are summarised in **Table 8-1**.

Age-Related Differences

For the under 5s, poisoning is the fourth most common cause of injury related hospital admission. The number of fatalities due to accidental poisoning by a pharmaceutical product is low, with only 28 deaths registered for the under 5s between 2001 and 2013 (see **Table 8-2**).

Most exposures in children younger than 6 years of age are asymptomatic. The toddler is a fearless, curious individual who explores the world by placing objects in his or her mouth (**Figure 8-1**). Because toddler ingestions are unintentional, and most non-food items ingested are not very palatable, poisonings in this age group often involve small volumes of a single substance. Exploratory ingestion by toddlers accounts for about 2% of attendances of pre-school children at emergency departments (EDs). The most common reasons for poisoning admissions are medicines (70%) and household/garden chemicals (20%). For examples of household and garden hazards see **Table 8-3**.

The majority of toddlers are initially asymptomatic; however, toddlers may also present with significant symptoms without a known history or witnessed ingestion. It is important that providers consider this possibility and survey the scene to better understand possible causes. Also, it is important to keep in mind, that the initially asymptomatic child may have dangerously high levels of a toxin in his or her body that may not become apparent until much later. In the absence of any apparent life threats it is absolutely imperative to obtain a thorough history before making a transportation decision.

Children under 5 years of age may swallow button (disk) batteries, which usually pass through the digestive tract without a problem but that can get stuck in the oesophagus or anywhere else in the body. If there is suspicion that a child has ingested a battery (or one is stuck in the nose, ear, or elsewhere), attempt to find out exactly what kind of battery it is and bring the child to the ED. While initially asymptomatic, symptoms such as vomiting (occasionally bloody), abdominal pain, discoloured stools, fever, diarrhoea and rashes develop when the battery begins to corrode

Table 8-1 Top 10 Toxbase Pages Accessed by Ambulance Clinicians

Rank	Agent	Number
1	Paracetamol	19,239
2	Ibuprofen	7,704
3	Codeine phosphate	6,069
4	Sertraline	2,748
5	Sodium hypochlorite	2,449
6	Diazepam	2,035
7	Tramadol hydrochloride	1,987
8	Aspirin (acetylsalicylic acid)	1,849
9	Citalopram hydrobromide	1,837
10	Mirtazapine	1,698

Source: National Poisons Information Service

Table 8-2 Severe and Fatal Pharmaceutical Poisoning in Young Children in the United Kingdom

	Deaths number (%)	PICU admissions (% of identified substances)
Region	England and Wales	UK
Study period	2001–2013	2002–2012
Source	ONS	PICANet
Benzodiazepines	0	22 (19%)
Methadone	16 (57%)	20 (17%)
Other opioids	1 (4%)	19 (17%)
Tricyclic and tetracyclic antidepressants	3 (11%)	13 (11%)
Iron and its compounds	1 (4%)	13 (11%)
Anticonvulsants (except benzodiazepines)	1 (4%)	6 (5%)
Heroin	2 (7%)	–
Others/unspecified	4 (14%)	108
Total	28	201

ONS, Office of National Statistics; PICANet, Paediatric Intensive Care Audit Network; PICU, paediatric intensive care units; 2,079,090 (excludes 108,923 cases of unknown age)
Source: Anderson, 2016.

and damages surrounding tissues. Children may also be asymptomatic when the battery is lodged in the oesophagus. Although battery ingestion can be fatal, most pass through the gastrointestinal tract in 2–7 days.

Children 6–12 years of age are less likely to ingest non-food articles or non-prescribed medicines. Although most exposures continue to be unintentional in this age group, intentional exposure begins to play a role, particularly among the older age group. Unintentional fatal exposures are mostly caused by smoke inhalation and carbon monoxide poisoning. Intentional exposure, non-fatal and fatal, is seen with solvent abuse (also known as "buzzing", "huffing", "sniffing", "tooting"), which is the intentional inhalation of volatile chemicals.

Among adolescents (13–19 years), toxic exposures are usually intentional, either as recreational abuse or as a suicide gesture or attempt. Intentional exposures lead to more ED visits and hospital admissions than unintentional exposures. In suicide attempts, adolescents usually ingest two or more substances, often in large quantities (**polypharmacy**) and the number of suicides in the 15–19 year old age group is increasing in the UK. Recreational abuse often involves alcohol in addition to another recreational drug. Many adolescents would have difficulty getting the resources to purchase illicit drugs were it not for the ever-evolving creative ways they find to get high. Solvent abuse usually involves common household products, such as industrial glue or liquid petroleum gas (butane and propane), which may be found in cigarette lighters, aerosols, petrol, and other products. These substances are inexpensive, easy to find in many homes, and give the teenager an easy-to-hide substance, because it would not normally seem out of place to have these items in one's home.

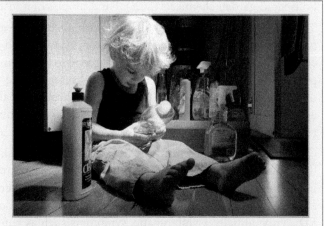

Figure 8-1 Toddlers are "oral explorers"; they will try to taste or swallow almost any substance.
© Image Source/age fotostock

Table 8-3 NPIS Age Related Poisoning Enquiries for Examples of Household and Garden Hazards 2016/17

Agent	Total number of patients exposed	Number of patients under defined age	Number of patients under 5 years old
Automatic dishwashing tablets (soluble film)	488		453
Automatic dishwashing tablets (traditional)	492		430
Automotive screenwash	255		66
Button batteries	54		20
Carbon monoxide	1081 (within an 18 month timeframe)	222 aged 12 years and under	
Iron	310 analysed	95 aged 15 years or under	36
Pesticides	973	423 aged 12 and under	

Source: National Poisons Information Service

Novel psychoactive substances (formerly legal highs) such as Spice are now being sold by street dealers in plain, clear bags with no branding. These can cause tachycardia, elevated blood pressure, and nausea. In 2016, 123 people in the UK are reported to have died as a result of using these substances; only four of these were under 20 years of age.

The drugs most commonly associated with death in people under 20 years old are opiates and amphetamines, and to a lesser extent cocaine, new psychoactive substances, antidepressants and benzodiazepine. It is always important to remember team member safety because some of these substances can cause delusional and violent behaviour in the teenage patient.

An unusual form of abuse involves deliberate intoxication of infants or young children, referred to as fabricated or induced illness. This condition is a complex form of deliberate poisoning of a child by a caregiver. In these cases, the caregiver frequently possesses more than average medical information and is trying to induce a state of illness in the child in an attempt to bring attention to himself or herself. Children with such exposures may be especially difficult to identify because the intoxication is secretive and often chronic. Child protection issues should be dealt with in accordance with local safeguarding guidelines.

Common Substances Responsible for Serious Poisonings in Children

Most poisonings occur in the home. Table 8-3 lists some common substances responsible for serious poisonings.

Summary of Age-Related Differences

Most toxic exposures in children are minor and involve household products. The most common patient is the toddler who unintentionally ingests a small quantity of a single agent and is asymptomatic. Another common patient is the

Case Study 1

A mother calls 999 because her 2-year-old toddler is drooling and having trouble breathing. On arrival at the home, you find a young boy crying but consolable by the mother. He has no abnormal airway sounds, no flaring, and no retractions. His skin is pink. The respiratory rate is 32 breaths/min, the pulse oximetry is 98%, and the heart rate is 120 beats/min. His lungs are clear. On further assessment, you note that the child has very red, swollen lips, and a mouth odour that smells like bleach. His mother states that she was doing the laundry when she received a telephone call and left her son briefly.

1. What are key aspects of the scene assessment?

2. Outline transport and management priorities.

adolescent who uses recreational drugs or who is making a suicide attempt or gesture. Adolescent exposures often consist of more than one drug and often involve large quantities. Common serious exposures in young children involve benzodiazepines, methadone, and antidepressants, whereas those in adolescents involve analgesics, alcohol, and recreational drugs. In England and Wales, opiates and amphetamines are the most common cause of death in the under 20s, according to ONS (2017). An unusual form of intoxication in young children involves fabricated or induced illness, a complex form of deliberate poisoning or abuse of a child by a caregiver. Any suspicion that this is the case requires a safeguarding referral.

Tip

Most patients with toxic exposures are toddlers or pre-school-aged children. There is usually only one poison involved, the exposure is usually small and unintentional, and the child is asymptomatic.

Pre-arrival Preparation and Scene Assessment

Sometimes at the time of dispatch the toxin has already been identified by the caregiver or another health care professional. In these cases immediately review Toxbase® or call the National Poisons Information Service (NPIS)—either directly or through operational control depending on the local service guideline. This will help clarify the toxicity of the agent and priorities in assessment and treatment. In other cases, where the dispatch involves a toddler or adolescent with a sudden change in behaviour, consider a toxic exposure.

On arrival, first perform the scene assessment. Note whether there are potentially hazardous toxins in the area or on the patient's clothes or skin and whether immediate patient decontamination is safe to perform. Assessment and management of overdose and poisoning is shown in **Table 8-4**.

The NPIS may assist in defining the risk and the need to mobilise other personnel (e.g., Hazardous Area Response Team). Pay close attention to scene safety when dealing with adolescents with sudden behavioural changes, because some common substances of abuse can lead to paranoia and sudden violent actions.

If there is a possible toxin or hazardous material, secure the scene and minimise the risk of toxic exposures through the skin, eyes, nose, mouth, or lungs of the ambulance clinicians by use of personal protective equipment. Use all your senses to gather information at the scene. Pay particular attention to your initial impression of the smell at the scene. Some dangerous toxins quickly overwhelm the sense of smell, rendering it useless after just a few sniffs ("olfactory fatigue/nose blindness"). Other toxins have an odour only at low levels, such as hydrogen sulphide. The "rotten egg" smell given off by this chemical overwhelms the sense of smell and one cannot smell it at high toxic levels. Other key smells include

Table 8-4 Assessment and Management of Overdose and Poisoning in Children

Overdose and Poisoning	
ASSESSMENT	MANAGEMENT
• Assess ABCD	• If any of the following **TIME CRITICAL** features present: - major **ABCD** problems - decreased level of consciousness—NB Most poisons that impair consciousness also depress respiration—**refer to altered level of consciousness guideline** - respiratory depression—refer to airway management guideline - hypotension <70 mmHg - cardiac arrhythmias—**refer to cardiac rhythm disturbance guideline** - convulsions—**refer to convulsion guideline** - hypothermia—**refer to hypothermia guideline** then: • Start correcting **A** and **B** problems. • Undertake a **TIME CRITICAL** transfer to nearest receiving hospital. • Continue patient management en route. • Provide an alert/information call.

Overdose and Poisoning	

• Substance	• Ascertain what has been ingested
	• Estimate the quantity.
	• Ascertain what, if any, treatment has been administered.
	• Document the time the incident occurred.
	• **NEVER** induce vomiting.
	• In the case of caustic/petroleum ingestion encourage the child to drink a glass of milk, if possible.
	• If possible take and handover to staff at hospital:
	  - a sample of the ingested substance
	  - medicine containers
	  - a sample of vomit—if present.
	• Consider non-accidental injury—refer to safeguarding children guideline.

• Chemical exposure	• If exposure to chemical substance is suspected—**refer to CBRNE guideline** for management.
• Oxygen	• Administer high levels of supplemental oxygen, particularly in cases of carbon monoxide poisoning or inhalation of irritant gases—**refer to oxygen guideline**. • Apply pulse oximeter. NB Supplemental oxygen may be harmful in cases of paraquat poisoning.
• ECG	• Undertake a 12-lead ECG.

• Respirations	• Monitor respirations.
	• Consider assisted ventilation if:
	  - SpO$_2$ is <90% after administering high levels of oxygen for 30–60 seconds
	  - respiratory rate is **<½ normal rate** OR **>3 times normal rate**
	  - expansion is inadequate.
	  - Opiates such as morphine or heroin can cause respiratory depression; consider naloxone - refer to naloxone guideline.

• Blood pressure	• Hypotension is common in cases of severe poisoning. • Monitor blood pressure.
• Intravascular fluid	• If fluid is indicated **refer to intravascular fluid guideline**.
• Blood glucose level	• Measure blood glucose. - Blood glucose levels <4.0 mmol/l need correcting - refer to glucose 10% guideline. NB Glucagon is often not effective in overdoses.
• Thermoregulation	• Hypo- or hyperthermia can occur.
• Mental health assessment	• In cases of attempted suicide undertake a rapid mental health assessment—**refer to mental disorder guideline**.
• Transfer to further care	• All children who have encountered a serious poisoning. • All children who have taken a deliberate overdose. (Even if the substance was harmless, they need to be transferred for a hospital-based assessment of their mental health). Following an accidental poisoning, it is possible for some children to be managed at home. This option may be considered when: • the substance is/verified on TOXBASE as harmless • the incident is/was accidental • the carers know to seek medical advice if the child becomes unwell • arrangements have been made to inform the health visitor or GP

Source: JRCALC, 2016.
© Association of Ambulance Chief Executives

bitter almonds (cyanide) and garlic (organophosphates, arsenic). Pay attention to confined spaces, and remember that some toxic gases are heavier than air and may affect children first or may only be in low-lying areas, such as cesspits or ditches.

Be aware of the possibility of a mass exposure to a toxic substance, either because of unintentional or deliberate action (e.g., bioterrorism). If a disaster or mass-casualty event is suspected, implement the major incident plan (see *Children in Disasters* chapter).

Next, look over the surrounding area. Bring any bottles, containers, or plastic bags containing possible toxins and samples of ingested plants or syringes to the ED along with the patient (**Figure 8-2**). If the caregiver refuses to let a poisoned child be transported to the hospital, a discussion with another clinician over the telephone may be helpful. If this strategy does not work, then request assistance from the police who in an emergency have the power to ensure a child's safety in accordance with the Children Act 1989.

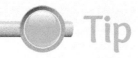

Tip

The adolescent who makes a suicide attempt or gesture should be assessed for mental capacity and transported to the ED for medical and psychological assessment. This is true even if the injury or immediate medical risk is assessed as trivial.

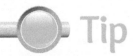

Tip

Bring bottles, containers, plastic bags, suspicious substances, plants, or syringes to the ED.

Think Point

Never forget about toxic hazards on scene. Watch out for absorbable toxins and protect skin and eyes by using gloves and other personal protective equipment.

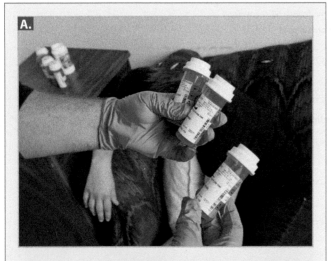

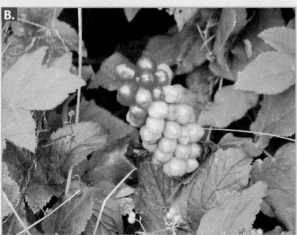

Figure 8-2 Bring any bottles or plant samples to the ED. **A.** Bottles and containers. **B.** The poisonous plant Lords and Ladies.

A: © Jones & Bartlett Learning. Courtesy of Glen Ellman; **B:** © Maigheach-gheal - geograph.org.uk (cc-by-sa/2.0)

Role of the National Poisons Information Service

In the UK, the National Poisons Information Service (NPIS) is a valuable resource for the prehospital professional when managing children with a toxic exposure. NHS professionals can contact the NPIS by telephone (0344 892 0111) or for online information (www.toxbase.org). The service is open 24-hours a day and provides information about the potential toxicity of an item, and can recommend home or hospital management. If necessary, enquirers can consult directly with a consultant clinical toxicologist.

Local protocols should define the circumstances when contact with the NPIS can be made either directly or through the operational control centre. Members of the public do not have access to Toxbase® or the NPIS telephone helpline.

Assessment of the Child With a Possible Toxic Exposure
General Assessment

After the rapid scene assessment and environmental evaluation for toxins, assess the child. Use age-appropriate techniques to approach the patient, as outlined in the *Paediatric Assessment* and *Using a Developmental Approach* chapters, and conduct a general assessment (paediatric assessment triangle (PAT)), a primary assessment, and then an additional assessment when appropriate. If the child is unstable, treat the physiological abnormalities detected in the general (PAT) and primary assessment, and then transport to hospital. En route do a reassessment and the additional assessment, if possible.

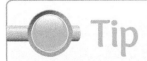
Tip

The National Poisons Information Centre (NPIS) has a key role in individual and community prevention and treatment of toxic exposures. Have the website (www .toxbase.org), user name and password and telephone number (0344 892 0111) posted near or on your telephone or tablet.

History is the best tool for overall assessment of risk and for determining urgency for treatment in paediatric poisoning. It is usually more accurate than a physical evaluation in determining the specific type of toxic exposure. In the first few minutes, the important questions are: (1) the identity of the agent; (2) the route of exposure (ingestion, inhalation, injection, absorption); (3) the time since the exposure occurred; and (4) the amount of the agent involved in the exposure, but if unknown, assume the worst case scenario. Using the acronym TART is a useful reminder: T = Toxin, A = Amount, R = Route, T = Time. See **Table 8-5**, TART Chart.

Special Considerations in the Primary Assessment

After the PAT, do the hands-on <C>ABCDEs to complete the primary assessment, and then immediately treat any physiological abnormalities. Special elements of the physical assessment that may help identify the type of poison include breath odour, vital signs, pupillary size, skin temperature, and skin condition. An odour of bitter almonds may be caused by cyanide, whereas garlic odour may be caused by organophosphates. Also, look for stains and powders on the skin or clothes. Use assessment information to match the patient's signs and symptoms with possible "toxidromes", identifiable clinical patterns of single-agent intoxications. **Table 8-6** outlines the signs and symptoms of important toxidromes in paediatrics. The drugs most commonly associated with death in people under 20 years of age are opiates and amphetamines, and to a lesser extent cocaine, new psychoactive substances, antidepressants, and benzodiazepines.

Airway

Clear, maintain, and control the airway in the child with a suspected toxic exposure who has altered mental status (AMS). This may happen in a child exposed to a sedative, hypnotic and anxiolytic such as a benzodiazepine, non-benzodiazepine alternative (e.g., zopiclone) or some antidepressants. Beware of the child who has ingested a caustic agent, such as caustic soda. This child may have severe burns of the oesophagus and present with drooling, dysphagia, and signs of upper airway obstruction. Have a suction unit on hand; if using it becomes necessary, do so gently with the appropriate device.

Breathing

Give 100% supplemental oxygen by a reservoir (non-rebreather) mask if there is AMS, respiratory distress, or a history of exposure to a toxic substance known to cause breathing problems. One example of this type of toxic exposure is hydrocarbon inhalation such as lighter fuel. Obtain pulse oximetry, but be aware that for some oxygen saturation monitors the reading is not accurate for some toxic exposures, notably carbon monoxide poisoning. Sedative or hypnotic drugs, opiates, and γ-hydroxybutyrate (GHB) may decrease the respiratory rate, whereas sympathomimetic agents (cocaine, amphetamines), phencyclidine (PCP, Angel Dust), and aspirin may increase the respiratory rate.

Close monitoring is essential to evaluate the adequacy of breathing so that intervention with a bag-valve-mask device with supplemental oxygen can be started without delay should breathing become inadequate.

Circulation

If the child has eaten or swallowed a possible cardiopulmonary toxin, place him or her on a cardiac monitor to watch for dysrhythmias. Medicines such as β-blockers, digoxin, or calcium channel blockers may decrease the heart rate, whereas sympathomimetic agents and anticholinergic agents (hyoscine, antihistamines) may increase heart rate. Skin can be warm and dry because of medicines such as antihistamines and anticholinergics, whereas the skin may be hot and sweaty from sympathomimetics, organophosphates, aspirin, and PCP.

Table 8-5 TART Chart			
Toxin	**Amount**	**Route**	**Time**
Name of substance Type (tablet, capsule, liquid, seed, root, flower, suppository, patch, etc.)	Milligrams or other amount if known. Include approximate number of tablets, seeds, amount of liquid, and so forth (note if any spilled on floor or clothes). Any vomitus? Take with you if possible.	By mouth, snorted, smoked, injected, rectal, skin absorption, eyes, nose, other.	Approximate time of first exposure or ingestion. Include duration and whether confined space, if applicable.

Table 8-6 Common Toxidromes

Toxidrome	Agents	Signs and Symptoms
Anticholinergics	Antihistamines, tricyclic antidepressants*	"Hot as a hare, red as a beet (hot dry skin, hyperthermia), blind as a bat (dilated pupils), mad as a hatter (delirium, hallucinations)"
Cholinergics	Organophosphates	DUMBELS: diarrhoea, diaphoresis, urination, miosis, bronchoconstriction, bradycardia bronchorrhoea, emesis, lacrimation, salivation
Opiates	Morphine, methadone	Hypoventilation, bradycardia, hypotension, miosis
Sympathomimetics	Cocaine, amphetamines	Tachycardia, hypertension, hyperthermia, mydriasis (dilated pupils), diaphoresis (sweating)
Specific Agents		
γ-Hydroxybutyrate	GHB, "date rape drug"	Initially drowsiness, dizziness, and disorientation; high doses result in bradycardia, hypoventilation, and apnoea
Cathinones and amphetamines	Mephedrone, methylone (M1), and MDPV; amphetamine itself (speed); and MDMA (ecstasy),	Euphoria, increased energy, intense visual perceptions Complications: hyperthermia, hypertension, seizures, dehydration, myocardial infarction, and intracerebral haemorrhage
Synthetic cannabinoids	Spice, "synthetic marijuana"	Elevated mood, relaxation, and altered perception; agitation, hallucinations, severe paranoia, seizures, vomiting, tachycardia, hypertension, and myocardial ischaemia

© Jones & Bartlett Learning

Disability

AMS is a common effect of many different chemical exposures. Recreational drug use with sedatives or hypnotics depresses the central nervous system (CNS). Sympathomimetic drugs may stimulate the CNS and cause excitement, agitation, paranoia, or hallucinations. Local guidelines may enable you to administer diazepam to manage some of the symptoms caused by use of these drugs. For example, diazepam can be used to relieve cocaine-related chest pain and has beneficial cardiac haemodynamic effects, as well as effects on neuro-psychiatric symptoms and a role in managing convulsions. Tricyclic antidepressants such as amitriptyline may cause coma, hypotension and cardiac arrhythmias, as well as convulsions, which once again can be managed with diazepam. In the comatose or unresponsive patient, always consider the other common causes of AMS, such as a head injury, seizure, or hypoglycaemia (which may accompany alcohol or β-blocker ingestion). Check the glucose level in any patient with AMS, even if toxins are suspected.

Exposure

Undress the child and look for evidence of toxic exposure to the eyes and skin. Many substances, such as hydrocarbons, irritate the eyes. Other toxic substances, such as hydrochloric acid, are caustic to skin. Organophosphate insecticides can be inhaled and also enter through the skin and can cause a severe cholinergic crisis with diaphoresis (sweating); urination; miosis (small pupils); bradycardia; bronchoconstriction; emesis; tearing; and salivation. The mnemonic DUMBELS (Table 8-6) helps identify signs of cholinergic drug intoxication. The mnemonic SLUDGE may also be used: Salivation, Lacrimation, Urination, Diarrhoea, Gastrointestinal upset and Emesis. These signs coupled with agitation and respiratory distress signal a severe exposure, as you will read in the *Children in Disasters* chapter.

Initial Management of Toxic Exposures

After the primary assessment, determine the need for treatment and transport of the poisoned child by combining the physical assessment with a risk assessment. The physical assessment is a way to determine the child's physiological stability and the overall urgency for treatment and transport. The risk assessment evaluates the probability of serious toxicity (early and delayed) from the exposure. Perform the risk assessment with knowledge of the identity of the drug involved, time since ingestion or exposure, the amount of poison involved and the child's weight (see **Table 8-7**). The operational control centre and the NPIS can help with the risk assessment.

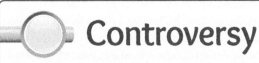

Controversy

If the child is stable and has a history of a single small ingestion of a low-risk agent, some services may allow the child to be discharged at home dependent on local protocol. Safety-netting can be used as appropriate for example safe-guarding referral, follow up visit by community team, etc. Although this approach may be medically sound, it eliminates an opportunity for assessment of psychosocial risk factors in the ED.

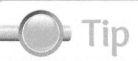

Tip

In suspected toxic exposures, perform risk assessment to determine the chances of serious toxicity.

Common toxic agents, such as aspirin, paracetamol, or iron, have predictable physiological effects that are determined by how much of the medicine was taken, time since exposure, and the weight of the patient. By collecting information and evidence at the scene, the prehospital professional serves an important role in later ED testing and treatment. Ask about *all* medicines (prescription and over-the-counter), preparations, and other substances that the child may have been exposed to. Caregivers may not realise that some topical preparations (e.g., creams for aches and pains or wart treatments) contain salicylate and can contribute to potential salicylate toxicity, especially when a child ingests aspirin or some common herbal preparations and oils, many of which also contain salicylates.

Sometimes the prehospital professional's risk assessment determines that a child has had a potentially lethal exposure, although the child is physiologically stable. Indeed, in a small child, one ingested tablet or teaspoon of some common medications can kill. **Table 8-8** lists potentially dangerous medicines where a tiny exposure (e.g., one tablet) may be toxic to a toddler. Treatment for exposure should be administered as per local policy.

Table 8-7 Risk Assessment

Assess the chances of serious toxicity from the following five pieces of information:
The agent involved and its toxicity, usually identified through consultation with the operational control centre or the NPIS
Amount of the toxin, in milligrams when possible
Child's weight
Route of exposure
Time since the exposure

© Jones & Bartlett Learning

Table 8-8 Potentially Lethal Toxic Toddler Ingestions

Medicine	Lethal Dose
Chloroquine	One 500-mg tablet
Glibenclamide	One 5-mg tablet
Imipramine	One 150-mg tablet
Propranolol	One 160-mg tablet
Theophylline	One 400-mg tablet
Verapamil	One 240-mg tablet

© Jones & Bartlett Learning

Case Study 2

You respond to a call for a 4-year-old that just ingested all of her expectant mother's iron tablets (approximately 30). On your arrival, the child is active and running around the room, but complaining that her "tummy hurts". She has no increased work of breathing, and her skin is pink. Her respiratory rate is 24 breaths/min, heart rate is 110 beats/min, and blood pressure is 90/60 mm Hg. Her physical examination reveals no abnormalities. The mother hands you the empty bottle of fruit-flavoured chewable vitamins. Reading the label, you learn that each vitamin contains 17 mg of iron.

1. Do you need to transport this child to the hospital?

2. Should you give activated charcoal?

Iron poisoning is a common cause of poisoning in young children. A NPIS study over 1 year (to January 2016) reported 301 individual patient enquiries from UK hospitals; 95 involved patients aged 15 or younger and 36 were for children under 5 years of age. Children's flavoured chewable vitamins usually have low amounts of iron (around 6 mg), but the common vitamins for expectant mothers have 15–17 mg of iron each. A young child can easily mistake children's orange chewable multivitamin tablets for sweets and eat excessive amounts. A dose of 20 mg/kg of elemental iron is potentially toxic (about 40 or more tablets for a 12 kg child) and > 50 mg/kg has been associated with severe toxicity. Gather up all bottles and assume that when tablets are missing, the child has eaten them until proved otherwise.

The Transport Decision: Stay or Go?

After the primary assessment, initial treatment, and risk assessment, consider whether to transport immediately, performing additional assessment and treatment on the way to the ED, or to stay on the scene. If the results of the physical assessment and the risk assessment reveal an asymptomatic child and the ingestion of a small amount of a single low-risk agent, consider discharging the patient at home after appropriate consultation with a clinician in the operational control centre or the NPIS. This is controversial because some ambulance services consider hospital transport necessary in all toxic exposure cases. Other services allow the NPIS to manage minor ingestions over the telephone.

If the physical assessment indicates that the child has any physiological abnormality, or if the risk assessment indicates that the toxic exposure is potentially harmful, transport the child and perform additional assessment on the way to the ED, if possible. The onset of symptoms varies with the substance involved. A child without symptoms on arrival of clinicians may have swallowed a lethal dose of a substance. For example, ingestions of paracetamol, a common over-the-counter medicine, may be extremely dangerous but cause no early symptoms. History from the scene is critical to the management in the ED.

Additional Assessment

If the child has no physical abnormalities and is asymptomatic, and if the risk assessment indicates no serious toxicity,

perform a complete assessment on scene. Additional assessment includes the focused history and physical examination and the detailed physical examination. Sometimes it is more appropriate to perform this additional assessment on the way to the ED. **Table 8-9** lists important history in a suspected toxic exposure, presented in the standard SAMPLE format. During the primary assessment and the risk assessment, the prehospital professional will have already obtained some of the SAMPLE history.

Summary of Assessment of the Child With a Possible Toxic Exposure

Every child with a toxic exposure needs a careful physical assessment and risk assessment. The physical assessment includes all of the features of the standard assessment. There should be an emphasis on the history, which is usually the most important part of the toxicological evaluation. Preparation begins on the way to the scene with dispatch information about the age of the patient, the type and potential toxicity of exposure, and the need for personal protective equipment. Preparation then continues with the scene assessment and environmental assessment. If multiple patients are involved, consider activating the major incident plan.

Table 8-9 The Paediatric SAMPLE for Toxic Exposures

Component	Explanation
Signs and symptoms	Time of suspected exposure Behaviour changes in child Emesis and content of vomitus
Allergies	Known medicine reactions or other allergies
Medications	Identity of suspected toxin Amount of toxin exposure (count tablets or measure volume) Tablet or chemical containers on scene Exact names and doses of prescribed medicines
Past medical problems	Previous illnesses or injuries
Last food or liquid	Timing of the child's last food or drink Type and time of home treatment
Events leading to the exposure	Key events leading to the exposure Type of exposure (inhaled, injected, ingested, or absorbed through the skin) Poison centre contact

© Jones & Bartlett Learning

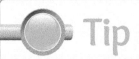

Tip

Most pre-adolescent paediatric poisonings do not require any treatment in the field.

After the physical assessment, the risk assessment helps determine if there might be serious toxicity based on the type of toxin involved, the amount of the toxin, the weight of the child, route of exposure, and the time since the exposure. The risk assessment gives important information about expected physiological effects, need for treatment, and timing of transport. The NPIS often plays a key role in helping decide about treatment and transport.

Toxicological Management

The prehospital professional has three possible options for toxicological management of serious or potentially lethal exposures: (1) decontamination to reduce local or systemic exposure to the toxin; (2) enhancement of elimination, or increasing the speed of removal of the toxin; or (3) antidote administration to reverse the actions of the poison directly. In most cases, documenting a thorough history, evaluating the risk assessment, and appropriate transport supporting the ABCs are usually the best treatment.

Decontamination

After the treatment and transport decision, consider decontamination. There are several ways to decontaminate, depending on the toxin and the type of exposure.

Skin

If there is a chance that the poison was **absorbed** through the skin, remove the child's clothing. The prehospital professional must protect his or her own skin and eyes by using gloves and protective gear. Flood the skin with large amounts of warm water for 15–20 minutes (if time allows and no apparent life threats take priority), avoiding harsh scrubbing, and be careful not to contaminate anyone else.

Eyes

Immediately wash out the eyes if there has been direct eye contact (**Figure 8-3**). **Alkali** burns with caustic agents, such as caustic soda, are the most dangerous. Flush the eyes for 20 minutes using normal saline or water. For example attach intravenous (IV) tubing to a bag of normal saline and flush the eye with the end of the IV tubing. If this is not possible, hold the patient's head and pour warm water into the eye from a cup. When the eyes are the main point of exposure, continue flushing during transport if possible.

Gastrointestinal Decontamination

Before any **gastrointestinal (GI) decontamination**, contact the operational control centre or the NPIS, depending on service protocol. In some cases, it may be beneficial to dilute mild **acid** or alkali ingestions by asking the alert patient to drink a glass of milk or water. Dilution is contraindicated

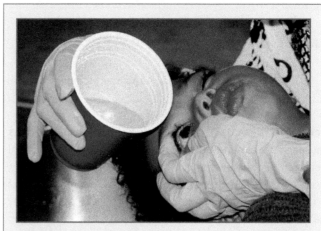

Figure 8-3 Immediately wash out the eyes if there has been direct eye contact.
© Jones & Bartlett Learning

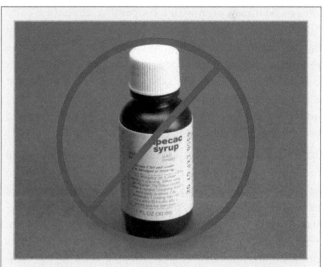

Figure 8-4 Inducing vomiting has no role in prehospital professional treatment of paediatric poisoning.
© Jones & Bartlett Learning

when there is absent gag reflex, airway compromise, diminished level of consciousness, or ingestion of a hydrocarbon or caustic (strong alkali or acid).

Ipecacuanha is an old remedy for ingestions, and although *no longer recommended for home, ambulance service, or hospital use*, it may have been given in the home by the caregiver. Make note of this and the time it was given. Induction of emesis (vomiting) with ipecacuanha for example is not recommended because there is no evidence that it removes significant amounts of ingested toxins from the stomach, it may increase the risk of aspiration, and it may cause prolonged emesis, delaying the administration of activated charcoal (**Figure 8-4**).

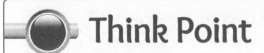

Think Point

Do not induce vomiting in a child with a suspected ingestion.

Activated Charcoal. Most high-risk ingestions in toddlers and pre-school children do not require any out-of-hospital treatment. In cases where GI decontamination is necessary, consider using activated charcoal. Activated charcoal is made from burned wood products. Its surfaces are "activated" by steam or chemical treatment, so the material can **adsorb** ingested toxins in the stomach and small bowel, and reduce bloodstream absorption of the toxins. Charcoal itself is not absorbed from the GI tract, nor is it metabolised. Activated charcoal has no odour or taste, other than the container it is presented in, but has a granular consistency that makes many children unwilling to drink it. Charcoal administration can be messy, even with a cooperative child. In a child with altered or deteriorating mental status, aspiration of charcoal can lead to serious pulmonary consequences. There are limited data on the use of activated charcoal in the prehospital setting, and the risks of prolonged scene time must be weighed against the potential benefits of rapid transport and early ED management. Some agents are not adsorbed by activated charcoal, as noted in **Table 8-10**.

Administration of Activated Charcoal. The actual amount of ingested substance is usually not known, and so the dose administered is empirical. For children under 12 years, activated charcoal 25 g is given, and 50 g if a large quantity of toxic substance has been ingested, and where there is a risk to life. For adults activated charcoal 50 g is administered. Activated charcoal begins working immediately, and it is most effective when given within an hour of ingestion (**Figure 8-5**).

Never force a child to take activated charcoal because this may lead to aspiration and pulmonary complications. If

Table 8-10 Toxins Poorly Adsorbed by Activated Charcoal
Boric acid
Cyanide
Ethanol
Ethylene glycol
Iron
Lithium
Malathion
Methanol
Petroleum distillates
Strong acids and alkalis

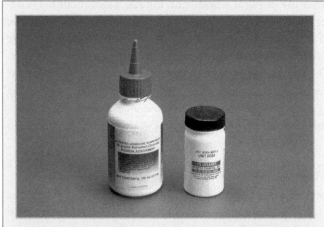

Figure 8-5 Activated charcoal is a treatment option for potentially serious ingestions of toxins that are adsorbed.
© Jones & Bartlett Learning

Think Point

Administration of activated charcoal can be difficult. Administration should not delay transfer to hospital, but may be indicated when transport time is long and risk assessment indicates severe toxicity.

Tip

The biggest problem with prehospital use of activated charcoal is the difficulty getting children to take it.

Think Point

Patients who have taken an overdose may not be fully conscious, and so will be unable to protect their own airway.

local service policy allows, the activated charcoal may be mixed with soft drinks or fruit juice to mask the flavour, and should be administered as per local guidelines.

Antidotes

Antidotes are available to reverse or treat the side effects of toxic ingestions. Prehospital providers carry several antidotes that may be life-saving for poisoned patients. Use these medicines with knowledge of the type of ingestion or exposure, patient's clinical status, and possible adverse effects associated with the antidote.

Naloxone is an antidote used frequently in adult patients with suspected opioid overdose. It can have a therapeutic and diagnostic effect in selected paediatric patients. If a child under 12 years old has signs of an opioid ingestion or overdose (bradycardia, coma, small pupils, respiratory depression), naloxone can be given at a dose relative to the patient's age as per the JRCALC guidelines. Although IV is the preferred route because it has a rapid onset of action, naloxone can be given intramuscularly (IM), intraosseously (IO), intranasally (IN), or subcutaneously (SC) in accordance with local protocol. The child may then awaken slightly or fully, with improvement in vital signs. The duration of action of naloxone is short, so repeat doses may be necessary if longer-acting opioids such as methadone are involved. When administering naloxone give the lowest effective dose and administer slowly. In adolescents chronically addicted to opioids, rapid administration of naloxone may induce undesired acute withdrawal symptoms. Have suction on hand in case vomiting occurs.

Flumazenil may be available and is an effective benzodiazepine antagonist, but must not be routinely used as an antidote for patients with AMS of unknown cause. One of the most common causes of AMS in children is the postictal state after a seizure. If flumazenil is given and the child has further seizures, benzodiazepines such as diazepam and midazolam will not be effective. Also, flumazenil may precipitate seizures if administered to the patient who is on chronic therapeutic doses of a benzodiazepine.

β-blockers are used for treatment of hypertension and adult cardiac disease. An overdose in children can cause bradycardia, hypotension, heart failure, and cardiogenic shock. Glucagon, a familiar medicine to prehospital professionals because of its role in treatment of hypoglycaemia, helps reverse toxicity from β-blocker overdose. Although there are no good paediatric studies, the suggested dosage of glucagon is a bolus of 50–150 micrograms/kg IV administered over 1–2 minutes followed by an infusion of 50 micrograms/kg/hour, titrated to clinical response. β-blocker overdose can

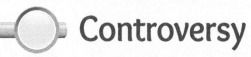

Controversy

The value of activated charcoal for out-of-hospital treatment of oral poisoning and overdose is unproven. Although activated charcoal has a possible advantage of early binding of toxins in the gut, there are potential complications, such as aspiration and bowel obstruction.

also cause hypoglycaemia in young children, so check the glucose level and treat hypoglycaemia if present.

Organophosphates

DUMBELS (Table 8-6) is the mnemonic that summarises the clinical hallmarks of organophosphate poisoning toxidrome. Treatment involves several steps:

1. Ensure your personal protection (use gloves and other protective clothing to prevent exposure).
2. Perform the primary assessment and ensure adequate oxygenation and ventilation.
3. Patients with clinically significant hypoxia, bradycardia, and/or hypotension require oxygen and atropine before decontamination.
4. Remove contaminated clothing and double-bag, seal, and store safely.
5. Decontaminate the patient. Decontaminate open wounds first and avoid contamination of unexposed skin. Flush the skin with large amounts of water for at least 10–15 minutes; include mucous membranes, moist areas such as skin folds, fingernails, and ears.
6. Flush exposed eyes with large amounts of warm water or saline.
7. Maintain a clear airway and ensure adequate ventilation. Give oxygen. Continuous suctioning of the airway may be required because of excessive secretions. Securing the airway and assisted ventilation will be necessary in severe cases.
8. Atropine helps reverse the "muscarinic" organophosphate effects (diarrhoea, urination, miosis, bronchoconstriction, bradycardia, bronchorrhoea, emesis, lacrimation, salivation). The initial paediatric atropine dose is 50–75 microgram/kg IV and is repeated every 5 minutes as necessary until the lungs are clear, heart rate is greater than 80/min, and blood pressure is adequate. Pupil size should not be used as an end point for atropinisation.
9. When available, specific antidotes should be administered as per local policy.

The likelihood of responding to a child involved in a nerve agent attack is far less likely than responding to a child poisoned by one of the many household or garden pesticide preparations containing organophosphates.

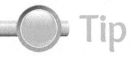

Tip

The National Poisons Information Service can refer calls to consultant clinical toxicology staff.

Summary of Toxicological Management

Most children with toxic exposures do not require treatment of any kind in the prehospital environment. If the child is asymptomatic, has ingested a small amount of a single low-risk substance, and there are no "red flags" for child abuse and neglect, consider cancellation of transport after consultation with a clinician in operational control or the NPIS. In other circumstances, when physical assessment and risk assessment together show physiological instability or possible toxicity, treatment is indicated. After managing the <C>ABCDEs, consider toxicological management by decontamination or, in special situations, administering an antidote. Perform skin and eye decontamination when indicated. Attempt GI decontamination for serious or potentially fatal ingestions based on local protocol. Activated charcoal is a useful binding agent for many types of toxic ingestions, but can only be safely administered to a cooperative child. Several antidotes carried by prehospital professionals may be diagnostic, therapeutic, and even life-saving. More advanced antidote therapies are best performed in the ED or hospital setting. Remember to educate the family or caregiver on poisoning prevention if circumstances allow, as discussed in the *Paediatric Assessment* chapter.

Medico-legal Issues

There are several scenarios where medico-legal issues play an important role in the management of toxicological emergencies in children. If the child and/or adult refuses treatment and transport to the hospital, it may be appropriate for another clinician to talk to him or her over the telephone. If this strategy does not work, then all essential steps to stabilise the child should be taken, and this may include requesting assistance from the police. If the police believe that the child would suffer significant harm, they may take the child to a place of safety in accordance with the Children Act 1989.

The child who makes any suicide attempt or gesture and refuses transport should be assessed for mental capacity and should be transported to the ED; the safety and welfare of the child is paramount. An individual who has attempted suicide will usually be emotionally distressed and so will be unable to make a competent decision. In some cases, the police may need to be called to protect the clinicians and other people from any threat posed, as well as to enable transport to hospital through their power to ensure a child's safety (see the *Medico-Legal and Ethical Considerations* chapter).

The adolescent can also present legal challenges because of issues such as the ability to consent, and illegal use of alcohol or recreational drugs. If an adolescent has taken a potentially toxic dose of medicine, or has life-threatening complications of drug use or overdose, then always act in the best interests of the child as explained in the *Medico-Legal and Ethical Considerations* chapter. Do not become involved in the legal issues of alcohol or drug use, but do consider any safeguarding concerns and make a referral if appropriate.

Case Study 3

You respond to a call about an unconscious female. On arrival, you find a group of college students surrounding one of their friends who "passed out" at a party. The patient is a 17-year-old girl who is lying on a couch, is unresponsive to voice, and is not moving. Work of breathing is normal, but her skin is pale. Her respiratory rate is 8 breaths/min and shallow, heart rate is 50 beats/min, and blood pressure is 110/70 mm Hg. Her pupils are 1 mm and sluggishly reactive. There is no evidence of head trauma. The remainder of her examination is negative. There is an empty vodka bottle on the kitchen counter.

1. What are your initial management priorities?

2. Can you treat and transport this patient without parental consent?

CASE STUDY ANSWERS

Case Study 1 — page 157

The sudden onset of mucous membrane changes in a previously healthy toddler is suggestive of a caustic (alkali or acid) ingestion. Laundry detergents and bleach are caustic, and most household-strength products cause irritation when swallowed. Treatment is usually unnecessary when only small amounts of household bleach have been ingested (less than 5 ml/kg of hypochlorite) and a small glass of milk is then recommended. Industrial-strength products with alkaline pH values can cause severe tissue damage and swelling of the lining of the mouth, pharynx, and oesophagus when ingested. All patients who have any signs of corrosive injury (hypersalivation, difficulty swallowing, retrosternal pain or haematemesis) or pulmonary irritation (cough, wheeze or dyspnoea) need to be referred to hospital.

Given the circumstances of this event, and the tell-tale odour on the child's breath, a bleach ingestion is most likely. Undertake skin and eye decontamination if indicated, and protect yourself with gloves and goggles.

Rapidly transport this child to the hospital, frequently reassessing his airway. Bring the bottle to the ED. Allow the child to sit upright in a position of comfort. Administer blow-by oxygen, because a face mask will not likely be tolerated. Contact with a clinician at the operations centre or the NPIS can provide information on potential complications to anticipate during transport, such as airway oedema, stridor, or wheezing. Do not give anything by mouth without advice, including charcoal or fluids to dilute the bleach, because this increases the risk of vomiting with the potential to further damage the oesophagus as the stomach contents are regurgitated.

The toxicity of bleach is related primarily to the oxidizing capacity of the hypochlorite ion and the pH of the solution. Because the exact nature of this product is unknown, it should be assumed to be highly corrosive. Given the oral mucous membrane findings, this child may undergo oesophagoscopy and bronchoscopy (fibre optic inspection of the oesophagus and airways while under anaesthesia) in theatre to assess the degree of damage and need for further treatment.

Case Study 2 — page 163

Although this child appears well, this is a potentially dangerous ingestion. Iron overdose can be a cause of fatality. There are four phases to an oral iron overdose. The initial phase begins with the ingestion and lasts 6 hours. Common signs and symptoms in mild ingestion include nausea and vomiting, abdominal pain, and diarrhoea. Stage 2 (at 6–12 hours) is the quiet phase during which the child with mild poisoning appears well, although in more serious cases there may be evidence of shock. It is not until stage 3 (more than 12 hours after ingestion) that in serious cases the child begins to show additional signs of toxicity, including GI haemorrhage, hypotension, AMS, and renal and hepatic failure. Stage 4 (2–5 weeks after ingestion) is the post-recovery phase, during which GI strictures can still occur. Because the extent of toxicity cannot be predicted from early symptoms, a cautious approach is warranted. Transport any child who has ingested iron-containing tablets to hospital for further evaluation unless the NPIS has been contacted and has determined that based on the nature and number of tablets taken this is a non-toxic ingestion. This is commonly the case with ingestion of children's multivitamins, where the concentration of iron is low; however, because children's vitamins are often manufactured to look and taste a lot like sweets, it is not unheard of for a toddler to ingest a full bottle of 60 colourful character vitamins, many of which can contain up to 6 mg of iron each. The ingestion of vitamins made for pregnant women, however, can be very serious, especially now that the more palatable fruit-flavoured chewables are becoming more and more popular for women with morning sickness and who are unable to swallow the larger traditional vitamin tablets with iron. Bring any bottles to the ED to ensure proper identification and risk assessment. Because iron is not absorbed by activated charcoal, do not attempt GI decontamination.

Case Study 3 — page 168

The first priority is to establish an effective airway and begin bag-valve-mask ventilation with 100% oxygen, because respiratory depression is present based on rate and depth of respirations.

Some questions to ask her friends include a SAMPLE history:

- Signs and symptoms: Did anyone see her before she passed out? Was she acting normally?

- Allergies: Any known medicine allergies or other reactions?

- Medicines: Does she take any medicines? Was she drinking any alcohol? Does she use illicit drugs? Did anyone see other drugs being passed around?

- Past medical problems: Does she have any medical problems?

- Last food or liquid: When was the last time anyone saw her with something to eat or drink?

- Events: Did anyone see her fall? When she passed out, did she hit her head?

The triad of respiratory depression, decreased level of consciousness, and pinpoint pupils is typical of opiate use. This can also be a mixed overdose, because there is evidence of alcohol on the scene. Consider naloxone, and transport the patient to the ED, supporting airway, breathing, and circulation as needed based on frequent reassessments.

As this girl is under 18 years old and has a life-threatening condition, you must act in her best interests and take her to hospital.

SUGGESTED READINGS

Resources

British Medical Association and Royal Pharmaceutical Society. *British National Formulary*. London: Pharmaceutical Press.

Department of Health and Home Office. Talk to Frank. Available at: http://www.talktofrank.com/. Accessed October 21, 2017.

National Institute for Health and Care Excellence. *Clinical Knowledge Summaries. Poisoning or Overdose* Available at: https://cks.nice.org.uk/poisoning-or-overdose#!scenario. Accessed October 21, 2017.

National Poisons Information Service. Toxbase. Available at: www.toxbase.org.

Public Health England. *Chemical Hazards Compendium*. Available at: https://www.gov.uk/government/collections/chemical-hazards-compendium#chemicals-m-to-o. Accessed October 21, 2017.

References

Anderson M et al. *Severe and Fatal Pharmaceutical Poisoning in Young Children in the United Kingdom*, 2016. Available at: https://webcache.googleusercontent.com/search?q=cache:szhXx4UG9EcJ:https://www.research.ed.ac.uk/portal/files/24585245/SeverePoisoningChildren_vADC_revision2210316.docx+&cd=1&hl=en&ct=clnk&gl=uk. Accessed 5 June, 2018.

Dijkstra B, and Gossman WG, *Disk Battery Ingestion*, StatPearls Publishing LLC, 2018.

EMC. Ferrous fumarate 210mg Tablets. Available at: https://www.medicines.org.uk/emc/product/2821/smpc. Accessed 19 June, 2018.

HM Government, Emergency Response and Recovery, 2013. Available at: https://www.gov.uk/government/uploads/system/uploads/attachment_data/file/253488/Emergency_Response_and_Recovery_5th_edition_October_2013.pdf. Accessed October 21, 2017.

Home Office and Sarah Newton MP. 2016. Headshops closed and offenders arrested after 'legal highs' ban. Available at: https://www.gov.uk/government/news/headshops-closed-and-offenders-arrested-after-legal-highs-ban. Accessed October 21, 2017.

National Institute for Health and Care Excellence, Emergency treatment of poisoning, 2018. Available at: https://bnfc.nice.org.uk/treatment-summary/emergency-treatment-of-poisoning.html. Accessed 21 October, 2017.

National Institute for Health and Care Excellence 2018. British National Formulary: Naloxone Hydrochloride. Available at: https://bnf.nice.org.uk/drug/naloxone-hydrochloride.html. Accessed 6 June, 2018.

New York State Department of Health. SEMSCO protocol guidelines; SLUDGEM+respiratory distress+agitation. National Registry EMT protocols.

NSPCC, 2018. A child's legal rights: Gillick competency and Fraser guidelines. Available at: https://www.nspcc.org.uk/preventing-abuse/child-protection-system/legal-definition-child-rights-law/gillick-competency-fraser-guidelines/. Accessed 19 June, 2018.

ONS, 2017. Deaths related to drug poisoning in England and Wales: 2016 registrations, 2018. Available at: https://www.ons.gov.uk/peoplepopulationandcommunity/birthsdeathsandmarriages/deaths/bulletins/deathsrelatedtodrugpoisoninginenglandandwales/2016registrations. Accessed: 5 June, 2018.

Re-Solve, 2017. FAQs—Volatile Substance Abuse. Available at: http://www.re-solv.org/faqs-volatile-substance-abuse/. Accessed October 21, 2017.

Samaritans, 2017. Suicide statistics report 2017. Available at: https://www.samaritans.org/sites/default/files/kcfinder/files/Suicide_statistics_report_2017_Final.pdf. Accessed: 5 June, 2018.

Teva UK Limited, 2018, Activated Charcoal: Patient Information Leaflet. Available at: http://www.tevauk.com/p/activated-charcoal-355. Accessed 6 June, 2018.

The Children Act 1989. https://www.legislation.gov.uk/ukpga/1989/41/contents. Accessed October 21, 2017.

Waseem M, 2010. Pediatric Salicylate Toxicity. Available at: http://emedicine.medscape.com/article/1009987-overview. Accessed October 21, 2017.

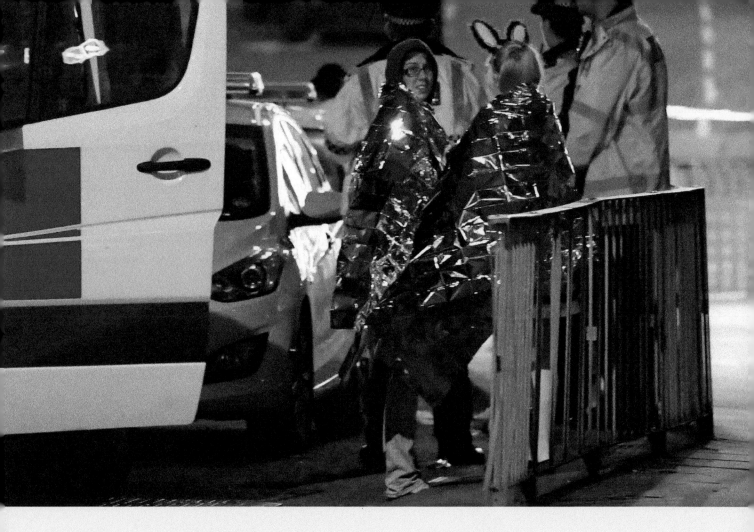

Learning Objectives

1. Define disaster and mass-casualty incident, providing examples of specific paediatric considerations in each.

2. Discuss the modifications required by prehospital professionals to accommodate the special needs of children during disasters and mass-casualty incidents.

3. Recognise the anatomical, physiological, and psychological features specific to children that increase their vulnerability and place them at special risk when disasters occur.

4. Differentiate the unique effects that chemical, biological, radiological, nuclear, and explosive events may have on children.

5. Discuss paediatric issues related to the assessment and management of specific types of toxic exposures.

Children in Disasters

Chapter 9

Introduction

Disasters have always been a dramatic part of human history, and community responses to disasters are a highly visible feature of modern emergency care systems. Indeed, catastrophic events have afforded a good deal of affirmation about the essential role of ambulance services, as well as highlighting its limitations. Disasters present unique difficulties to prehospital professionals, and children present additional complex challenges because of their special anatomical, physiological, psychological, and transportation needs. There is limited data on the types and frequencies of children's injuries and illnesses during disasters, and additionally there are limited national guidelines on disaster triage, treatment, and transport of children. However, in such uncommon circumstances, chaos and an overwhelmed operating system are common, so planning and preparation are imperative. Hence, all prehospital professionals must have a basic understanding of the unique paediatric issues in disasters, and all emergency services must possess a thorough, well-rehearsed disaster response plan that addresses children. Some disasters, such as school mayhem, may primarily victimise children; the horrific idea of prehospital professionals responding to a scene that involves their own children, or children in the community whom they know, is also a distinct possibility. After such an event trauma incident management has become an integral part of long-term disaster response.

What Is a Disaster or Major Incident?

Major Incidents pose a significant local impact but may often also have a nationwide, or regional impact. The definition of a major incident is the same irrespective of the size or location of the event. The Cabinet Office released an updated definition in 2016 which states: "*An event or situation, with a range of serious consequences, which requires special arrangements to be implemented by one or more emergency responder agencies*". They further outline:

- "emergency responder agencies" describes all category one and two responders as defined in the Civil Contingencies Act (2004) and associated guidance

- a major incident is beyond the scope of business-as-usual operations, and is likely to involve serious harm, damage, disruption or risk to human life or welfare, essential services, the environment or national security

Case Study 1

Your town has been subjected to torrential rains for 4 days. Minor flooding has occurred, but it has been controlled thus far. You are dispatched to a primary school where wind gusts have blown out windows and, reportedly, 12 children have been injured. While en route, you are notified that a nearby dam has just broken; this is very close to the school, and tens of thousands of gallons of water are pouring into the surrounding neighbourhoods each minute. Your station has a total of three ambulances, and one of those is already out of town on a routine transfer.

1. What are your incident management priorities?

2. What are your specific concerns for the paediatric patients?

- a major incident may involve a single-agency response, although it is more likely to require a multi-agency response, which may be in the form of multi-agency support to a lead responder

- the severity of consequences associated with a major incident are likely to constrain or complicate the ability of responders to resource and manage the incident, although a major incident is unlikely to affect all responders equally

- the decision to declare a major incident will always be a judgement made in a specific local and operational context, and there are no precise and universal thresholds or triggers. Where Local Resilience Forums and responders have explored these criteria in the local context and ahead of time, decision makers will be better informed and more confident in making that judgement.

(Source: JESIP, available at: http://www.jesip.org.uk /definitions)

A bus crash in a large city may not have as much of an impact on that ambulance service (and wider health economy) as the same incident in a small rural town which may see casualty numbers exceeding the community's response capabilities.

Disasters are community emergencies that disrupt normal function and threaten the safety of citizens. Because the UK health economy is designed primarily around the care of adults, the infrastructure for the care of children in a disaster in most communities is likely to be challenging, with fewer hospital beds, fewer specialists, and less experience with paediatric critical illness or injury.

A mass-casualty incident (MCI) is an event that generates more patients than available resources to care for them using routine procedures. An MCI may require multiple resources and additional help from another Ambulance Trust. In some circumstances, an MCI may have an enormous impact on the service. The UK Civil Contingencies Act 2004 brings together local responders, here responders will work together to ensure plans, procedures and agreements are in

Table 9-1 Common Natural and Man-Made Disasters

Natural	Man-Made
Earthquake	Hazardous material spill
Hurricane	Significant fire
Tornado	Biological exposure
Flood	Chemical exposure
Blizzard	Nuclear exposure
Wildland fire	Structural failure
Disease epidemic	Terrorism

© Jones & Bartlett Learning

place to ensure care can be provided in the event of a mass casualty incident. Some of the mutual aid agreements in place will support the moving of patients to other areas of the country to support the delivery of care.

There are two basic types of disasters: natural and man-made. **Table 9-1** lists common examples. Natural disasters are events caused by environmental perturbations, such as earthquakes, severe storms, flooding, wildfires, and natural epidemic disease outbreaks. Man-made disasters result from human errors, such as toxic spills, structural collapses, or malicious intent, such as terrorism or mass shootings. Regardless of origin, disasters typically cause a significant increase in the incidence of paediatric injuries and illnesses.

Specific paediatric considerations in disasters and MCIs include the current lack of a universally accepted routine paediatric response and management plan, let alone a disaster response plan. NHS Ambulance Trusts have a responsibility for the coordination of first responders. Additionally, there is significantly less essential paediatric equipment on ambulances and first responder units and less paediatric training for emergency medical personnel.

NHS Ambulance Trusts are nationally funded with key performance indicators which allow the comparing of different Trusts. On the whole, UK Ambulance Trusts operate under the Joint Royal College Liaison Committee guidance (JR-CALC) for the delivery of care and administration of prescription only medications (POMs) for paediatric patients.

Roles of the Prehospital Professional in a Disaster

Pre-disaster Planning

Emergency services are a vital resource in pre-disaster preparedness and response. Prehospital professionals might be called on before a disaster to assist in evacuating hospitals, nursing homes, and other specific skilled care facilities and to provide medical staffing for evacuation shelters. After an MCI, clinicians are responsible for providing medical care to those in need and, where necessary, arranging transportation to hospital. The ambulance service will work with partner agencies (including the wider NHS) through the Local Resilience Forums (LRF) to ensure appropriate and necessary information is cascaded and shared.

Planning and preparation for such events are indispensable to the successful functioning of emergency services before, during, and after a disaster. The most effective plans are often those that closely match an agency's daily activities. Unfortunately, because children are an infrequent part of a clinician's daily encounters, the child's needs are often only a small consideration in most pre-disaster plans. Therefore, it is essential to include hospital-based paediatricians, nurses, and other personnel with expertise in paediatric illness and injury in the development process for pre-disaster planning.

Phases of Disaster Response

Disaster response can be subdivided into three phases. The first phase is the activation phase. This occurs at the time of notification and initial response, and includes initiation of an Incident Management System and scene assessment. This is followed by the implementation phase, during which there is initial treatment, stabilisation and transport of the injured. Finally, the recovery phase occurs; following the withdrawal of all emergency personnel on scene there will be a return to normal (or a new normal) operations and post-incident debriefing.

Overall Response Strategy

Disasters often overwhelm prehospital professionals and the emergency services. Prehospital professionals must recognise that the incident will probably exceed their individual capabilities and should immediately activate an appropriate response plan with a pre-established unified command and management structure. Within the UK, the Civil Contingencies Act 2004 sets out how planning and preparation for incidents of this nature should occur, ensuring the Local Resilience Forums have plans in place for high risk locations and activities within their area. While each responding emergency service will be responsible for their own command and control, the Joint Emergency Service Interoperability Program (JESIP) clearly sets out how each agency should interact and work seamlessly together, sharing risk with each other, (see **Figure 9-1**).

This system provides structure and continuity for efficient management of the event. The goal in a disaster response is to do the most good for the most victims, and these actions allow optimal organisation of the response.

Prehospital professionals must refrain from rushing into the scene and becoming victims themselves. This task is even more daunting when the victims are children and the impulse to help is powerful. Remember that you cannot help if you become ill or injured. Use appropriate personal protective equipment (PPE) on every call when there is a potential that the rescuer may come in contact with contaminated patients. Chemical, biological, and radiological incidents require specific and specialised equipment. Only specially trained and equipment responders should be entering a hazardous environment leaving unprotected responders to manage the patients once they have been decontaminated. The JESIP website gives guidance on the new Initial Operational Response (IOR) guidance where patients will

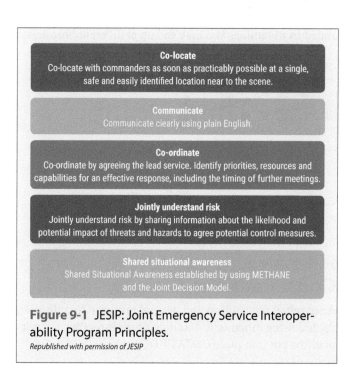

Figure 9-1 JESIP: Joint Emergency Service Interoperability Program Principles.
Republished with permission of JESIP

be decontaminated using dry decontamination processes, however, for certain chemicals it may still be necessary to use wet decontamination processes on patients.

What Is JESIP?

"Initially JESIP was a two year programme (Joint Emergency Services Interoperability Programme) which ran from 2012-2014. It was primarily about improving the way the Police, Fire & Rescue and Ambulance services work together when responding to major multi-agency incidents.

What JESIP produced was much needed practical guidance to help improve multi-agency response. The *Joint Doctrine: the interoperability framework* sets out a standard approach to multi-agency working, along with training and awareness products for organisations to train their staff.

Whilst the initial focus was on improving the response to major incidents, JESIP is scalable. The five joint working principles and models can be applied to any type of multi-agency incident and in fact could be utilised in a multitude of environments where organisations need to work together more effectively.

The programme initiated the largest and most successful joint training initiative across the emergency services. Now JESIP is about all services integrating the JESIP ways of working and models into all policies, procedures until staff use JESIP as a matter of course."

Source: JESIP, 2018.

Prehospital professionals must also exercise the highest vigilance in securing communications between victims and families. This is especially important for children during disaster triage, treatment, and transport, as they often get separated from families and may end up at different hospitals.

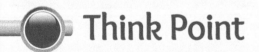

Think Point

Prehospital professionals must refrain from rushing into the scene and becoming victims themselves. Injured and dead rescuers are not able to save anyone.

Paediatric Response Considerations

After initial recognition and general response to a disaster, the following mnemonic describes procedures that will normally be put into place CSCATTT:

- Command
- Safety

- Communication
- Assessment
- Triage
- Treatment
- Transport

Attention is given to pre-disaster planning as an essential component to an organised response.

Planning

Before a disaster occurs, having the appropriate resources and training to treat paediatric patients is essential. Response vehicles should have paediatric supplies, including a range of paediatric airway equipment, paediatric-sized cervical collars, intraosseous needles, smaller gauge intravenous (IV) catheters, and methods to control hypothermia. In addition, having a system in place for patient tracking and reunification is essential, given the likelihood of family separation.

Ambulance Parking Point

Depending on the size of an incident an Ambulance Parking Point may be established. Prehospital ambulance professionals should meet at this assigned location where the Ambulance Parking Officer will be recording their arrival, as required the ambulance will either be called forward to treat patients or to collect and convey a patient to hospital. This ensures a quick and systematic deployment. For the incident management system to function properly, all prehospital professionals need to co-ordinate their efforts to ensure appropriate and timely patient care.

Triage

Triage is the process of prioritising patients based on the severity of their injuries and available resources. The goal of triage in the disaster setting is to make a daunting task manageable. The paediatric population can be challenging, because many patients are non-verbal, frightened, and separated from family members, and they may have injuries with which rescuers are unfamiliar (e.g., crush injuries, bomb blasts, chemical or radiological exposures). Proper triaging of paediatric patients requires standardised triage algorithms.

The Simple Triage and Rapid Treatment (START) triage system is one recognised method for triage of adult disaster patients. The START triage system categorises patients by colour and allows the prehospital professional to quickly classify each patient according to physiological status and urgency for treatment. It is difficult to apply the START concept to young children because this system uses adult vital sign measurements and requires that victims have the ability to verbally communicate and ambulate.

The JumpSTART triage system was devised as a modification of the START triage system for use in children younger

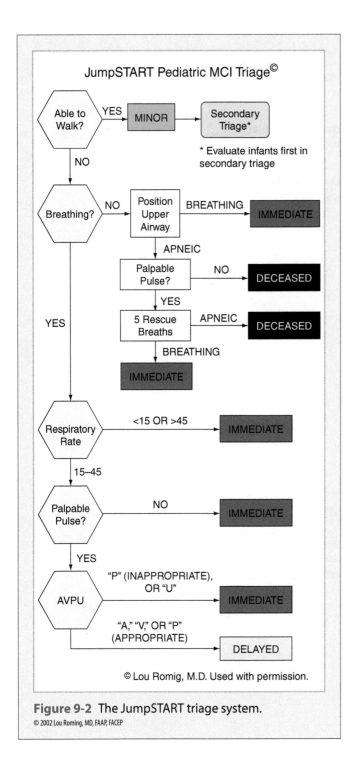

JumpSTART Pediatric MCI Triage©

Able to Walk? — YES → MINOR → Secondary Triage*

* Evaluate infants first in secondary triage

NO ↓

Breathing? — NO → Position Upper Airway → BREATHING → IMMEDIATE

APNEIC ↓

Palpable Pulse? — NO → DECEASED

YES ↓

5 Rescue Breaths — APNEIC → DECEASED

BREATHING ↓

IMMEDIATE

Breathing? YES ↓

Respiratory Rate — <15 OR >45 → IMMEDIATE

15–45 ↓

Palpable Pulse? — NO → IMMEDIATE

YES ↓

AVPU — "P" (INAPPROPRIATE), OR "U" → IMMEDIATE

"A," "V," OR "P" (APPROPRIATE) → DELAYED

© Lou Romig, M.D. Used with permission.

Figure 9-2 The JumpSTART triage system.
© 2002 Lou Roming, MD, FAAP, FACEP

presence of spontaneous breathing, respirations less than 15 or greater than 45 breaths/min, palpable peripheral pulse, and appropriate response to painful stimuli on the alert-verbal-pain-unresponsive (AVPU) scale.

Patients who are able to walk should be assigned to the green category for "minor" and are not in immediate need of treatment. Those breathing spontaneously, with a peripheral pulse and an appropriate response to painful stimuli, should be assigned to the yellow category for "delayed" treatment. Children who have apnoea responsive to positioning or rescue breathing, have respiratory failure, are breathing but do not have a palpable pulse, or have an inappropriate pain response should be assigned to the red category for "immediate" intervention. Children who are apnoeic and without a pulse, or apnoeic and unresponsive to rescue breathing, should be assigned to the black category and considered deceased or expectant deceased.

Another more recently developed triage system currently in use in other parts of the world is the Sort, Assess, Life-saving interventions, and Treatment and/or transport (SALT) triage system (**Figure 9-3**). This guideline has the advantage of being applicable in adults and children. It describes four sequential activities that take place. (1) Global sorting of patients using voice commands often works for older children who can understand and follow a command to move to another location, but young children may not be able to respond. (2) Individual assessment and assignment of a priority category follows, starting with the individuals who were unable to respond first. (3) Life-saving interventions that can be quickly applied may include rescue breaths for children who do not respond to positioning of the airway. (4) Finally, provision of treatment or transport completes the process.

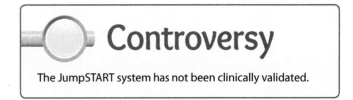

Controversy

The JumpSTART system has not been clinically validated.

Within the UK some Ambulance Trusts use the SMART Triage Tape, which allows the responder to lay the tape next to the child, which helps to easily calculate the child's age and weight.

There are a variety of triage algorithms available, and no current recommended paediatric standard. All prehospital professionals within a service should be familiar with the method used by their service, and trained in its use. This system optimally should account for children in a disaster.

Treatment

Treatment of paediatric patients in disaster situations varies greatly depending on the specifics of the disaster, the

than 8 years of age or less than 45 kg. This triage system uses important assessment characteristics of infants and children to distinguish them from older patients. Jump-START uses breathing as the cornerstone for triage decisions (**Figure 9-2**).

As in the START triage system, there are four triage categories in the JumpSTART system, designated by colours corresponding to different levels of urgency for treatment. Decision points include: ability to walk (except infants),

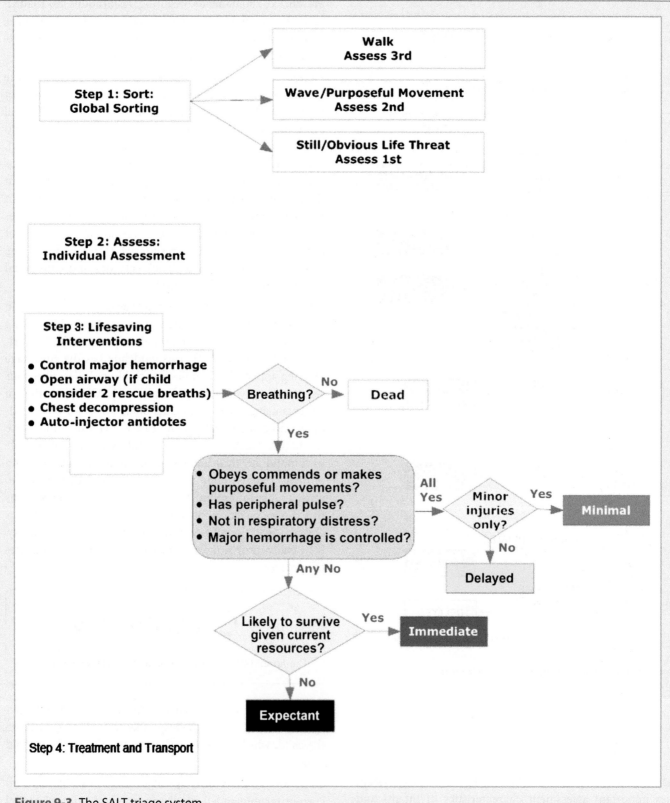

Figure 9-3 The SALT triage system.

exposure of the patient, and the availability of resources of the responding agencies. Treatment should always include removing the patient from the source of the threat or agent as quickly as possible, with due consideration to hot zone (contaminated area), warm zone (where full decontamination occurs), and cold zone (safe area); secondary threats; and the prehospital professional's safety.

After the patient is moved to safety, depending on the exposure, decontamination may be necessary. <u>Decontamination</u> is the physical process of removing or neutralizing potentially harmful substances from patients, personnel, equipment, and supplies. A person may become contaminated by contacting vapours, mists, solids, or liquids from a specific source or from others already contaminated. *Decontamination should be performed whenever an individual is actually or potentially contaminated with a hazardous substance.* Decontamination is designed to minimise the amount of a hazardous material that is available for absorption through a victim's skin and prevent contamination of the rescuers. Because of children's proportionally greater body surface area, and skin that is less keratinized and more permeable, they have an increased likelihood of systemic toxicity from agents that contact their skin; this underlies the importance of rapid decontamination in the paediatric population. Therefore, time is a critical consideration in effective decontamination of skin exposed to chemical agents. Even if large amounts of time have elapsed since the initial exposure, perform decontamination on the patient to eliminate any remaining agent and mitigate the risk of exposure to others.

Families are likely to be kept together during this process. Keeping families together reduces the risk of secondary contamination to emergency responders.

Because children lose body heat faster than adults, special care is indicated during decontamination because they are at an increased risk for hypothermia when exposed to the environment. Appropriate planning can ensure that there is warming equipment, and paediatric-sized clothing and blankets available after decontamination is complete.

When the number of patients exceeds the number of ambulances available for transport, designate and assign treatment areas and attempt to keep families together. After these patients have arrived at the treatment area, conduct a secondary triage to determine if the patient's initial triage status has changed. Essential medical equipment is vital to maintaining a functional treatment area. Each of the different triage divisions—red, yellow, green, and black—should have its own treatment area. The most experienced providers should treat the red and yellow designated patients.

Transport and Tracking

Early identification of patients by first responders in combination with patient tracking technology should be part of every disaster plan and drill. There are many patient tracking devices available. Coordination with regional resources (e.g., ambulance services and hospitals) is critical to ensuring compatibility and access.

The Loading Officer's duty is to get patients into ambulances and routed to appropriate hospitals. The Loading Officer must be flexible to ensure patients are transported to the most appropriate facilities. Prehospital professionals must be cognisant of destination policies and guidelines, so that children go to the hospitals best prepared for paediatric emergencies or for specific injuries, such as trauma and burns. Do not give paediatric patients priority for transport just because they are children. Assign transport priority based on the specific patient's condition.

Reuniting Children With Their Families

Although child and parent separation should be minimised during disaster response, one should anticipate and prepare for this situation. The parents and caregivers that children depend on may also be injured and incapacitated. For those paediatric victims and caregivers who require transport, it is necessary to track patients to ensure reunification.

Natural Disasters
Earthquakes

In Europe there are very few seismically active fault lines. Faults are seams in the Earth's crust along which geologic plates slide. An earthquake is a sudden, rapid shaking of the earth caused by the breaking and shifting of rock beneath the Earth's surface along these fault lines. This shaking can cause buildings and bridges to collapse; disrupt gas, electric, and telephone service; and sometimes trigger landslides, avalanches, flash floods, fires, and huge destructive ocean waves (tsunamis). Ground movement during an earthquake is seldom the direct cause of death or injury. Most earthquake-related injuries result from collapsing walls, flying glass, and falling objects.

Damage from earthquakes can be extensive, and multiple types of injuries may occur. These injuries usually include blunt and multisystem trauma. *Seismic events have been known to also trigger illnesses, especially asthma.* The lack of appropriate shelter exposes children to environmental elements, such as stray animals, insects, hazardous chemicals, and exposed building materials. The additional psychological stress caused by earthquakes may also contribute to increases in domestic violence and child abuse.

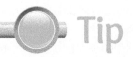

Tip

A natural disaster and environmental disturbance, such as an earthquake, often causes a major increase in paediatric respiratory ailments, especially asthma.

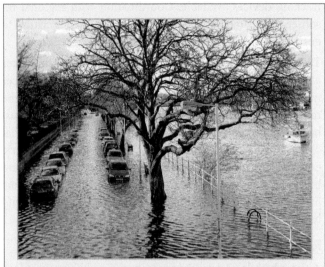

Figure 9-4 Flooding is a yearly concern in many areas of the country.

Floods

Several environmental events can cause flooding, including heavy rains, rapid snow melt, and coastal storm surges (**Figure 9-4**). Flooding is usually somewhat predictable, and river flooding typically has a more gradual development. Therefore, family dislocation can be anticipated and plans can be implemented so that families are not separated unexpectedly. However, separation can occur during flash flooding. In recent years there have been a number of flooding incidents within the UK that have had a wide-reaching impact. These have ranged from fluvial flooding through residential and shopping areas to coastal flooding, which has affected many different groups of people.

Following the flooding in 2007 the UK Government commissioned report from Sir Michael Pitt to review the different flooding incidents across the country, the Pitt Review 2007. These flooding incidents were seen as the country's largest peacetime emergency since World War II. Flooding, irrespective of where it occurs, or whether it is fresh or salt water flooding, can cause significant damage to property resulting in the loss of both personal possessions and community cohesion. These 2007 floods saw over 50,000 properties flooded with 7,000 people needing to be rescued by the emergency services from some form of flood water.

Even people whose properties weren't damaged by flooding were still affected by the flooding. Many lost mains water and power supplies; some for only a few days, others for much longer. The utility losses brought their own challenges for those who hadn't been flooded, especially for ill and infirm people who still lived outside of a care community, with some having to be transported to other locations where there was either fresh running water or power to ensure their wellbeing.

An additional public health consequence of flooding is contamination of the drinking water that is still flowing and outbreaks of disease. Because of their small size and relatively low fluid reserve, children are at a greater risk of dehydration from vomiting and diarrhoea associated with drinking contaminated water.

Flooding can occur at any time of the year and following periods of hot dry weather the impact can be both unexpected and devastating as the water simply runs off the hard ground and into the rivers, resulting in fluvial flooding happening significantly quicker than people may have been expecting.

Severe storms differ from one geographic region to another. Coastal areas in the US are subject to hurricanes, whereas inland regions often experience more tornado activity. Luckily the UK very rarely suffers from either hurricanes or tornados, however, our weather can result in significant rainfall and flooding which can result in devastation. The UK has fewer extreme weather events such as blizzards and hurricanes than many other parts of the world but communities can still find they are either isolated or adversely affected by these events. Prehospital professionals must be aware of the potential for paediatric patients to experience cold-related emergencies during severe storms, because infants and young children have a higher body surface area-to-weight ratio and lose heat more quickly than adults when their skin is wet or cold.

As an island the UK is very susceptible to tidal surges; where strong land-bound winds occur at the same time as spring tides there is a significant risk of tidal flooding. The East of England has seen a number of tidal surges over the years, some of which have caused significant damage to property and infrastructure. The 2013 tidal surge floods resulted in the East Coast of the UK being battered by strong winds and high seas. The high tides reached levels not seen since 1953 and resulted in many people having to be evacuated, some even losing their homes to the devastation the waters brought with them. Across the UK severe storms can lead to structural damage, loss of power, communication outages, isolation and flooding. These events place children and the elderly at high risk of injury from environmental conditions and structural damage. There are also the added problems of asthma exacerbations, respiratory ailments, gastroenteritis, and emotional crises over family separation. Depending on the time of day the event occurs, there may be heavy concentrations of children in schools, child care facilities, and other locations. Younger children will have little understanding of the events, and they may be primarily focused on separation from loved ones. Being separated from their caregivers, and not comprehending the current events, make the management of their emotional needs difficult. *Emergency responders must anticipate these emotional crises and have a plan in place to establish communications and restore unity of families as quickly as possible.*

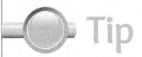

Emergency responders must anticipate emotional crises in children who are separated from their families during a disaster and have a plan in place to establish communications and restore unity of families as quickly as possible.

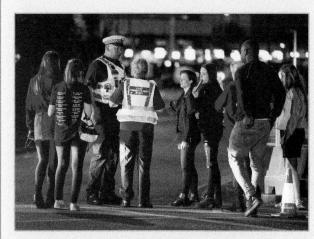

Figure 9-5 The Manchester Arena terrorist attack.

Disease Epidemics

Every year there are significant communicable disease outbreaks. Sometimes, the paediatric population is at the heart of these outbreaks. These outbreaks include infections such as influenza, chicken pox, measles, and hepatitis. Sometimes new viruses, especially influenza, may attack a community and greatly elevate requirements for prehospital and hospital services. Occasionally, the prehospital professional may be at risk for disease transmission from contact with an infected patient.

Many children will have received inoculations as they have grown up to help protect against diseases such as measles. However, many of the illnesses brought by stagnant water will not be covered by childhood inoculations. Without proper medical care, this can lead to children becoming dehydrated and extremely unwell.

Within the UK the guidance on immunisation is provided by Public Health England and the latest recommendations and guidance for Healthcare Professionals Immunisation Practitioners is provided in a document called "The Green Book".

Man-Made Disasters

Man-made disasters include hazardous material incidents; structure failures; and criminal activities such as acts of terrorism or aggression. Terrorism is an emerging threat in all regions of the world. Children are frequent targets, sometimes precisely because of the psychological impact of death and injury of vulnerable victims by the perpetrators.

Criminal Activity and Terrorism

A troubling trend is the targeting of children by their peers for criminal acts. These disasters may generate horrific mass casualties.

In the UK there have been only a limited number of attacks on schools, one of the most notable being the shootings at Dunblane Primary School near Stirling in Scotland in 1996. During this attack 16 pupils and 1 teacher were killed.

More recently there have been a number of arrests of pupils or ex-pupils who have been preparing to carry out attacks at UK schools. In October 2017 two youngsters were arrested after plotting a mass shooting attack on a school in North Yorkshire.

Following the number of high profile terrorist attacks, and failed attacks, within the UK during 2017 the government issued new advice and guidance specifically aimed at young people during a terrorist attack. This included the "Run Hide Tell" message in a format more akin to the understanding of younger people, along with more direct advice about not standing and filming an attack but to getting to safety.

On 22 May 2017 a terrorist attack occurred at the Manchester Arena as fans were leaving a concert by a singer with a large pre-teen and teenage following (**Figure 9-5**). Many of those killed and injured were children; however, some were the adults either accompanying the youngsters or those waiting in the foyer to collect people from the concert. In all, 23 people lost their lives and it is believed over 500 were injured. Many of the injuries resulted from flying debris and shrapnel from the bomb.

Hospitals within the surrounding area were used to deliver care to those injured in the attack and this included a local Specialist Paediatric Hospital. The impact on many of the injured young people lasted for significantly longer than a single visit to an ED, with some patients having to undergo numerous operations to ensure they were well enough to leave. Some received life-changing injuries and many youngsters were left with both physical and mental scars from this attack.

These events can have an extensive impact on children, including those not directly involved in the disaster suffering from post-traumatic stress disorder (PTSD), separation anxiety, and agoraphobia.

Hazardous Materials Exposures

In daily life, hazardous materials are everywhere (**Table 9-2**). Examples of these hazards include chemicals used in cleaning, refrigeration, swimming pool maintenance, fuels, and agricultural products. Many of these materials are present in schools and other public facilities, and in homes. Additionally, illegal activities, such as methamphetamine laboratories, use materials that are highly explosive and toxic,

Table 9-2 Examples of Common Hazardous Materials

Diesel fuels	Insecticides
Petrol	Fertilisers
Motor oil	Propane
Herbicides	Natural gas
	Fireworks

which may cause burns and serious injuries to bystanders including children.

Structural Failures

Buildings, bridges, and platforms sometimes fail. These collapses typically cause multiple injuries. Victims may be hysterical and confused, and individuals may be buried under other victims. Children can be the primary victims, especially when structural failures involve schools or recreational facilities.

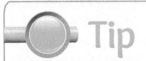

Children have a proportionally greater body surface area and thin skin, which makes them more susceptible to injury from burns, chemicals, and absorbable toxins.

Recently there have been a number of attacks where acids were used as a weapon, either randomly or in a targeted manner. The potency of the chemical used varies; however, these attacks have resulted in many people suffering lifelong injuries. The most common part of the body to be affected is the face because it is rarely covered up and as such it is not unusual for an acid attack to leave someone blind or to scar their face, making them almost unrecognisable.

Acid attacks and the NHS – in numbers

14 – victims treated in one of England's 23 specialist burns centres in all of 2014.

20 – victims treated in specialist burns centres in the first six months of 2017.

22 – average number of days these victims need to spend in a specialist burns unit.

£34,500 – estimated cost of NHS care for victims needing specialist burns treatment, eye care, rehabilitation and mental health support.

408 – reported acid attacks in the 6 months to April 2017 according to the National Police Chiefs Council – all attacks require urgent medical attention.

21 – percentage of victims (where age was recorded) who are under 18.

Source: National Ambulance Resilience Unit Available from: https://naru.org.uk/acid-attacks-nhs-offers-public-advice-respond/

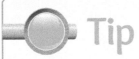

A new and troubling trend is the targeting of children, sometimes by their peers, for school and terrorism.

Vulnerable Paediatric Physiological and Psychological Characteristics in Disasters

Because of their unique anatomy and physiology, children are especially vulnerable to the effects of disasters. In addition, their immature behavioural and psychological characteristics place them at higher risk for immediate injury and longer-term effects. **Table 9-3** summarises vulnerable physiological and psychological characteristics of children that place them at high risk during disasters.

Physiological Considerations

Children have a higher respiratory rate compared to adults, which makes them more vulnerable to large quantities of inhaled chemical or biological agents. Additionally, their shorter stature lowers their "breathing zone," potentially making them more susceptible to inhalation injuries from chemicals or fires

Table 9-3 Vulnerable Paediatric Characteristics

Paediatric Characteristic	Special Risk During Disaster
Respiratory	Higher minute volume increases risk from exposure to inhaled agents. Nuclear fallout and heavier gases settle lower to the ground and may affect children more severely.
Gastrointestinal	May be more at risk for dehydration from vomiting and diarrhoea after exposure to contamination.
Skin	Proportionally greater body surface area and thinner skin make them more susceptible to injury from burns, chemicals, and absorbable toxins. Also, hypothermia is more likely.
Endocrine	Increased risk of thyroid cancer from radiation exposure.
Thermoregulation	Less able to cope with temperature problems with higher risk of hypothermia.
Developmental	Less ability to escape environmental dangers or anticipate hazards.
Psychological	Prolonged stress from critical incidents. Susceptible to separation anxiety.

where the materials are denser than air. Their increased respiratory rate also increases insensible fluid loss, further placing them at risk for dehydration. The characteristics of a paediatric patient's airway make them more susceptible to compromise. These features include a smaller-diameter airway that may easily become occluded with mucus, oedema, or secretions.

Compared to adults, children have less fluid reserve and smaller circulating blood volumes, making them more prone to dehydration. Causes of dehydration include heat exposure, burns, vomiting, and diarrhoea. An increased metabolism, compared to that of adults, often causes children to metabolise medications differently; this characteristic may require the prehospital professional to adjust medications and dosages when administering antidotes.

Children with special health care needs (CSHCN) include children who may have chronic physical, developmental, behavioural, or emotional conditions that require health-related services beyond those required by children generally. In a disaster, these children may be at an increased risk for suboptimal outcomes. Each carer (family member or hospital) will have detailed information summarising the child's critical medical information required for optimal care and support. This information should be kept with the child and their carer when transported. See the *Children With Special Health Care Needs* chapter for more information on CSHCN.

Emotional Responses of Children

Response to a disaster or MCI must include an assessment of the emotional state of a child and the child's caregivers. The mental health needs of children also must be recognised in the incident management system and when planning for disasters. *Appropriate mental health personnel with paediatric expertise have an important role in the aftermath of disasters, to help ensure adequate stress management and counselling services.* Reuniting children with their caregivers is key to child-family-centred care. Child and caregivers' emotional responses may range from fear and anxiety to depression, grief, and symptoms of post-traumatic stress. Children may be especially vulnerable to post-traumatic stress reactions. Paediatric aspects of shelter management need to be considered if children are separated from their caregivers. Each child will respond differently to a disaster, depending on his or her age, maturity, previous experience, and cultural background. However, children of all ages experience anxiety from disasters. Younger children may interpret the disaster as a personal danger to themselves and those about whom they care.

Effects of Chemical, Biological, Radiation, Nuclear, and Explosive Disasters on Children

Chemicals

Millions of different chemicals in the world are potentially detrimental to human health (**Table 9-4**). Chemicals are

Table 9-4 Common Chemicals Detrimental to Human Health

Alcohols, including antifreeze and windscreen washer fluid	Washing tablets
Ammonia	Laundry soap
Asbestos	Pesticides
Bleach (laundry)	Rodent poison
Chlorine	Sulphuric acid
Drain and oven cleaners	Toilet bowl cleaner
Hydrocarbons, including furniture polish, gasoline, lighter fluid, and paint thinner	

transported throughout the country daily by lorries, trains, and planes with a potential for unintentional or deliberate population exposure. Additionally, chemical weapons are an important consideration for the prehospital provider, causing injury, death, and disease.

When chemical spills are identified, officials trained to work with hazardous materials (HazMat) are a key resource for identification of the toxicity, relative risk, decontamination procedures, and specific treatments required.

Assessment and Treatment of Specific Chemical Agents

Nerve Agents

Nerve agents are extremely toxic and have very rapid effects. Common agents include tabun, sarin, soman, VX, and organophosphates. The nerve agent, either as a gas, aerosol, or liquid, enters the body through inhalation or transdermally (through the skin). These two characteristics have a greater effect on children because of their faster respiratory rates and larger skin surface area-to-mass ratio. Poisoning may also occur through consumption of liquids or foods contaminated with nerve agents. All nerve agents produce toxic effects by preventing the proper operation of the chemical that acts as the body's "off switch" for glands and muscles. Without an "off switch", the glands and muscles are constantly being stimulated, causing the victim to tire and no longer be able to sustain breathing. Because of the extremely rapid onset of symptoms, it is likely that children exposed to these agents will develop symptoms before adults who are exposed to the same event.

The initial signs and symptoms of a nerve agent exposure include frontal headache, eye pain, miosis (pupil constriction), runny nose, anorexia (loss of appetite), nausea, excessive sweating, tightness in the chest, and heartburn. If the patient is exposed to large amounts of a nerve agent, abdominal cramps, vomiting, profuse sweating, dyspnoea (shortness of breath), diarrhoea, drooling and tearing, increased urinary frequency, involuntary urination or defecation, or excessive bronchial secretions with bronchospasm may occur. Children are more prone to dehydration because of gastrointestinal fluid losses, further complicating their management. Additionally, apnoea, seizures, paralysis, and coma may ensue. Bradycardia is typical (although tachycardia may occur).

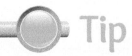

Symptoms of nerve gas exposure are often remembered as the mnemonic "DUMBELS": diarrhoea, diaphoresis, urination, miosis, bradycardia, bronchorrhoea, bronchospasm, emesis, lacrimation, salivation.

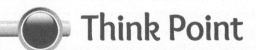

Inhalation of nerve gas may occur without the knowledge of the victim.

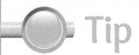

Children may be more susceptible to nerve gas because of their faster respiratory rates and larger skin surface area-to-mass ratio.

Treatment for nerve agents includes decontamination and use of atropine, pralidoxime (2-PAM), and benzodiazepines. These can all be given intramuscularly (IM) with effective absorption. Use antidotes only for severe exposures exhibiting the signs and symptoms listed previously. Treat skin contact after resuscitation by undressing and decontaminating the patient with copious amounts of water. The initial paediatric atropine dose is 50–75 microgram/kg IV and is repeated every 5 minutes as necessary until the lungs are clear, heart rate is greater than 80/minute, and blood pressure is adequate. The National Poisons Information Service recommends the intravenous loading dose of pralidoxime chloride is 30 mg/kg body weight over 20 to 30 minutes. DuoDote® is an auto-injector which is available to prehospital practitioners in the UK and delivers atropine 2.1 mg and pralidoxime chloride 600 mg by intramuscular injection. In severe, life-threatening paediatric cases local guidelines may allow the device to be used in older children. For children who cannot be treated with DuoDote®, then atropine and

diazepam may be administered according to local guidelines. Personnel who are wearing PPE may find children challenging to care for, because it is difficult for rescuers to perform procedures while simultaneously having to battle their own environmental conditions. In addition, prehospital personnel wearing PPE may frighten children and render the assessment more complicated.

Cyanide

Cyanide is a rapidly acting, potentially deadly chemical that can exist in various forms. Cyanide can be a colourless gas or may be found in a crystallised form. Cyanide sometimes is described as having a "bitter almond" smell, but it does not always give off an odour; if it does, it has been found that not everyone can detect this odour. Cyanide is released from natural substances in some foods and in certain plants. It is in cigarette smoke and the combustion products of synthetic materials, such as plastics (e.g., in house fires). Patients may be exposed to cyanide by breathing air, drinking water, eating food, or touching soil that contains cyanide. The extent of poisoning caused by cyanide depends on the amount of cyanide a patient is exposed to, the route of exposure, and the length of time that a patient is exposed.

Cyanide is highly toxic by inhalation, ingestion or dermal or eye exposure. Cyanide prevents the cells of the body from using oxygen. When this happens, the cells die. Cyanide is more harmful to the heart and brain than to other organs, because the heart and brain require more oxygen compared to other areas. Children may be exposed to cyanide by breathing it, eating foods that contain it or absorbing it through their skin. Patients may have some or all of the following symptoms of cyanide poisoning within minutes:

- Mild Poisoning: Nausea, dizziness, drowsiness, hyperventilation, and anxiety.
- Moderate Poisoning: Reduced conscious level, vomiting, convulsions, and hypotension.
- Severe Poisoning: Coma, fixed dilated pupils, cardiovascular collapse, respiratory failure, and cyanosis.

Toxicity may be delayed for several hours following a spill on the skin.

Cyanide is highly volatile, and removing the patient from the environment is often all that is needed to decontaminate them. Even though cyanide inhibits cellular oxygen usage, administration of 100% oxygen via a high flow mask with a rebreather mask is still useful and should be employed. Most cases of cyanide poisoning respond to these simple steps. If the child is soaked from a spill they should be resuscitated before decontamination. Remove any particulate matter from the skin and wash with soap and water under low pressure for at least 10–15 minutes. Pay particular attention to mucous membranes, moist areas such as skin folds, fingernails and ears (National Poisons Information Service).

Following assessment of the severity of the poisoning in symptomatic patients, then an antidote may be appropriate and this should be administered in consultation with the National Poisons Information Service (see the *Toxic Emergencies* chapter).

The cyanide antidotes administered to children in the UK are:

- Mild Poisoning: intravenous sodium thiosulfate;
- Moderate Poisoning; intravenous sodium thiosulfate or hydroxycobalamin;
- Severe poisoning: Intravenous dicobalt edetate solution over 1 minute followed by glucose 10%. If there is only a partial response or the patient relapses after recovery, a further dose of dicobalt edetate should be given. If a second dose of dicobalt edetate is administered there is a danger of inducing cobalt toxicity but only if the diagnosis is not cyanide poisoning.

Alternatively, intravenous hydroxocobalamin or sodium thiosulphate may be administered.

An important distinction by the prehospital provider is determining if the exposure in question was from a nerve agent or from cyanide, given the different immediate antidotes required in each scenario. One important distinction is that patients exposed to nerve agents are more likely to have cyanosis, altered vision with miosis, copious secretions, and bronchospasm.

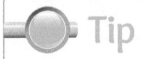

Patients may have symptoms within minutes of exposure to a small amount of cyanide by breathing it, absorbing it through their skin, or eating foods that contain it.

Pulmonary Intoxicants

Pulmonary intoxicants produce pulmonary oedema. The most widely known agents are phosgene and chlorine. Patients typically exhibit eye, nose, throat and lung irritation, dyspnoea, and chest tightness. In most cases, patients have shortness of breath caused by pulmonary oedema hours after the exposure. Without supportive treatment, including decontamination and advanced airway management, patients may progress to respiratory failure.

Blister agents

Blister agents (vesicants) are chemicals that cause blistering of the skin, irritation and inflammation of the eyes and airways, and vomiting and diarrhoea. Exposure to blister agents can be through inhalation, absorption, or ingestion. The most common blister agents are lewisite and sulphur mustard (mustard gas). Blistering usually occurs hours after

Table 9-5 Biological Agents That Pose a Threat to Humans

Anthrax	Plague
Botulism	Ricin
Cholera	Smallpox
Influenza	Tularemia

contact. Sulphur mustard has no immediate effects, while lewisite causes immediate irritation to the eyes, skin, and upper airways. Within minutes, lewisite liquid causes pain and burning on any surface with which it comes in contact.

Treatment for these chemicals includes decontamination with large amounts of water under low pressure for at least 10–15 minutes, eye irrigation (remove contact lens), airway control, and oxygen administration. Blisters should be dressed in the same way as burns. Lewisite contains arsenic and hospitals may use chelation agents such as DMPS and DMSA in symptomatic patients.

Biological Agents

There are many different biological agents that can pose a threat to humans (**Table 9-5**). They can be as common as influenza or as lethal as plague. Biological weapons used by terrorists can cause widespread disease and death. Typical agents that may be used as weapons include anthrax, smallpox, botulism, and plague. Terrorists could use these agents because they are fairly easy to purchase or formulate. An added incentive is that some of the agents are extremely contagious and can be spread to a large number of people, which very often includes children in schools and child care facilities.

Assessment and Treatment of Specific Biological Agents
Biological Pathogens

Biological pathogens, released intentionally, accidentally, or naturally occurring, can result in disease or death. Human exposure to these agents may occur through inhalation, cutaneous exposure, or ingestion of contaminated food or water. After exposure, physical symptoms may be delayed and are sometimes confused with naturally occurring illnesses. Biological agents may persist in the environment and cause problems sometime after their release.

Smallpox

In December 1979, the Global Commission for the Certification of Smallpox Eradication declared the world free of smallpox and this declaration was ratified by the World Health Assembly in May 1980. Because of the global eradication of smallpox, with the last endemic case in 1977, and the subsequent discontinued use of the vaccine, a large segment of the population remains unvaccinated. This population at risk includes children and young adults. Smallpox is caused by the variola virus. The incubation period is about 12 days (range, 7–17 days) after exposure. Initial symptoms include high fever, fatigue, and head and back aches. A characteristic rash, most prominent on the face, arms, and legs, follows in 2–3 days. The rash starts with flat red lesions that evolve at the same rate. Lesions become pus-filled and begin to crust early in the second week. Scabs develop, then separate and fall off after about 3–4 weeks. The majority of patients with smallpox recover, but death occurs in up to 30% of cases. Smallpox is spread from one person to another by infected saliva droplets; this exposure is usually through a susceptible person having face-to-face contact with the ill person. Persons with smallpox are most infectious during the first week of illness, because that is when the largest amount of virus is present in the saliva. Airborne, droplet, and contact precautions are essential and should be initiated immediately, wearing gowns, gloves, FFP3 respiration protection, and eye protection. Exposed lesions should be covered with a sheet, and the patient should wear a mask. For exposed individuals, vaccination with vaccinia within 4 days from exposure may prevent development of the disease. Those who have come in contact should be observed for 17 days after the last exposure, with fever being the criterion for isolation in a negative-pressure room.

Within the UK smallpox is a reportable disease under the Public Health (Control of Disease) Act 1984. This means that healthcare professionals have a duty to ensure any patient they are treating who is diagnosed as having smallpox is reported to Public Health England.

In response to the threat of a bioterrorist release of smallpox, in 2003 the Department of Health published Guidelines for Smallpox Response and Management in the Post-eradication Era (Smallpox Plan). This outlines the vaccination of response teams who could safely manage and diagnose suspected cases of smallpox. In 2003–2004 more than 300 healthcare and ambulance workers were vaccinated, along with a small number of staff in laboratories designated to receive specimens from suspected cases.

An information pack entitled Smallpox Vaccination of Regional Response Groups: Information for Health Care Workers Administering or Receiving the Smallpox Vaccine has been developed specifically for non-emergency vaccination of such first responders. It includes information on administration and types of vaccine. It also has guidance on pre-vaccination screening and exclusion criteria and on work restrictions following vaccination.

Anthrax

Anthrax is an acute infectious disease caused by the spore-forming bacterium *Bacillus anthracis*. Anthrax most commonly occurs in hoofed mammals but can also infect humans. Symptoms of disease vary depending on how the disease was contracted, but usually occur within 7 days after exposure. The serious forms of human anthrax are inhalation anthrax, cutaneous anthrax, and intestinal anthrax. Initial symptoms of inhalation anthrax infection may resemble a common cold. After several days, the symptoms may progress to severe breathing problems and shock. Inhalation anthrax is often fatal. The intestinal disease form of anthrax may follow the consumption of contaminated food and is characterised by an acute inflammation of the intestinal tract. Initial signs of nausea, loss of appetite, vomiting, and fever are usually followed by abdominal pain, vomiting of blood, and severe diarrhoea. For inhalational and gastrointestinal anthrax, direct person-to-person spread of anthrax is extremely unlikely; however, with cutaneous anthrax, contact precautions should be employed. The use of gloves when in contact with skin lesions, hand washing, and cleaning and sterilizing equipment is required. In situations where risk of exposure to spores exists, decontamination of patients is recommended with providers wearing gloves, gown, and mask when handling contaminated clothing or other fomites.

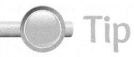

Tip

The serious forms of human anthrax are inhalation anthrax, cutaneous anthrax, and intestinal anthrax.

Plague

Plague is an infectious disease of animals and humans caused by the bacterium *Yersinia pestis*. *Y. pestis* is found in rodents and the fleas that feed on them in many areas around the world. Pneumonic plague occurs when *Y. pestis* infects the lungs. The first signs of illness in pneumonic plague are fever, headache, weakness, and a cough productive of bloody or watery sputum. The pneumonia progresses over 2–4 days and may cause septic shock and, without early treatment, death. Person-to-person transmission of pneumonic plague occurs through respiratory droplets, which can infect those who have face-to-face contact with the ill patient; therefore, droplet precautions must be used.

Ricin

Ricin is a potent protein synthesis inhibitor derived from the beans of the castor plant (*Ricinus communis*). The beans are available worldwide, and the toxin is fairly easily produced. When inhaled as a small particle aerosol, this toxin may produce pathological changes within 8 hours and cause severe respiratory symptoms (chest tightness, shortness of breath, cough), fever, and myalgias. Within 36–72 hours, cyanosis with pulmonary oedema and respiratory failure occurs. When ingested, ricin causes severe gastrointestinal symptoms with vomiting and bloody diarrhoea. Ingested ricin exposure may eventually lead to hallucinations, seizures, and low blood pressure, followed by vascular collapse and death. Treatment is supportive depending on the symptoms, and early diagnosis may be difficult. Decontamination should occur at the site of release before transport in the warm zone with a full chemical-resistant suit, gloves, surgical mask, and eye and face protection, such as a face shield and goggles. Clothing that has to be pulled over the head should be cut and double-bagged, and there should be soap and water decontamination of the skin, and irrigation to the eyes for 10–15 minutes with disposal of contact lenses. Once decontaminated, ricin cannot be transmitted from person to person; therefore, standard precautions should be used.

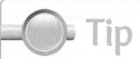

Tip

Plague is an infectious disease carried by rodents and their fleas in many areas around the world.

Botulism

Botulinum toxins are created by *Clostridium botulinum*, an anaerobic bacterium found commonly in soil. Botulism is the result of exposure to these toxins and can occur naturally through the ingestion of contaminated food or through bioterrorism exposure. The toxins act primarily at the neuromuscular junction, preventing the release of acetylcholine and ultimately leading to flaccid paralysis. The toxin effects can take from 24 hours to several days to manifest, and patients exhibit eyelid droop, dilated pupils, blurry vision, slurred speech, difficulty swallowing, dry oral mucosa, flaccid paralysis, and respiratory failure. The distinguishing factors from nerve agent exposure are the lack of initial muscle fasciculations, the dilation of the pupils, dry mucus membranes, and the period from exposure to onset of symptoms.

Infants are particularly susceptible to botulism because of the potential for colonisation of their gastrointestinal tract with the bacteria. This spore-forming bacterium can be introduced through environmental dust or by honey products. Therefore, it is recommended to avoid giving honey to children under 1 year of age. Treatment for this exposure is primarily supportive care with ventilator support. However, there may be benefit in using botulinum antitoxin, which is best given during the latent period after exposure. After the symptoms are recognised, this therapy may only reduce the further progression of symptoms. Botulism is not contagious, and standard precautions should be used for patient care.

Specific Treatment of Biological Disease
Radiation

Radiation disasters, although rare, can occur wherever radioactive materials are used, stored, or transported. Nuclear power plants, hospitals, universities, research laboratories, industries, road networks, railways, and shipping yards are all possible sites. Radioactive materials are dangerous because of the harmful effect certain types of radiation have on the cells of the body. The longer a person is exposed to radiation, the greater the risk. Children are more susceptible to radiation injury because of their rapidly reproducing cells. Radiation weapons include nuclear and "dirty" bombs. Radiation cannot be detected by sight, smell, or any other sense.

Nuclear

A dirty bomb, also known as a radiological dispersal device (RDD), consists of a conventional explosive, such as dynamite packaged with radioactive material that is meant to scatter when the bomb explodes. A dirty bomb can kill or injure by means of the initial blast of the conventional explosive or by airborne radiation and contamination (hence the term "dirty").

A nuclear bomb uses the power of nuclear fission or fusion to produce an intense pulse or wave of heat, light, air pressure, and radiation. In a nuclear blast, injury or death may occur as a result of the blast itself or as a result of debris thrown from the blast. Victims may experience moderate to severe skin burns, depending on their distance from the blast site. Those who look directly at the blast may experience eye damage, ranging from temporary blindness to severe burns on the retina. Individuals near the blast site may be exposed to high levels of radiation and develop symptoms of radiation sickness.

There are two types of exposure from radioactive materials from a nuclear blast: external exposure and internal exposure. External exposure occurs when patients are exposed to radiation outside of their body from the blast or its fallout. Internal exposure occurs when patients eat food or breathe air that is contaminated with radioactive fallout. Both internal and external exposure from fallout can occur miles away from the blast site.

Protection from radiation exposure can be attained by using a shield, minimising exposure time, and maximising the distance from the source. Depending on the type of radiation emitted, different shielding may be required, with alpha particles being stopped by a sheet of paper, beta particles by a layer of clothing or less than an inch of substance, and gamma rays by less than an inch of lead. Because PPE cannot protect against high energy, highly penetrating forms of radiation associated with most radiation emergencies, first responders should wear direct-reading personal radiation dosimeters to monitor radiation doses and stay within recommended dose limits for radiation workers.

External decontamination of radioactive particulate can be accomplished by removal of all clothing, warm soap water irrigation, wound debridement with foreign body removal, oral rinsing, and eye and ear irrigation. A radiation survey meter should be used to monitor the decontamination progress, and there may be the need to clip hair if washing was insufficient to remove the radioactive particulates. The goal is to reduce radiation level to no more than two times background radiation level. Care should be made to avoid the contamination of vehicles and equipment through on-site decontamination, and hospitals should not be used as decontamination centres. The management of internal radiation exposure varies by the radioactive element involved. Because radioactive fallout does enter the ecosystem and the foods that are consumed, radioactive iodine is a concern. In these cases, prophylactic treatment with potassium iodide prevents the radioactive form of the element from being absorbed into the thyroid gland, because children are vulnerable to late carcinogenic effects, especially of the thyroid.

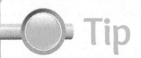

Tip

Perform decontamination whenever an individual is possibly contaminated with a hazardous substance.

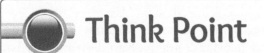

Think Point

Be sure children do not become hypothermic after decontamination. Immediately dry them and give them warm clothes.

Explosives

Explosive devices are frequently used for terrorism. Children are at risk for blast injury because of their size and susceptibility to head and abdominal injuries. The blast wave, flying debris, and injuries from being thrown may have deadly results.

Trauma Incident Management

A Trauma Incident Management (TrIM) team can provide support and counselling for prehospital professionals who have been exposed to stressful incidents in the course of their work. The need for this may be especially acute after dealing with paediatric patients in disasters.

Summary

Disasters are fortunately a rare occurrence, but when they happen they will likely involve children, either directly or indirectly. Preparation is the key to providing the best care possible. Planning and preparing in line with the Civil Contingencies Act and with partner agencies (normally via a Local Resilience Forum (LRF)) will help ensure the responding team have the appropriate resources, personnel, and communications to work with and support both the presenting patients and partner responding agencies. When children are triaged in a disaster scenario, there are several different triage methods used, which vary regionally. The JumpSTART triage system is one standardised method that takes into consideration the distinctive features of young children. Another recognised triage approach is the SALT triage system. However, these systems have not been validated; therefore, there is no nationally recognised recommendation.

Because of their physiological, anatomical, and psychological differences, children present a unique challenge to the prehospital professional. Natural and man-made disasters necessitate that emergency responders pre-plan their response and rehearse their roles in an ever-changing world.

Case Study 2

You are dispatched to a large hotel in the town centre at 7:00 AM. On arrival, you find two adult and three paediatric patients, all tourists from another part of the UK. They all have some level of respiratory distress, chest tightness, and coughing. The adults complain of weakness and joint pain; two of the children and one adult are cyanotic, especially around their lips. They state the only thing they can relate this to is being sprayed with an aerosol can in the underground at 10:00 PM last night by a group of protesters. The patients state they thought it was just air in the aerosol can. There was no odour or colour. They also state that there are 36 of them travelling together, but the others have not shown up for breakfast as planned.

1. Would you suspect a biological or chemical agent in this case?

2. How would you treat and transport these patients?

CASE STUDY ANSWERS

Case Study 1 — page 174

Your first action should be to confirm your position is safe and to identify all other potential initial responders. Ask for an official determination about whether the school is in a flood zone, and consider the necessity of an evacuation order. Initiate the Incident Management System and identify a casualty collection point at the nearest safe location. Begin rescue and evacuation operations (where safe to do so). Implement your Major Incident plan and activate your mutual aid agreements as necessary. Ambulance Control will, where necessary, notify local medical facilities of the Major Incident, and ensure the necessary notifications are made to other appropriate agencies.

During your assessment of the children, determine the severity of injuries and triage them using an appropriate standardised technique. Provide psychological support to the children by remaining calm, and attempt to reunite families when possible. Paediatric patients require additional care to maintain thermal balance during a weather-related emergency. Providing blankets and protection from the wind and rain is an important aspect of caring for these patients.

Case Study 2 — page 188

These patients may have been exposed to a toxic agent, dispersed in the aerosol spray. Most likely it is a toxin (e.g., ricin), because many chemical agents work within minutes of contact, and biological agents require time to incubate. Ricin is a mid-spectrum toxic agent derived from a biological organism, which causes a chemical poisoning.

Begin by donning PPE including gowns, gloves, and masks. Treatment should commence by first securing the scene to contain the spread of the potential disease. Have someone trustworthy attempt to make contact with the other guests from the group and determine if additional concerns exist. Contact medical control to determine the best location for transport of the patients. Make sure to notify other emergency responders, such as the police, because events of terrorism are first and foremost a crime scene. Determine if additional notifications must be made to the wider health economy or other governmental agencies. Refer to JESIP guidance for more information about patient decontamination.

SUGGESTED READINGS

Textbooks

Fleisher GR, Ludwig S. *Textbook of Pediatric Emergency Medicine*. 6th ed. Philadelphia, PA: Wolters Kluwer Lippincott Williams & Wilkins; 2010.

Hogan D, Burstein J. *Disaster Medicine*. Philadelphia, PA: Lippincott Williams & Wilkins; 2002.

Joint Royal Colleges Ambulance Liaison Committee, Association of Ambulance Chief Executives. *JRCALC Clinical Practice Supplementary Guidelines 2017*. Bridgwater: Class Professional Publishing; 2016.

Other Resources

Cabinet Office. The Pitt Review. http://webarchive.nationalarchives.gov.uk/20100702215619/http://archive.cabinetoffice.gov.uk/pittreview/thepittreview/final_report.html Accessed 3rd April 2018.

Department of Health. Emergency Care Ten Years On: Reforming Emergency Care. http://webarchive.nationalarchives.gov.uk/20130104180720/http://www.dh.gov.uk/en/Publicationsandstatistics/Publications/PublicationsPolicyAndGuidance/DH_074239 Accessed 3rd April 2018.

Department of Health. Guidelines for Smallpox Response and Management in the Post-eradication Era (Smallpox Plan). http://webarchive.nationalarchives.gov.uk/20081212100021/http://www.dh.gov.uk/en/Publicationsandstatistics/Publications/PublicationsPolicyAndGuidance/DH_4070830. Accessed 3rd April 2018.

Department of Health. Smallpox Vaccination of Regional Response Groups: Information for Health Care Workers Administering or Receiving the Smallpox Vaccine. http://webarchive.nationalarchives.gov.uk/20081205012453/http://www.dh.gov.uk/en/Publicationsandstatistics/Publications/PublicationsPolicyAndGuidance/DH_4009816. Accessed 3rd April 2018.

Department of Health. The acutely or critically sick or injured child in the District General Hospital: A team response. http://webarchive.nationalarchives.gov.uk/+/http://www.dh.gov.uk/en/Consultations/Closedconsultations/DH_4124412. Accessed 3rd April 2018.

JESIP. Aide Memoire for All Staff. http://www.jesip.org.uk/uploads/media/pdf/Aide_Memoires/JESIP_Aide_Memoire_All_Staff.pdf. Accessed 3rd April 2018.

National Ambulance Resilience Unit. Management of Hazard Group 4 viral haemorrhagic fevers. https://naru.org.uk/wp-content/uploads/2015/11/VHF_guidance_updated_7_Sept_15.pdf. Accessed 3rd April 2018.

National Ambulance Resilience Unit. National Ambulance Service Guidance for Preparing an Emergency Plan. https://naru.org.uk/wp-content/uploads/2013/02/NARU-AACE-PEP-GUIDANCE-v8Fas.pdf. Accessed 19th June 2018.

NHS England. Emergency Preparedness, Resilience and Response (EPRR). https://www.england.nhs.uk/ourwork/eprr/. Accessed 3rd April 2018.

Public Health England. Immunisation Against Infectious Disease: The Green Book. https://www.gov.uk/government/collections/immunisation-against-infectious-disease-the-green-book Accessed 3rd April 2018.

Public Health England. Infection control precautions to minimise transmission of acute respiratory tract infections in healthcare settings. https://www.gov.uk/government/uploads/system/uploads/attachment_data/file/585584/RTI_infection_control_guidance.pdf. Accessed 3rd April 2018.

Public Health England. Smallpox and vaccinia: the green book, chapter 29. https://www.gov.uk/government/publications/smallpox-and-vaccinia-the-green-book-chapter-29. Accessed 3rd April 2018.

Public Health England. Health matters: preventing infections and reducing antimicrobial resistance. https://www.gov.uk/government/publications/health-matters-preventing-infections-and-reducing-amr/health-matters-preventing-infections-and-reducing-antimicrobial-resistance. Accessed 3rd April 2018.

Romig L. *JumpSTART Pediatric MCI Triage Tools*. Team Life Support. 2011. http://www.jumpstarttriage.com. Accessed December 10, 2012.

Royal College of Paediatrics and Child Health. Children's Attendance at a Minor Injury/Illness Service (MIS). https://www.rcpch.ac.uk/sites/default/files/asset_library/Publications/C/MIS.pdf. Accessed 3rd April 2018.

UK Government. Civil Contingencies Act 2004. https://www.legislation.gov.uk/ukpga/2004/36/contents. Accessed April 3, 2018.

UK Government. Public Health (Control of Disease) Act 1984. http://www.legislation.gov.uk/ukpga/1984/22. Accessed 3rd April 2018.

World Health Organization. *Psychosocial Consequences of Disasters—Prevention and Management*. Geneva: WHO, Division of Mental Health; 2002.

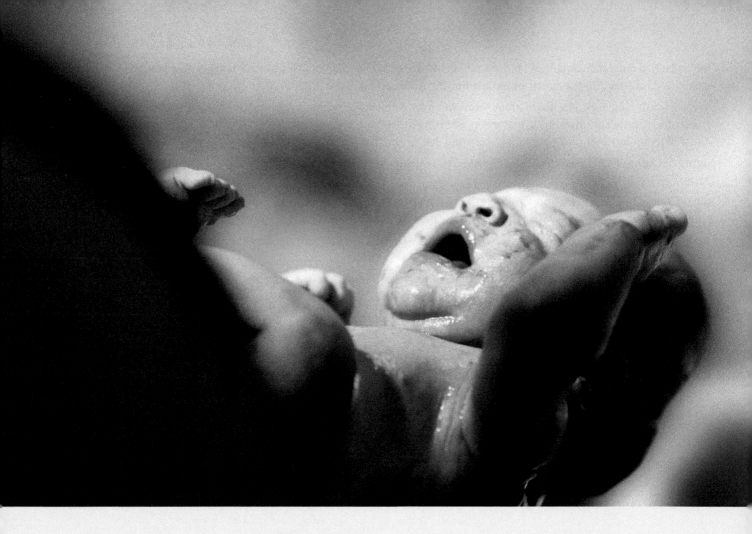

Learning Objectives

1. Describe the components of the patient history and examination that would identify pregnant patients at risk for birth outside of a hospital setting.

2. List potential maternal, fetal, and newborn risk factors that may adversely affect the health of the mother or child during or immediately after the birth.

3. Compare and contrast when it is appropriate to initiate transport of a pregnant patient to a hospital for birth versus when it is appropriate to prepare for birth in the prehospital setting.

4. Describe how to prepare for a birth, and provide post birth care to the mother and newborn.

5. Recognise the conditions and identify the correct interventions when complications jeopardise the health of the mother or newborn during childbirth.

6. Explain the indications and technique for assisting in the transition from intrauterine to extrauterine life.

7. Identify situations in which a newborn infant might require vascular access for drug and fluid administration.

Emergency Birth and Newborn Stabilisation

Introduction

Clinicians may be called to assess a patient in labour or assist with childbirth in the prehospital setting. In the past it was very common for babies to be born at home with the assistance of midwives, however, from 1965 to 1975 there was a dramatic rise in hospital birth. By 1975 home births had fallen to below 5% and have remained at this low level ever since. With the overwhelming trend toward childbirth in a hospital setting, only 2.3% of women had a planned home birth in 2015, as the Office for National Statistics 2016 data show.

As a physiological process, birth is unpredictable in its nature, and ambulance clinicians may be the only trained clinicians available when birth occurs rapidly and unexpectedly. The clinicians may encounter pregnant patients in active labour in a vast array of settings. Prehospital professionals may be called to assist with transport when labour or pregnancy are unrecognised or concealed.

Birth in the Prehospital Setting
The Clinician's Capabilities, Scope of Practice, and Legal Pitfalls

The birth of an infant is not a common procedure in the out-of-hospital setting, so the level of anxiety for both the labouring patient and the attending clinician is often high. Most newborns require only minimal assistance to make the transition to life outside the uterus. Clinicians should remain aware that although most babies require minimal resuscitative efforts, complications during birth have the potential to cause devastating, lifelong neurologic impairment or even death for the child. Limited training, equipment, scope of practice, and experience may prevent the clinicians from recognising serious complications of pregnancy or birth until it is too late to prevent injury to the mother or child. With the high level of anxiety this often causes clinicians to make rash decisions to "scoop and run" rather than stay and utilise the space of the home environment. Although uncomplicated childbirth is arguably a basic level skill, many neonatal or maternal complications outlined in this chapter require advanced interventions. Paramedic skill level should be requested when prehospital childbirth is imminent.

Case Study 1

You are responding to a local residence for a 22-year-old female reported to be in labour. The woman explains that this is her second pregnancy and she has been having contractions for 4 hours, which are now becoming more frequent and intense. She states that she was in labour for 5 hours with her first child, and she thinks it is almost time. She also states that her "waters have broken". The woman tells you that she has taken time to clean up after her waters broke, but now thinks it may be too late.

1. What questions will help you decide whether to transport immediately or to birth on scene?

2. What physical findings would tell you to prepare for birth on scene?

Ethical Considerations and the Clinician's Professionalism

The goal of every birth is a healthy mother and child. Not every childbirth attended by clinicians produces a viable, healthy newborn. For example, extreme fetal prematurity is a situation where full resuscitative efforts may not be appropriate. Clinicians periodically encounter these situations without the benefit of prior diagnosis and often without the opportunity to discuss resuscitation decisions with the child's parents in a controlled environment. When faced with this situation, clinicians should delicately balance ethical responsibilities to the patient with the professional requirement to adhere to the ambulance service policy and procedures as well as regulations pertaining to initiation and termination of resuscitation.

Complications During Pregnancy

A wide variety of conditions can adversely impact the health of the mother and fetus during pregnancy. These conditions have the potential to create complications for the mother or newborn during or after birth. Clinicians should consider these conditions when weighing the risks and benefits of performing a birth in the prehospital setting versus initiating prompt transport to a maternity facility for birth. Many complications, such as placenta praevia, cannot be managed in the prehospital setting. When known complications exist that are definitely beyond the ability of clinicians, it is often better to begin transportation immediately.

Pre-term Labour

Pre-term labour refers to labour beginning before the 37th week of gestation. Technologic advances allow newborns as young as 22–24 weeks to survive, although often with severe, lifelong complications. Between 24 and 37 weeks, each additional week of gestation reduces the impact or severity of complications on a newborn. Clinicians may encounter patients in labour with a gestational age less than 22–23 weeks; in many instances, the infant will not survive a prehospital birth. Older pre-term infants require immediate assistance from the clinicians. Treatment of a woman in pre-term labour is largely supportive until definitive care can be reached. If an infant is born before 37 weeks, clinicians should expect a vast array of complications roughly proportional to the degree of prematurity.

Post-term Pregnancy

If the fetus remains in the uterus past 40 weeks, the pregnancy is said to be post-term. After 42 weeks the uterus and placenta are unable to support the physiological and environmental needs of the growing fetus, which is why most labours are artificially started after 41 weeks to prevent fetal demise. After 40 weeks meconium may be released into the amniotic fluid. Meconium is the baby's first bowel movement and is a thick tar-like substance that can cause problems if inhaled prior to or during birth.

Multiple Pregnancies

Most multi-fetal (more than one fetus) pregnancies are diagnosed during antenatal care. Every maternal assessment should include questions about the possibility of multiple pregnancy, especially if birth is believed to be imminent. Clinicians should consider every multiple pregnancy a high-risk pregnancy. Breech presentation, umbilical cord prolapse, premature labour, and a variety of other maternal and fetal conditions are more common when more than one fetus is present.

Antepartum Haemorrhage: Placenta Praevia and Placental Abruption

At the beginning of pregnancy, the placenta may become implanted either partially or completely over the cervical os (opening) at the base of the uterus. This is placenta praevia (**Figure 10-1**). If placental rupture occurs, either from cervical dilation or mechanical shearing factors, bleeding can be

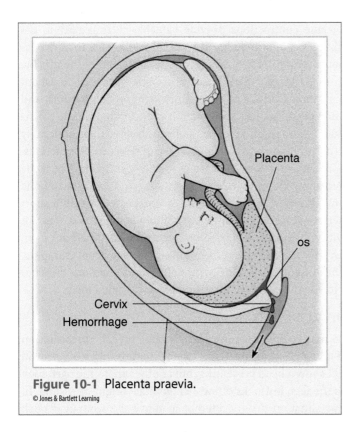

Figure 10-1 Placenta praevia.
© Jones & Bartlett Learning

Table 10-1 Determining Whether Birth Is Imminent
Questions
Is this your first birth?
If you have given birth before, how long was the labour?
Do you feel the "urge to push"?
Physical Findings
Is the child's head visible?
Is the head or scalp visible at the perineum during contractions?

© Jones & Bartlett Learning

massive and is usually painless. Patients with a placenta over or close to the cervical os require a cesarean section for the birth of the baby. A placental abruption is the shearing of the placenta from the uterine wall in a normally sited placenta. This can be due to trauma or assault.

Profound haemorrhage can be fatal for mother and fetus if the bleeding occurs prehospital and these patients cannot safely give birth in the prehospital environment. Transport of patients in labour should begin immediately.

Triage of a Patient in Labour

Clinicians must be capable of deciding whether a patient can safely be transported to a hospital for birth or if it is more prudent to prepare for an imminent birth outside the hospital. The goal of every clinician should be to transport the patient in labour to a hospital before childbirth occurs if there are no signs of imminent birth.

If birth is to occur outside of a maternity unit, then the advice of the booked unit should be sought. In certain areas it may be possible to request that midwives still attend birth imminent or babies born before arrival (BBAs).

Maternal History

Clinicians should obtain a brief, focused patient history when assessing a patient suspected to be in labour. Many factors help determine whether birth is likely or if complications should be expected. Ultimately, the answer to key

questions helps determine whether the clinician should anticipate a prehospital birth (**Table 10-1**):

1. How many times has the patient given birth? Typically, the time in active labour is longer for first-time mothers (primipara) than for women who have had prior births (multipara). If this is not a first birth, ask the woman the length of her previous labours. A history of short labour with prior pregnancies may repeat itself. Unless there is a long period between pregnancies, expect each successive labour to be shorter than the previous.

2. Does the patient feel the need or urge to push? Most pregnant patients experience this sensation as birth becomes imminent, usually within 30 minutes, often sooner. Women with the urge to push require consent to be gained for inspection of the perineum and preparation for birth of the newborn.

3. How many weeks pregnant is the woman? The gestation of the fetus will again be an important factor in decisions to move the woman to a hospital facility for birth. The lower the gestational age, the more likely the fetus is to need resuscitation and require assistance with airway and breathing support.

4. Are there any known complications that would prevent birth such as transverse lie of the fetus, placenta praevia, or an extensive type 3 FGM (female genital mutilation)?

If time permits, clinicians should inquire about maternal medical history (including medications and allergies), whether abnormalities were identified during antenatal care and any complications during previous births. Other factors, such as rupture of membranes, colour of fluid, the possibility of multiple gestation, and prior newborn anomalies, should also be included when obtaining a patient history. History may be obtained while simultaneously performing a physical examination or preparing the environment and equipment for birth.

Maternal Physical Assessment

Every patient encountered by clinicians requires a primary assessment to identify any immediate threats to life. This assessment includes airway patency, the quality of respirations and perfusion, and an assessment of level of consciousness. In many instances, immediate threats to life can be excluded if a patient is awake, speaking appropriately in full sentences, while demonstrating good skin colour and strong pulses. Any deviation from these findings suggests a potential threat to life and must be further evaluated before proceeding to a more focused assessment related to the pregnancy.

The clinician needs to perform a brief visual inspection of the perineum with consent only if an imminent birth is suspected. Look for the visible appearance of the fetal head at the vaginal introitus (**Figure 10-2**). Crowning is a sign that happens much later in the birth process as the widest part of the head is born, not the first presence of the head on the perineal area. If the presenting part is visible it means the birth is imminent and the woman must not be moved. If the woman has already been moved to the ambulance and en route to hospital, then the vehicle should be stopped at the nearest safe place.

If the baby's head is not immediately visible, inspect the mother's perineum during a contraction and note if the head becomes visible. If the baby's head is visible at the perineum with contractions, prepare for birth. Inspection of the perineum should be deferred if imminent birth is unlikely and the patient is able to reliably report the absence of any pressure, unusual sensation (including the urge to defecate), or fluid discharge (blood or amniotic fluid) in the vaginal area. The presence or suspicion of any of these items requires a visual inspection of the perineum by the clinicians.

Amniotic fluid, released from the vagina before birth, should be examined for the presence of meconium (fetal stool), a dark-green viscous substance visible in the normally clear amniotic fluid. Meconium may indicate fetal distress and increases the risk that the infant will require resuscitation after birth.

Uterine contractions provide valuable clues regarding the likelihood of a prehospital birth. Most patients in active labour demonstrate obvious contractions readily identifiable through simple visual observation of a patient. The patient may show periods of discomfort, panting respirations, and often verbalise that a contraction is occurring. Gentle palpation of the abdomen reveals a uterus that becomes noticeably firm during a contraction and relaxes between contractions. When contractions increase in intensity and duration, while becoming closer together (<2 minutes from the start of one until the start of the next), birth is expected within a short period of time. It is always possible for patients to present with subtle contractions, occasionally described as back pain, urge to defecate, or even abdominal or menstrual cramping. The absence of classic, obvious uterine contractions does not exclude the potential for imminent prehospital birth.

Breech Birth

Four percent of term births are breech presentation (**Figure 10-3**). Inspection of the perineum with a breech will not show a head presenting, but another anatomic part, such as the feet, buttocks or swollen genitals might be visible. In this situation do not attempt to move the woman if birth is imminent. It is much safer for the woman to give birth and then transport the mother and newborn according to local procedures. The JRCALC algorithm for management of breech birth is presented in **Figure 10-4**.

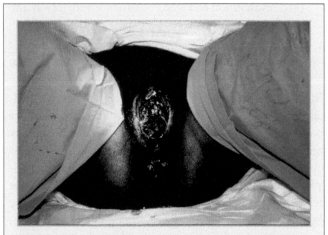

Figure 10-2 Use the presence or absence of the presenting part to help decide whether to transport or prepare for delivery.
© Jones & Bartlett Learning

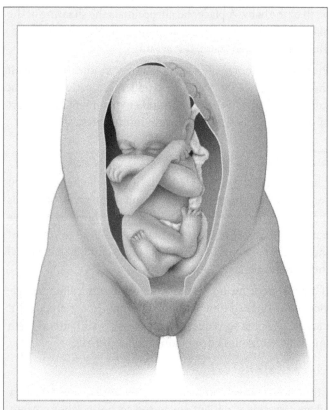

Figure 10-3 Breech birth.
© Jones & Bartlett Learning

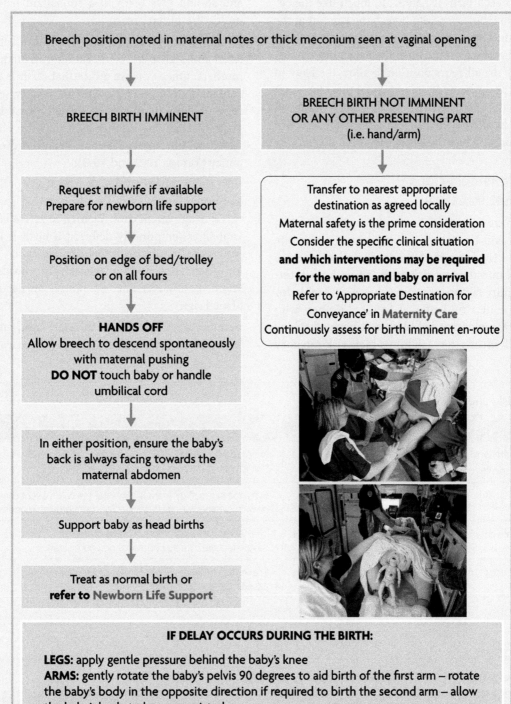

Breech position noted in maternal notes or thick meconium seen at vaginal opening

BREECH BIRTH IMMINENT

BREECH BIRTH NOT IMMINENT OR ANY OTHER PRESENTING PART (i.e. hand/arm)

Request midwife if available
Prepare for newborn life support

Transfer to nearest appropriate destination as agreed locally
Maternal safety is the prime consideration
Consider the specific clinical situation **and which interventions may be required for the woman and baby on arrival**
Refer to 'Appropriate Destination for Conveyance' in Maternity Care
Continuously assess for birth imminent en-route

Position on edge of bed/trolley
or on all fours

HANDS OFF
Allow breech to descend spontaneously with maternal pushing
DO NOT touch baby or handle umbilical cord

In either position, ensure the baby's back is always facing towards the maternal abdomen

Support baby as head births

Treat as normal birth or
refer to Newborn Life Support

IF DELAY OCCURS DURING THE BIRTH:

LEGS: apply gentle pressure behind the baby's knee
ARMS: gently rotate the baby's pelvis 90 degrees to aid birth of the first arm – rotate the baby's body in the opposite direction if required to birth the second arm – allow the baby's body to hang unassisted
HEAD: support the baby with one arm and use the other hand to aid flexion of the back of the baby's head while delivering baby

DO NOT PULL ON THE BABY
DO NOT CLAMP AND CUT THE UMBILICAL CORD DURING THE BIRTH

Figure 10-4 JRCALC algorithm for management of breech birth.

From: Joint Royal Colleges Ambulances Liaison Committee and Association of Ambulance Chief Executives: 2017. Clinical Practice Supplementary Guidelines. Bridgwater: Class Professional Publishing.

The key to the breech birth is hands off, much like the cephalic presentation; however, with breech the key is that the whole birth is hands off completely and allow gravity to assist in the birth. The mother should birth the baby in the standing or preferably the all-fours position to allow the baby to be born without any assistance. It is vital that the fetus is not held or touched as it is birthed because any intervention will prevent the fetal head from engaging into the pelvis and also stimulating the baby to breathe while it is still in utero.

Transport Considerations for the Patient in Labour

When women have their initial antenatal appointment in pregnancy they will be booked in with either a midwife or a consultant. Those booked for midwife-led care are women who fall into the low-risk category, with no countering co-morbidity factors, meaning they are suitable for birth at home or in a midwife-led facility. Women who are booked for a consultant-led birth will have some co-morbidity, which means they fall into a high-risk category

and should give birth in a consultant-led facility with a multi-disciplinary team.

In many areas midwifery services will still attend BBAs and assist ambulance crews in dealing with birth and post-natal mothers. Once you are aware that birth is imminent then contact should be made with midwifery services and ask for a midwife to attend the scene if possible. If this is not possible, then the mother and newborn should be transferred to the appropriate facility according to the local policy (**Tables 10-2** and **10-3**).

Vital signs remain a valuable part of any prehospital patient assessment and should be monitored at appropriate intervals during patient care. Women in active labour may have vital signs temporarily deferred if birth is imminent, personnel are limited, or the primary survey is initially negative for life-threatening abnormalities. This needs constant reassessment, however, does not replace the need or importance of vital signs.

Because of the position of the vena cava, pregnant patients are at risk of hypotension when placed in a supine position.

Table 10-2 Risks and Benefits of Birth on Scene

Benefits	Risks
• At least one additional clinician to assist with the birth • Nobody is needed to drive the transport vehicle at this time	• No progress toward definitive care if complications develop or additional trained personnel or equipment are needed
• Possible helpful assistance from patient's family or bystanders	• Bystanders or patient's family may interfere with patient care, disrupt privacy, or otherwise distract clinicians from providing optimal care
• No vehicle movement, noise, or road hazards to undermine patient care	• The scene may pose safety hazards to the clinicians or patient; may not have adequate climate control for newborn care
• Possibly more room to assess patient and assist in the birth of the newborn	• Scene may have less room, more obstacles, or poor lighting, which make assessment and birth more difficult

© Jones & Bartlett Learning

Table 10-3 Risks and Benefits of Initiating Prompt Transportation

Benefits	Risks
• Movement toward definitive patient care where trained personnel, specialised equipment, and a controlled environment are available	• One less clinician to assist with patient care (this may be mitigated in certain situations if a 3-person training crew is in attendance)
• Patient may have increased privacy in the transport vehicle, without detrimental interference from bystanders or family members	• Limited or no assistance available from family or bystanders
• May avoid safety risks and uncontrolled environmental temperature that may have been present on scene	• Vehicle movement, noise, and road hazards may undermine patient care efforts
• May have more room to assess patient and the newborn than was available on scene • May have better lighting; resuscitation equipment immediately available	• May have less room or less access to the patient for assessment and birth • Restricted maternal position

© Jones & Bartlett Learning

In the supine position, the uterus can compress the inferior vena cava, which can result in decreased cardiac output by up to 40%. This is primarily a complication during the third trimester. Whether placed on an ambulance stretcher or, if following trauma, a longboard, the pregnant patient should be in the lateral position if she has to lay flat and is unable to sit up to displace the uterus from her inferior vena cava and promote optimal blood return to her heart. Stretcher and longboard straps should not be placed over the pregnant patient's gravid abdomen. Place straps or seat belts above and below the patient's abdomen instead during transport.

Table 10-4 Resuscitation-Oriented History: Three Essential Questions
1. Do you have twins or multiple fetuses?
2. When are you due?
3. What colour is the amniotic fluid?

© Jones & Bartlett Learning

Tip

The "urge to push" experienced by most women at the end of labour is a sign that birth is imminent, usually within 30–60 minutes, and the woman should not be moved.

Tip

A large number of out-of-hospital births are pre-term, and the need for resuscitative efforts rises with the number of weeks of prematurity.

Summary of Triage of Patient in Labour

The responses to the key previously asked questions (see Table 10-1), along with visual assessment of the perineum, provide the essential information to triage a labouring woman. Other findings obtained from the maternal history and physical examination influence the decision whether to initiate transport or prepare for birth on scene.

Preparation for Birth
Resuscitation-Oriented History

Many factors in the mother's medical history affect the outcome of the baby and help predict the need for resuscitation of the newly born. However, once the decision has been made to stay on scene, only three questions are pertinent for the immediate safety of the baby (**Table 10-4**).

1. Is there more than one **fetus** present? If twins or multiple newborns are expected, prepare for more than one birth. This may mean finding extra equipment, preparing an

additional warm environment, and planning the management of the first baby while catching the second. This usually requires calling for an additional ambulance, with a paramedic if there is not one on scene.

2. When is your due date? A significant number of out-of-hospital births are pre-term (less than 37 weeks **gestation**), and the further from the expected due date, the greater the chances of the newborn requiring resuscitation. Knowing the due date is important for preparing the right resuscitation equipment for airway management and breathing support.

3. What colour is the **amniotic fluid**? Greenish colour in the amniotic fluid is a sign of passage of **meconium**, which is fetal stool. Meconium is released by the fetus during periods of intrauterine stress, especially hypoxia. It can also be a normal feature of the post-mature fetus, after 40 weeks especially.

Assembling Equipment

If the triage decision is to remain on scene, get the appropriate equipment ready. **Table 10-5** lists the essential ambulance equipment that is recommended in the national maternity pack guidance. **Figure 10-5** shows an example of an obstetric pack.

Case Study 2

You are called to a residence by a woman in labour who has no transportation to the hospital. On arrival you find the woman lying on the floor screaming, "It's coming!" She tells you that this is her sixth baby and the last one came "really quick". Her water broke 30 minutes ago and it was clear. Your visual inspection shows the baby's head is visible and the mother has an urge to push.

1. What three questions are most appropriate to ask at this time to best prepare for birth?

2. What equipment should be prepared for the birth?

Table 10-5 Contents of a Maternity Pack (National Standard, Clinical Practice Guidelines, JRCALC)

Number	Item
1	Sterile disposable umbilical scissors
2	Soft hooded towels
1	Maternity pad
1	Baby hat
4	Umbilical clamps
1	Large plastic bag (to store the **placenta**)
2	Identity bracelets (one for mother and one for baby)
2	Disposable plastic aprons
1	Baby nappy (newborn size)
1	Yellow clinical waste bag
1	Twist tie for the waste bag
1	Sticky label (for the placenta bag)

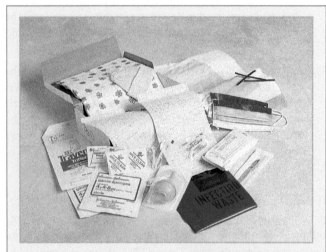

Figure 10-5 An example of an obstetric pack.
© Jones & Bartlett Learning

Warming the Environment

Avoiding hypothermia is a vitally important part of newly born patient care. Before birth, make the room or ambulance as warm as possible. Turn up the heat until it is uncomfortable for an adult. Air blowing across the newly born can lead to heat loss, so turn off all fans. If the setting allows, consider having a family member warm towels in the dryer, or on a radiator in anticipation of the birth.

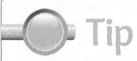

Tip

The presence of meconium increases the risk of resuscitation needs in the newly born.

Positioning of the Mother

Birth is a natural physiological event. However, when it happens unexpectedly prehospital in the presence of ambulance clinicians, it is often seen as an emergency, and the clinician needs to remember that for the woman and her family the birth of a baby is also a highly personal and emotional event. Establish a plan for positioning for birth with the mother, but let her stay in a comfortable position and covered before birth.

The evidence points to the safest position for birth being that of the woman in an upright position, i.e., a standing, squatting or all-fours position. Being in an upright position allows for the pelvic outlet space to increase in diameter and is proven to decrease the time in labour and to decrease the need for interventions.

Infection Prevention and Control

Ensure as far as possible infection prevention and control measures are taken. Although birth is not a sterile procedure, care needs to be taken to ensure the procedure is as clean as possible. Ensure where possible clinicians have washed their hands and have access to several pairs of gloves. The use of disposable incontinence sheets are most helpful in preventing the birthing fluids causing damage to beds or floors, making the clean-up process after the birth easier as well.

Assisting in the Birth

Most mothers birth themselves without any assistance at all. Although the clinician may attempt to coach the birth, as described next, only minimal interference with this natural process is necessary in most cases, with no hands on or contact at all required.

Most births follow this progress:

1. Encourage the mother to push with her contractions when she has the urge to bear down. At the crowning stage, as the widest part is being born encourage small breaths, or little pushes to reduce the risk of perineal tearing. Once the head is born, there is a natural break in contractions. This is to allow the restitution of the fetal head, and this remains a "hands off" process.

2. Next, with the head born DO NOT feel the infant's neck for the umbilical cord. It is not necessary to lift it over the baby's head. This procedure is not required because the

nuchal cord (a cord 360° around the neck) will not prevent the baby from being born, and the procedure has been removed from the birth guidelines. With the next contraction the baby will be born. If the woman is in a standing or upright position, it is important to keep the hands poised ready to catch the infant as the anterior shoulder emerges from behind the mother's symphysis pubis. If the mother is upright then placing a pillow or something soft between the mother's legs for the infant to be born on will help.

3. The newborn should be placed immediately skin-to-skin with the mother if she is receptive to this but must be thoroughly dried off with a dry warm towel, which is then removed. This removes amniotic fluid, prevents heat loss, and stimulates the newborn to breathe. Remove damp towels or blankets from around the baby, place the baby against mother's chest or abdomen skin-to-skin, and cover with clean, dry towels or blankets.

4. The cord must be left alone and unclamped until it has stopped pulsating and has gone flat white and opaque. This can take anything from 5 to 30 minutes. During this time do not hold the baby higher than the mother's breast before clamping the cord, otherwise there is a higher possibility of fetal to placental transfusion.

5. Clamp the cord in two places, ONLY once it has stopped pulsating, 15–20 cm from the umbilicus. Cut the cord between the two clamps (**Figure 10-6**).

6. The last step in the birth process is the delivery of the placenta. This generally occurs spontaneously 15–20 minutes after birth. If the placenta is not expelled 30 minutes after the baby then transfer to hospital should be sought. Do not pull on the umbilical cord to expedite the process.

Separation of the placenta from the uterus is often signalled by a "gush of blood" from the vagina. This can be up to 500 mls, but the normal loss is somewhere between 200–300 mls. This is completely normal and the mother does not need cannulation or fluid administration unless the loss is over 500 mls or the woman is clinically showing signs of shock. Place the placenta in a plastic bag labelled with the mother's name and transport it with the woman for midwife inspection of its completeness.

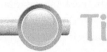

Tip

Birth of the placenta can be encouraged by the mother in the squatting position and encourage her to push with uterine contractions

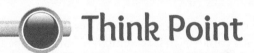

Think Point

Do not hold the baby higher than the breast before clamping the cord.

Maternal and Newborn Complications During Vaginal Birth
Umbilical Cord Prolapse

Disruption of the oxygen and nutrients supplied to the fetus through the umbilical cord can cause devastating injury to the fetus, including fetal death. On rare occasions, the umbilical cord may enter the vaginal cavity before or simultaneously with a birthing fetus. The umbilical cord becomes compressed and the fetal blood supply is compromised. During assessment the umbilical cord will be visible at the vaginal opening. When recognised in the prehospital setting, unless the presenting part is visible and advancing, then transportation should commence immediately to a facility capable of performing an immediate cesarean section. Umbilical cord prolapse is more common in patients with premature rupture of membranes, premature birth, multiple gestation, multiparity, and fetal breech presentations.

If the woman has no contractions or urge to push, then the loop of cord must have minimal handling to prevent spasm. If the loop is so long that replacement would not be feasible, then the advice would be to support the cord loop with a dry pad and the woman's underwear. If the cord is not long, i.e., less than 3 inches in loop, then the JRCALC guidelines permit the clinician, **one** attempt only to perform a replacement manoeuvre. This is as follows:

1. The woman should be informed of the importance of the procedure and a chaperone should be present.

2. Lay her flat on her back with a cushion under her head, keeping her covered when possible to preserve her dignity.

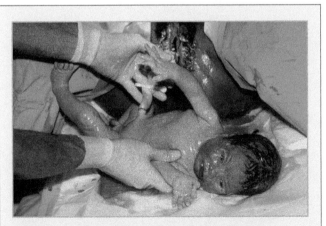

Figure 10-6 Tie or clamp the cord in two places (approximately 3 and 4 inches from its insertion into the baby) ONLY once it has stopped pulsating. Cut the cord between the two ties or clamps.

© Jones & Bartlett Learning

3. Using a gloved hand, two fingers in a downward movement, push the cord inside the vagina just pushing inside at the introitus, not up into the uterus.

4. Once the cord is replaced, replace her underwear with a dry pad also.

5. Remember this manoeuvre can only be used once, so it is recommended this is done once the woman is on the ambulance, because it is not recommended the woman sits onto a carry chair due to the pressure this will place onto the exposed cord. So it is permissible for her to walk a short distance, i.e., from the house to the ambulance.

6. Once the cord is replaced, then the woman should be placed in the exaggerated left lateral position with her hips raised by using a pillow, or if available vacuum splints; see **Figure 10-7**.

Nuchal Umbilical Cord

During the birth, clinicians should NOT assess for the presence of a nuchal cord, which is the umbilical cord wrapped 360° around the neck of the baby at birth. Although it is more common to have the umbilical cord wrapped around the newborn's neck only once, it is possible for the umbilical cord to wrap around the neck more than once. In the presence of a nuchal cord the "somersault manoeuvre" should be utilised at the point of the fetal shoulders birthing (see **Figure 10-8**).

This manoeuvre involves lifting the baby upward toward the pubis in order to untangle the newborn from its cord. The clinician must never be tempted to clamp and cut the cord prior to the birth of the fetal shoulders, in case they fail to be born in the following contraction and a shoulder dystocia is diagnosed. This could be fatal for the fetus.

Meconium

Meconium is fetal stool passed in the uterus. It can be thin and watery or thick and sticky. If the newly born is vigorous

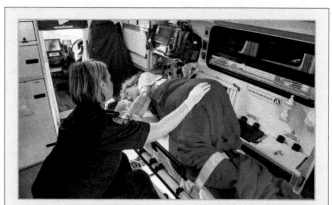

Figure 10-7 Maternal positioning during transport to hospital.
© Class Publishing

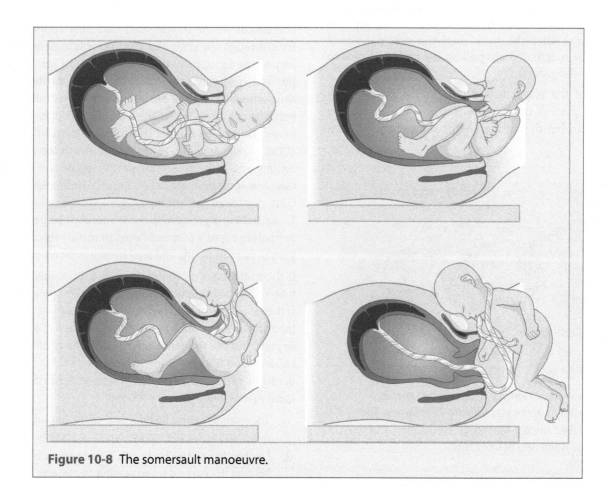

Figure 10-8 The somersault manoeuvre.

(normal respiratory effort, muscle tone, and a heart rate >100 beats/min), then no further action is required.

There are two main reasons for the passage of meconium. The first is physiological, where the infant who is post-dates, i.e., over 40 weeks, passes meconium through a physiological cause. This type of meconium is normally thin and watery, turning the amniotic water a pale yellow or greenish colour. The second cause of meconium release is acute distress, normally hypoxia driven. In these situations the amniotic water will be thick and dark green, often described as "pea soup". This type of meconium release will normally mean the newborn will require resuscitation at birth.

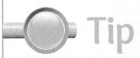

Tip

In the presence of meconium always have a newborn life support (NLS) area prepared if possible before birth.

Shoulder Dystocia

Shoulder dystocia is the mechanical entrapment of a fetus by the maternal symphis pubis, after the fetal head has successfully birthed (**Figure 10-9**). The baby may not be born without hands-on assistance. The following description is the process for the birth (Clinical Practice Guidelines, JR-CALC, 2017):

1. The initial treatment is the McRoberts manoeuvre (**Figure 10-10**), which has two assistants hyper-flex the maternal thighs against the woman's abdomen rotating the pelvis anteriorly, bringing the woman's bottom up off the birthing surface, with the attending clinician applying axial traction to the fetal head for 30 seconds.

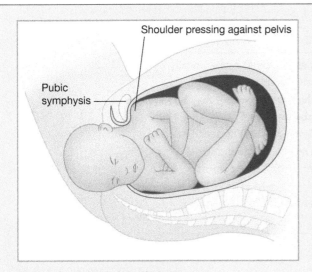

Figure 10-9 Shoulder dystocia
Adapted from http://emedicine.medscape.com/article/1602970-overview

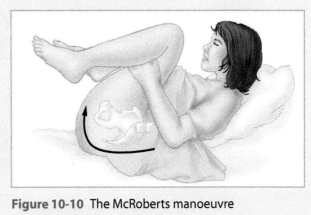

Figure 10-10 The McRoberts manoeuvre
© Jones & Bartlett Learning

2. If this is unsuccessful in facilitating the birth, then continuous suprapubic pressure needs to be applied. This is applied in the direction of the fetal face to try and compress the diameter of the shoulders. Care must be taken that it is in the right direction because misplaced pressure could result in the diameter of the shoulders increasing, and this would make the compaction worse, done for 30 seconds.

3. If that has still not led to the birth, then apply further suprapubic pressure intermittently, as if you were performing CPR. Again this is in the direction of the fetal face to compress the diameter again for 30 seconds.

4. If the birth has still not occurred, then the woman needs to be rolled over into the "all fours" position. This movement may help to shift the fetal shoulder and again axial traction applied to facilitate the birth for 30 seconds.

5. If the baby is still not born after these manoeuvres, then it is time to leave. Rapid removal from the scene is needed.

6. If the woman is upstairs, she will not be able to sit on a carry chair and again will have to walk out of the property to the awaiting ambulance.

Figure 10-11 outlines the JRCALC algorithm for management of shoulder dystocia.

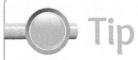

Tip

A real-life experience: A woman was in a tiny upstairs bedroom and the baby was not born despite all the manoeuvres described in this chapter. The clinician grabbed a dressing gown from behind the door and told the woman to put it on, tying it over the bump. This not only protected her dignity but the clinician got her to pull the hem of the gown up between her legs as she descended backwards down the stairs. This created a sling incase the baby made an appearance half way down the stairs, which it did and was safely caught in the gown. The mother made it safely to the bottom of the stairs, much the relief of the crew.

REQUEST A MIDWIFE IF AVAILABLE AND PREPARE FOR NEWBORN LIFE SUPPORT
Position the woman in the McRoberts position
For a solo clinician – ask the woman to hold her legs and push with her next contraction

If shoulders do not release:
Attempt to deliver the baby
- With your hands on the baby's head apply gentle 'axial' traction, keeping the baby's head in line with its spine for up to 30 seconds

Undelivered?

Apply suprapubic pressure with the woman in the McRoberts position
- Identify the position of the fetal back and place assistant on that maternal side
- Using a CPR grip, apply continuous pressure downwards and lateral for 30 seconds (2 fingers above symphysis pubis)
- Encourage the woman to push **OR** attempt gentle 'axial' traction to deliver baby

Undelivered?

- Attempt intermittent 'rocking' suprapubic pressure for 30 seconds and encourage woman to push
- Or attempt gentle 'axial' traction to deliver baby

Undelivered?

- Change the woman's position to 'all fours' and encourage her to push
- Or attempt gentle 'axial' traction to deliver baby

Undelivered?

- Walk the woman to the ambulance and anticipate the birth during transfer
- Convey in a lateral position with legs separated by a blanket to protect the baby's head
- Reassure the woman and provide Entonox as required.

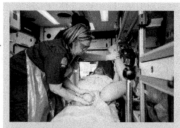

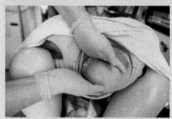

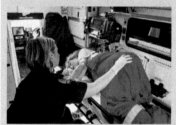

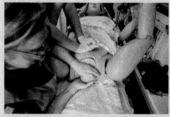

Baby born
Refer to Care of the Newborn

Transfer to the nearest appropriate destination as agreed locally
Maternal safety is the prime consideration
Consider the specific clinical situation **and which interventions may be required for the woman and baby on arrival**
Refer to 'Appropriate Destination for Conveyance' in Maternity Care
Pre-alert stating the obstetric emergency shoulder dystocia
Keep a log of the time each intervention is attempted

Figure 10-11 JRCALC algorithm for management of shoulder dystocia.

From: Joint Royal Colleges Ambulances Liaison Committee and Association of Ambulance Chief Executives: 2017. Clinical Practice Supplementary Guidelines. Bridgwater: Class Professional Publishing.

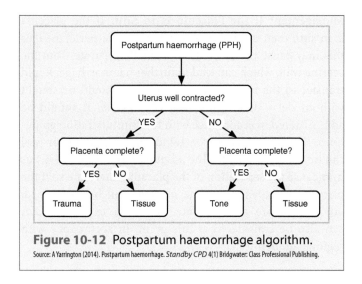

Figure 10-12 Postpartum haemorrhage algorithm.
Source: A Yarrington (2014). Postpartum haemorrhage. *Standby CPD* 4(1) Bridgwater: Class Professional Publishing.

Postpartum Haemorrhage

The most common postpartum maternal complication and leading cause of maternal death worldwide is excessive bleeding after birth. Usually, pregnant women will lose between 200–300 ml of blood with a normal vaginal birth. A postpartum haemorrhage (PPH) is a blood loss of 500 ml or more within 24 hours of birth (**Figure 10-12**). Because estimating blood loss is difficult, one must monitor the postpartum mother's vital signs carefully.

There are 4 causes of a PPH, which are known as the 4 Ts:

- Tone
- Tissue
- Trauma
- Thrombin

By eliminating each one in turn you will determine the cause for the PPH and be able to find the appropriate management.

Tone. Uterine atony (poor tone of the uterus) is the cause of 70–90% of PPHs. Usually, the uterus contracts after birth, occluding the spiral arteries that have provided the blood supply to the placenta during pregnancy. In order to control the blood loss from an atonic uterus, the upper portion of the uterus (called the fundus) must be massaged to encourage the uterine fibres to contract. To perform uterine massage see treatment and management of PPH below.

Trauma. Trauma to the genital tract during the childbirth occurs in approximately 85% of birth. These are wide ranging in terms of severity, from small tears that only involve the skin of the perineum, to deeper tears that affect the muscle layers. Due to an abundant vascular supply, 20% of PPHs are caused by tears. The bleeding can originate from the tear or ruptured vessels within suturing of the perineum, but direct external pressure with a maternity pad or gauze is the mainstay of prehospital management.

Tissue. If there is any tissue left behind after the birth, such as placenta or membrane, the uterus will continue bleeding in order to remove them. This mechanism is responsible for around 10% of PPHs. Retained products may be expelled during fundal massage, causing clots and tissue to be expelled. This is nothing to worry about! The completeness of the placenta and membranes is important, so keep the placenta with the mother so it can be checked to ensure it is complete.

Thrombin. Clotting problems are rare, responsible for only 1% of PPHs. The most serious is disseminated intravascular coagulopathy (DIC), an extremely rare complication, where there is a systemic increase in coagulation and clot formation, with simultaneous impairment of clotting factors and platelets, leading to abnormal and uncontrolled haemorrhage.

Treatment and Management of Postpartum Haemorrhage (PPH)

The management of the PPH has to be done in a step-wise manner gradually working upward to the worst case scenario. The management depends upon whether the placenta has been delivered or remains in situ.

Management If the Placenta Has Delivered. The most common cause of PPH is uterine atony. This is also the easiest to reverse if the placenta is out, by using uterine massage. Uterine massage must not be performed if the placenta is in situ.

To perform uterine massage, first you need to feel for the uterine fundus. This is performed by placing the left-hand just above the umbilicus and then moving behind and downwards towards the symphysis. The contracted uterus should feel hard and firm and sit just below the umbilicus; however, if the uterus feels soft and boggy, then the process of "rubbing up" a contraction should be performed. The fundus of the uterus is massaged in a circular motion in order to encourage the uterus to contract. This process may be quite uncomfortable and entonox can be offered for pain relief. This procedure should only be performed if the placenta has been delivered. While performing uterine massage, clots may be expelled from the vagina. This is to be expected because any tissue retained needs to be expelled. So don't stop if you get clots—carry on its working. Remember the next T: tissue.

If the uterus has been massaged and contraction achieved, careful monitoring should be observed, because if the uterus has lost tone, it is more likely to happen again.

If you are in a service that carries uterotonic or oxytocic drugs, this is when you would administer them. You must check a blood pressure prior to the administration of syntometrine, and if the woman has a BP above 140/90, you must not administer it as this will cause further hypertension. If her BP is low enough for syntometrine, give 1 ml IM. Following its administration, observe blood loss and keep performing uterine massage. If after 15 minutes the syntometrine has not worked to reduce the bleeding, then administer 800 micrograms (mcg) of misoprostol sublingually if available.

Cannulation with a wide bore cannula should be obtained and fluid therapy administered in relation to her BP. If there is ongoing and further bleeding, then tranexamic acid (TXA) should be considered for administration in accordance with service policy.

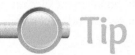

> Syntometrine belongs to the class of drugs known as uterotonics, i.e., they make the uterus contract. In midwifery they are used almost routinely to manage the third stage of labour in "active" management. Each 1 ml ampoule contains 500 micrograms ergometrine maleate and 5 IU oxytocin.

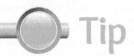

> Misoprostol is a prostaglandin E1 analogue, which works by assisting an atonic uterus to contract, producing the same physiological changes as when the uterus contracts naturally, therefore reducing the bleeding and blood lost.

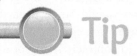

> TXA was included in the management of PPH due to the information brought to light following the WOMAN trial.
>
> The trial, which was published in April 2017, included over 20,000 women from 21 diverse geographical locations worldwide was the largest randomised controlled trial involving women with the clinical diagnosis of PPH.
>
> It showed that with a package of care including oxytocics and TXA administered within 4 hours of a woman experiencing a PPH there was a dramatic improvement in the maternal death statistics. This could have a massive impact on the care given to women, especially in developing countries where haemorrhage is the biggest killer of women. Of the 14 million women who suffered a PPH globally, 100,000 women died in 2015, and 99% of these were in a developing country.

Management If the Placenta Is In Situ. If the placenta is in situ, then uterine massage is not to be performed, as this may cause the placenta to partially separate from the uterine wall, which can lead to further haemorrhage. Rapid transfer to the nearest obstetric facility should be sought without delay. If syntometrine is available, it should be administered in accordance with the administration guidelines. If syntometrine is contraindicated, then misoprostol can be used if available. The administration of these drugs may cause the separation of the placenta, therefore so if the placenta is expelled, uterine massage can be performed, but not before the placenta has been expelled. TXA can also be considered at this point, in accordance with regional guidelines.

Summary of Vaginal Birth

Birth is a natural process that usually does not require any intervention. The birth attendant must simply control the environment and support the woman. A history of prematurity, multiple fetuses, or meconium-stained amniotic fluid suggests higher probability of a depressed newborn, more likely to need support in transition or resuscitation. Review the steps for assisting a birth while on the way to the scene. Have the equipment ready, control the temperature of the environment, and position the mother to facilitate childbirth and care of the newly born. Consider calling a second team if multiple births or complications are anticipated.

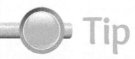

> Encourage the mother to breastfeed the active, vigorous infant. Not only is this good for the baby but it will encourage the release of oxytocin, and this will encourage the uterus to remain contracted and help with maternal bonding.

Immediate Care of the Newborn

A well organised plan guides clinicians through the optimal care of the newborn infant. **Table 10-6** lists the five essential steps to care for every newborn in every setting. Clinicians should keep every infant warm and dry, maintain a patent airway, and support newborn respiratory and circulatory function when indicated. Most term newborns do not require any ALS interventions.

Vigour is an immediate assessment of a newborn infant's appearance. This determination is based on the quality of

Case Study 3

On arriving at the home of a family who had called 999 for a birth imminent, you find a woman lying on the floor who has just given birth to an apparently term female. The infant is lying on the floor, still attached to the umbilical cord. The newborn infant is blue and is not crying or moving.

1. What are the steps in the resuscitation of this newborn?

2. What is the role of vascular access?

respirations or crying, skin colour, and muscle tone. This rapid visual assessment gives clinicians an immediate indication of the clinical status of a newborn infant and guides the approach to assistance in the transition or if resuscitation is required, although it should be noted that 90% of newborns do not require such interventions. The APGAR score (**Table 10-7**) is a numerical representation of vigour obtained at 1 minute and again at 5 minutes after birth, after initiating transition measures, such as drying and stimulating the baby.

Dry and Warm the Baby

At birth the baby is covered in amniotic fluid and can lose a lot of heat through evaporation unless immediately dried. Heat

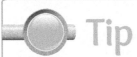

Perform the initial steps of drying, warming, and positioning on all newborns, whether active or depressed.

loss drastically increases the metabolic demand and oxygen consumption. Remove wet towels or blankets from around the baby after drying and replace them with clean, warm, dry towels. This should take no more than 5–10 seconds.

Open the Airway

Open the airway by head positioning. Use of a suction catheter should only be considered if the airway appears obstructed with blood clots or thick particulate meconium. Suction is very rarely required and care must be taken when doing this because suctioning of the nasopharynx may cause an exaggerated vagal response.

A newborn's head is larger than an older child's or an adult's compared to its overall body size, which leads to flexion of the neck in a supine position. This may cause airway occlusion. Extend the head slightly and place a towel under the infant's shoulders to place the airway in a neutral position if the baby is not crying vigorously.

Table 10-6 Organised Approach to Assessment and Care of the Newly Born

Dry and warm the baby
Place the head into the neutral position
Assess breathing
Assess heart rate
Assess colour

© Jones & Bartlett Learning

Table 10-7 APGAR Scoring

Sign	0	1	2
Appearance: Colour	Blue or pale	Acrocyanotic (hands and feet blue only)	Completely pink
Pulse: Heart rate	Absent	<100 bpm	>100 bpm
Grimace: Reflex irritability	No response	Grimace	Crying or active withdrawal
Activity: Muscle tone	Limp	Some flexion	Active motion
Respiration	Absent	Weak cry; hypoventilation	Good; crying

AAP, The APGAR Score, *Pediatrics* Vol. 117 No. 4 April 1, 2006, pp. 1444–1447

Assess Breathing

Most babies will be crying, indicating adequate respiratory effort. Breathing effort may be slightly irregular in normal newborns. Grunting is a sign of increased work of breathing. Gasping occurs pre-arrest and indicates the need for assisted ventilation.

An apnoeic baby, with no visible respiratory effort, requires immediate treatment. Most apnoeic newborns start breathing simply with tactile stimulation. If the baby is completely apnoeic or only has gasping, ineffective respiration after drying, further stimulation is not likely to improve respiratory effort. Begin positive pressure ventilation giving 5 initial inflation breaths. Ensure that rise and fall of the chest is noted. Due to the presence of fluid within the lungs in-utero the initial 2–3 breaths may not show rise and fall, but continue to provide 5 full breaths. The initial inflation breaths are different from ventilation breaths because inflation breaths are slower, over 2–3 seconds. This initial resuscitation should be started without supplemental oxygen attached to the bag-valve-mask device. This represents a huge paradigm shift from decades of resuscitation procedures. Supplementary oxygen, if needed, should be titrated to achieve a pre-ductal oxygen saturation on the commencement of chest compressions (see table in Neonatal Resuscitation Algorithm).

Treatment of an Infant Born to a Mother on Opiates. A special situation occurs when the prehospital professional encounters a newborn with respiratory depression after birth by a drug-addicted mother. Do not give naloxone (Narcan) to the baby if the mother is addicted to opiates. Reversal of opiates may precipitate acute withdrawal symptoms and seizure activity. Assist ventilation with bag-valve-mask and follow the NLS guidelines with rapid transfer to definitive care.

Assess Heart Rate

Bradycardia in a newly born is usually caused by hypoxia, not primary cardiac disease. The crying, active baby usually has an adequate heart rate. Assess heart rate carefully in a baby who is not active or who requires assisted ventilation. This is accomplished by auscultation over the mediastinum.

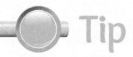

You may encounter pregnant women who have not received antenatal care, or who are addicted to drugs. If the pregnant woman is under the influence of drugs or alcohol then effectively so is her baby because these substances will pass the placental barrier. With such women, it can be difficult to determine how long they have been in labour and what complications they have in addition to their drug addiction. Be prepared for anything.

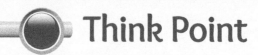

Do not give naloxone to the newborn if the mother is addicted to opiates.

This can be assisted with the use of an ECG as well as a correctly placed SpO_2 probe on the right hand.

Tachycardia (heart rate >160 beats/min) may also be present in a newborn. Severe physiological stress, such as maternal infection or newborn hypovolaemia, may cause an increased fetal heart rate.

Assess Colour

Skin colour assessment in newborns has several unique features. In utero, the fetus depends on the placenta for delivery of oxygen, and blood oxygen concentrations are very low compared to conditions after birth. Therefore, before the initiation of respiration after birth, the infant appears cyanotic.

If the cyanotic newborn is apnoeic, following drying and tactile stimulation begin the 5 positive-pressure inflation breaths. If the baby is breathing, but appears blue, determine if the cyanosis is central (on the trunk and face) or peripheral (limited to the hands and feet). This difference helps with decision making and therapy. If central cyanosis is present, a pulse oximeter with an infant probe should be applied to the right hand, to confirm hypoxia. When hypoxia is present (see table for expected SpO_2 following birth), administer supplemental oxygen by a mask held loosely over the baby's face and titrate to pre-ductal SpO_2.

Peripheral cyanosis, bluish skin colour present only in the extremities, is also termed acrocyanosis. This is a common finding in newborns through the first 24–48 hours of life and requires no therapy.

Infant colour and pulse quality provide an indication of overall perfusion status. Hypovolaemia, shock, and congenital cardiovascular defects may present with central cyanosis, poor overall skin colour, delayed capillary refill, or absent peripheral pulses. Persistent infant bradycardia, tachycardia, or alterations in perfusion may represent a severe condition requiring intervention and transport to definitive care.

General Principles of Newborn Resuscitation

Newborn resuscitation is in 90% of newborns only a mere assistance in the transition from intrauterine to extrauterine life. This is why the 2015 NLS guideline change from the Resuscitation Council also includes a change in title. The full title of the guideline is "Resuscitation and Support of Transition of Babies at Birth". This new title represents the

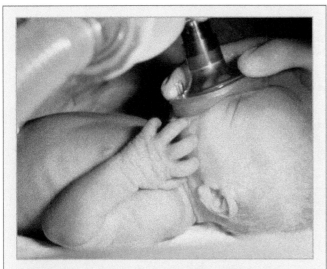

Figure 10-13 Using a bag-valve-mask device on a newborn.
Courtesy of David J. Burchfield, MD.

uniqueness of the baby at birth in that the vast majority of newborns do not require any form of the resuscitation described; they merely need the assistance of stimulating them to support in the transition.

The initial steps of transitioning are completed on every newborn. They include:

1. Dry the baby, remove all wet items, and keep the baby in a warm environment.

2. Perform as assessment of colour, tone, breathing, and heart rate.

When the baby remains depressed after initial drying and warming, begin assisting transition. Use the following sequence:

1. If respiratory effort is absent or gasping, give 5 positive pressure inflation breaths over 2–3 seconds each (**Figure 10-13**). Remember that you are looking to see rise and fall of the chest, and not further to reduce the risk of barotrauma, and this may not be seen in the apnoeic infant until the 2nd or 3rd breath.

2. If the chest wall does not move, then reassess the airway. Check the head position, consider a two-person jaw thrust or inspection and the possibility of an airway adjunct, and repeat these steps until the chest is moving. DO NOT move on to performing chest compressions until the chest wall has moved.

3. Assess heart rate after 30 seconds of adequate ventilation. If less than 60 beats/min, begin chest compressions. Compressions should be delivered a depth of one-third the anteroposterior diameter of the chest. The "two thumb encircling hand" technique is recommended (compressions using two thumbs with fingers encircling the chest and supporting the back). Deliver 90 compressions and 30 ventilations (120 events) per minute with a 3:1 compression to ventilation ratio (**Figure 10-14**).

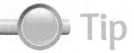

Tip

Good ventilation usually reverses bradycardia.

4. Reassess heart rate after 30 seconds. Continue compressions and positive-pressure ventilation until heart rate is more than 60 beats/min. Positive-pressure ventilations should be continued until the heart rate is more than 100 beats/min.

Specific Newborn Complications
Meconium Aspiration

A child born with any degree of meconium-stained amniotic fluid, who appears active and without respiratory distress, needs only standard care of the newborn. Never suction the airway of crying babies—allow them to clear this themselves. Do not allow prolonged suctioning to delay assisted ventilation or other critical resuscitation measures. Overly aggressive suctioning may cause vagal stimulation and lead to bradycardia and apnoea.

Treatment of Meconium Aspiration in a Non-Vigorous Newborn. If meconium is present and a newborn is not considered vigorous, initial steps of resuscitation should occur. Positive-pressure ventilation should be initiated if the baby is not breathing effectively. Routine intubation for tracheal suctioning is not required.

Pre-term Infants

Premature infants are at risk for a vast array of complications, which increase in likelihood and severity as the degree of prematurity increases. Many of these complications, such as acute respiratory distress syndrome, bronchopulmonary dysplasia, or intraventricular haemorrhage, cannot be adequately managed in the prehospital setting because of the medications or procedures required. In the event of these pre-term babies being born prehospital, clinicians need to provide the warmest environment possible during resuscitation and transport. As outlined in JRCALC 2017, babies born at less than 28 weeks must **not** be placed in plastic bags. Keeping the baby warm is vital. This can be achieved by drying thoroughly and keeping the baby wrapped in towels or blankets. Support ventilations as needed with bag-valve-mask ventilation for those with ineffective respiratory effort and carry out the NLS as required. The more pre-term the infant the more support they are likely to require.

Congenital Disorders
Choanal Atresia

Infants are occasionally born with a complete nasal obstruction (**Figure 10-15**). In severe, untreated cases, this condition may cause newborn death from hypoxia. Unless

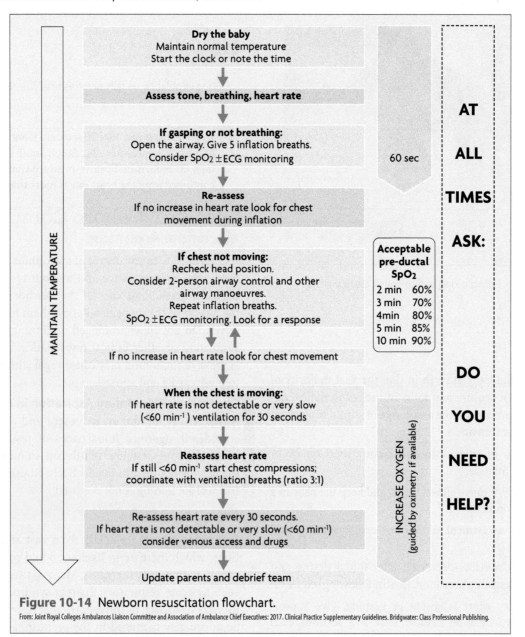

Dry the baby
Maintain normal temperature
Start the clock or note the time

Assess tone, breathing, heart rate

If gasping or not breathing:
Open the airway. Give 5 inflation breaths.
Consider SpO2 ±ECG monitoring

Re-assess
If no increase in heart rate look for chest
movement during inflation

If chest not moving:
Recheck head position.
Consider 2-person airway control and other
airway manoeuvres.
Repeat inflation breaths.
SpO2 ±ECG monitoring. Look for a response

If no increase in heart rate look for chest movement

When the chest is moving:
If heart rate is not detectable or very slow
(<60 min^{-1}) ventilation for 30 seconds

Reassess heart rate
If still <60 min^{-1} start chest compressions;
coordinate with ventilation breaths (ratio 3:1)

Re-assess heart rate every 30 seconds.
If heart rate is not detectable or very slow (<60 min^{-1})
consider venous access and drugs

Update parents and debrief team

MAINTAIN TEMPERATURE

60 sec

INCREASE OXYGEN
(guided by oximetry if available)

AT ALL TIMES ASK:

DO YOU NEED HELP?

Acceptable pre-ductal SpO2

2 min	60%
3 min	70%
4min	80%
5 min	85%
10 min	90%

Figure 10-14 Newborn resuscitation flowchart.

From: Joint Royal Colleges Ambulances Liaison Committee and Association of Ambulance Chief Executives: 2017. Clinical Practice Supplementary Guidelines. Bridgwater: Class Professional Publishing.

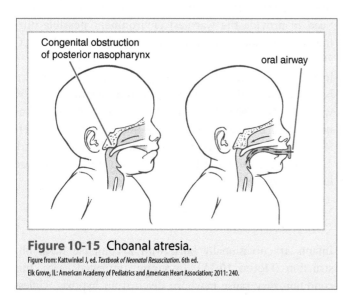

Congenital obstruction
of posterior nasopharynx

oral airway

Figure 10-15 Choanal atresia.

Figure from: Kattwinkel J, ed. *Textbook of Neonatal Resuscitation.* 6th ed.
Elk Grove, IL: American Academy of Pediatrics and American Heart Association; 2011: 240.

crying, newborn infants breathe exclusively through their nasal passages. Patients with choanal atresia may present with profound respiratory distress that resolves during crying episodes. If prehospital clinicians suspect this condition, place an oral airway to assist with respiratory efforts. The respiratory distress should improve. Monitor SpO$_2$ levels and support with oxygen therapy as required and transport to definitive care rapidly.

Pierre Robin Syndrome

Pierre Robin syndrome is another potential cause of airway obstruction in newborn infants (**Figure 10-16**). An under-developed mandible causes the tongue to obstruct the posterior pharynx. This can usually be treated in the prehospital setting by turning the infant onto his or her stomach (prone) for rapid transport to definitive care.

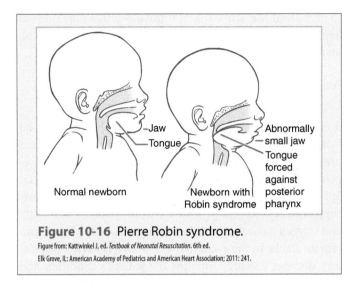

Figure 10-16 Pierre Robin syndrome.

Figure from: Kattwinkel J, ed. *Textbook of Neonatal Resuscitation*. 6th ed. Elk Grove, IL: American Academy of Pediatrics and American Heart Association; 2011: 241.

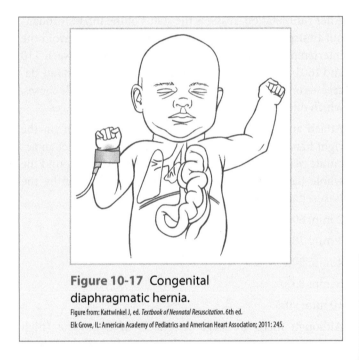

Figure 10-17 Congenital diaphragmatic hernia.

Figure from: Kattwinkel J, ed. *Textbook of Neonatal Resuscitation*. 6th ed. Elk Grove, IL: American Academy of Pediatrics and American Heart Association; 2011: 245.

Congenital Diaphragmatic Hernia

It is possible for infants to be born without a completely intact diaphragm. The stomach or intestines may migrate into the chest cavity, collapsing lungs or inhibiting ventilation. Clinicians should suspect congenital diaphragmatic hernia when an infant presents with a flat (scaphoid) abdomen and respiratory distress (**Figure 10-17**). Prolonged bag-valve-mask ventilations force additional air into the infant's stomach, worsening respiratory distress. Treatment in the prehospital setting requires prompt endotracheal intubation and OG tube to decompress stomach if the skill is available to the clinician. Prompt transport and cautious bag-valve-mask technique may be the only intervention available.

Congenital Cardiovascular Defects

Approximately 1% of infants are born with a congenital cardiovascular defect. Defects may involve several different parts of the heart and one or more of the great vessels in the chest. Diagnosis is often impossible without the assistance of a paediatric cardiologist or similar specialist, but certain cues may alert the clinician to infants with these conditions. Cyanosis, shock, pulmonary oedema, and altered peripheral pulses occur in infants with cardiovascular defects and may present across the full spectrum of severity. Clinicians should initiate immediate transport to definitive care whenever a congenital cardiovascular defect is suspected. Many types of defects present with persistent cyanosis that cannot be corrected in the prehospital setting, even with optimal resuscitation measures. Conversely, resuscitation with high concentrations of oxygen may actually worsen many of these conditions by altering the pulmonary circulation and vascular resistance. Clinicians are often limited to basic supportive care and prompt transport of infants with suspected cardiovascular defects.

Shock

Shock at birth is most commonly caused by asphyxia (severe hypoxia in the uterus or during birth) and acidosis. Blood loss during birth caused by umbilical cord avulsion or fetal-placental transfusion is an uncommon cause of shock in the newly born. Signs and symptoms of shock, whatever the cause, include abnormal appearance (lethargy, hypotonia), abnormal colour (pallor, mottling), tachycardia, and prolonged capillary refill time. Hypothermia may also mimic these findings.

Treatment of Shock. Because intrauterine or perinatal asphyxia is the most common cause of depression in the newly born, initial resuscitative efforts should ensure adequate oxygenation and ventilation. Volume resuscitation is rarely needed. In exceptional circumstances where hypovolaemic shock is suspected, consider placing an IV or IO line, and refer to JRCALC for dosage guidelines. Fluid resuscitation should be limited in premature infants, because giving volume too rapidly has been associated with intraventricular haemorrhage.

Vascular Access. Vascular access is rarely needed in newborn infants in the prehospital setting because resuscitation is largely focused on airway management and breathing. In reality, establishing vascular access is challenging in infants and its benefits must be carefully weighed against prolonged on-scene time and potential complications. IV access may be attempted in the antecubital fossa or the saphenous vein at the ankle. IO infusion is an alternative.

Newborn Hypoglycaemia. The depressed newborn or premature baby is at risk for hypoglycaemia, but this complication is unlikely to develop in the first 30 minutes of life. If a newborn is well it does not require a blood glucose test. The only newborns who require a blood glucose level test are newborns who require resuscitation at birth. Hypoglycaemia in a baby with no other risk factors is a reading of <1.0 mmol/l; however, a compromised newborn may be hypoglycaemic with a reading of <2.5 mmols/l or if symptomatic then an urgent review must be sought as per JRCALC guidelines.

If the clinician is concerned that the infant may be hypoglycaemic but is active, is in no respiratory distress, and has a suck reflex, allow the infant to breastfeed if the mother wishes to.

Signs of hypoglycaemia in the newborn include:

- Jitteriness
- Irritability
- Lethargy
- Apnoea episodes
- Convulsions (JRCALC 2017)

Summary of Resuscitation of the Newborn

A variety of newborn conditions present with airway, respiratory, or cardiovascular compromise. The primary treatment of the depressed newborn involves reversal of hypoxia with immediate bag-valve-mask inflation breaths. If the child does not improve, following effective rise and fall of the chest and effective ventilation, then begin chest compressions on the scene before transport. Initiate oxygen administration during newborn resuscitation only once CPR is being performed. Shock is rare, and is most commonly the result of asphyxia. Hypovolaemia is an uncommon cause of shock in the newly born. If hypovolaemic shock is suspected, transport immediately and initiate volume resuscitation by IV or IO access.

Transport Considerations

Depending on local policy, clinicians may need to transport healthy infants who have had an uncomplicated birth in the prehospital setting or critical infants in continued cardiopulmonary arrest. The degree of monitoring and ongoing intervention depends entirely on the clinical status of the patient. All infants require a warm environment. Every infant needs to be secured during transport in a manner that will not cause devastating injuries if the transport vehicle is involved in a collision during the transport (see Chapter 15). Transportation and the degree of intervention by the clinician will depend upon local policy and community midwifery services that are available to come out to the property and discharge on scene.

Healthy Infant

The active, term infant requires no intervention, be sure the child is restrained as per local policy. Encourage the mother to breastfeed the active infant if possible. This may prevent hypoglycaemia and promote maternal–infant bonding, uterine contraction, and decreased uterine bleeding.

Newborn With Complications

Oxygen Therapy

It is not appropriate to give supplemental oxygen to all infants. Infants with congenital cardiovascular defects and preterm infants should receive only limited amounts of oxygen during transport and should be titrated to pre-ductal SpO_2 levels. Most infant conditions do not require any supplemental oxygen, provided that the infant's heart rate and oxygen saturation can be continuously monitored and remain stable. In the event that a newborn is having respiratory distress, carefully monitor the patient's condition and provide only the oxygen necessary titrated to SpO_2 levels.

Monitoring

After resuscitation, reassess the status of the infant throughout transport. Place cardiac leads on the chest to avoid the interference from moving limbs. A heart rate between 110 and 160 beats/min is normal in a newly born. If heart rate decreases or increases unexpectedly, search for possible causes, which often include airway or respiratory compromise.

Attach an infant pulse oximetry probe to a finger on the right hand, for a pre-ductal reading. If unable to get an accurate reading, the probe may have to be placed around the whole hand. Normal saturation levels as outlined by the Resuscitation Council UK are:

2 min: 60%

3 min: 70%

4 min: 80%

5 min: 85%

10 min: 90%

Although there are negative effects of hyperoxia (high oxygen saturation) in the newly born infant, if the baby is respiratory compromised, the prehospital goal should be to ensure adequate oxygenation through administration of supplemental oxygen and assisted ventilation according to recorded observations.

Hypothermia

Hypothermia develops quickly in newly born infants. Oxygen demand triples when skin temperature drops by 1 degree. Signs of hypothermia are similar to those of shock. Keep the baby warm during transport. National standard maternity packs state there should be a hat available to cover the infant's head. Turn the heat on in the ambulance even at the risk of discomfort to the mother and crew. Prior to transport, place the baby on the mother's bare chest (skin-to-skin contact) and cover both of them to maintain the infant's temperature.

Transport Destination

It is impossible to account for all potential variables when discussing transport destination. When choosing a receiving hospital, clinicians should consider the condition of the mother and newborn, patient preference, transport times, and the obstetric and neonatal capabilities of the potential receiving hospitals. In obstetric emergency situations it may be appropriate to bypass a smaller midwife-led unit or birthing centre to take the infant to a larger tertiary care centre where specialty services are immediately available. In other instances, clinicians may choose the closest unit.

Summary

Clinicians are in the unique position to provide assistance to patients in labour outside the hospital setting, assist with birth, and provide immediate life-saving care to compromised newborns. Decisions and interventions performed by clinicians have a potential to impact the health and lives of a pregnant mother and her baby.

CASE STUDY ANSWERS

Case Study 1 — page 194

First decide whether to transport the mother to the nearest hospital or to prepare for the birth. Ask if this is a first pregnancy. If the mother has given birth before, how long was the labour? Does the mother feel the urge to push? If the mother feels the urge to push, then examine for the presence of the presenting part. If the baby is not visible, wait and examine again during the next contraction.

If you decide to manage the birth at the scene, obtain a resuscitation-oriented history. Are twins present? What is the due date? What colour was the amniotic fluid when the membranes ruptured? These questions assist you in preparation.

If the child is crowning at the perineum, open the delivery pack, familiarise yourself with the contents, and make sure all necessary equipment is present. Warm the environment and get clean towels to dry the baby. Get or make a hat to place over the child's head to reduce heat loss once born and dried. Assist the mother into a comfortable position for her to give birth in; standing, squatting or all fours are the best.

Case Study 2 — page 199

If time allows, review the procedure for birth while on the way to the address. On arrival, first plan for appropriate positioning of the mother. Discuss the position with the patient ahead of time so that she understands the plan for the birth. The woman should be encouraged into a comfortable position for her and encourage her to be mobile and if possible not lay flat on her back to avoid supine hypotension.

Obtain resuscitation-oriented history. Are twins present? What is the due date? What colour was the amniotic fluid when the membranes ruptured?

Clear amniotic fluid implies there is no meconium. Meconium is released by the fetus in conditions of stress. Although the presence of clear fluid does not rule out the possibility of a depressed newly born, it is a reassuring sign and increases the chances of an active child who will need only the initial steps of standard newly born care.

Equipment prepared should include the delivery pack, a neonatal resuscitation area and plenty of towels (warm if possible) should be readily available.

Case Study 3 — page 207

The baby is in acute distress and needs immediate intervention. Thoroughly dry the baby, position her on her back, with the head in the neutral position, a shoulder roll may help this. If possible logistically leave the cord intact and provide the initial 5 inflation breaths observing for chest rise. Assess the baby's colour, tone, breathing and heart rate. It the chest has not risen, inspect the airway and suction only if necessary with the use of a paediatric laryngoscope blade. An oralpharangeal airway (OPA) may be inserted if the baby lacks tone. If the initial inflation breaths had not made the chest rise, then repeat the initial 5 inflation breaths.

If the chest had risen on the first 5 inflation breaths, then assess again the baby's colour, tone, breathing and heart rate, if the heart rate is absent or less than 60 ventilate for 30 seconds. After 30 seconds of adequate assisted ventilation, assess the heart rate. If the heart rate is less than 60 beats/min, cut the cord if it has not been already and begin chest compressions. Administer three compressions followed by one bag-valve-mask ventilation. The encircling technique is the method most favoured for delivery of the compressions and oxygen must now be introduced according to the baby's SpO_2 readings.

If the infant does not respond to these efforts with improvement in tone, colour, and heart rate, then preparations to move the baby should now be made.

Optimal cardiopulmonary resuscitation requires three individuals: one to assist ventilation, one to administer chest compressions, and one to prepare the equipment and attach monitoring.

ALS | Although vascular access is not usually needed for newly born resuscitation, this baby is also at high risk for hypoglycaemia and hypotension during transport and may benefit from IV access. Attempt an IV or IO line in transport. Check the capillary glucose and treat accordingly. Because further resuscitation may be necessary, secure the infant to the stretcher and transport with continuous ECG and oxygen saturation monitoring. Consider transport to a facility with the correct level of neonatal intensive care. This baby is likely to need ongoing critical care and remember the baby may be taken to ED for stabilisation prior to admission to the neonatal unit, depending on local protocol.

SUGGESTED READINGS

Textbooks

American Academy of Family Physicians. *Advanced Life Support in Obstetrics Provider Manual*. Kansas: AAFP; 2012.

American Academy of Orthopaedic Surgeons. *Emergency Care and Transportation of the Sick and Injured*. 10th ed. Burlington, MA: Jones & Bartlett Learning; 2011.

JRCALC *Clinical Practice Supplementary Guidelines*. Bridgwater: Class Professional Publishing; 2017

Woollard M, Hinshaw K, Simpson H, Wieteska S, (eds). *Pre-hospital Obstetric Emergency Training*. Oxford: Wiley-Blackwell; 2009.

Articles

Davis, A (2013). Choice, policy and practice in maternity care since 1948. http://www.historyandpolicy.org/policy-papers /papers/choice-policy-and-practice-in-maternity-care-since-1948. Accessed 19 March, 2017.

Say L, Chou D, Gemmill A, Tunçalp Ö, Moller AB, Daniels J, Gülmezoglu AM, Temmerman M, Alkema L. Global causes of maternal death: a WHO systematic analysis. *Lancet Glob Health*. 2014;2(6):e323–333.

Smith LA, Price N, Simonite V, Burns EE. Incidence of and risk factors for perineal trauma: a prospective observational study. *BMC Pregnancy and Childbirth*. 2013;13(1):59.

The Lancet (2017) WOMAN: reducing maternal deaths with tranexamic acid. *The Lancet*, 389(10084):2081.

WOMAN Trial Collaborators (2017) Effect of early tranexamic acid administration on mortality, hysterectomy, and other morbidities in women with post-partum haemorrhage (WOMAN): an international, randomised, double-blind, placebo-controlled trial. *The Lancet*, 389(10084):2081.

Wyckoff MH, Aziz K, Escobedo MB, et al. Part 13: Neonatal Resuscitation: 2015 American Heart Association Guidelines Update for Cardiopulmonary Resuscitation and Emergency Cardiovascular Care. *Circulation*. 2015;132(suppl 2):S543–S560.

Resources

Emc (2018), *Syntometrine Ampoules*. https://www.medicines.org.uk/emc/product/865. Accessed 7 February, 2018.

FIGO. *Treatment of Postpartum Haemorrhage with Misoprostol*. FIGO: London; 2012.

MBRRACE-UK. *Saving Lives, Improving Mothers' Care – Lessons learned to inform maternity care from the UK and Ireland Confidential Enquiries into Maternal Deaths and Morbidity 2013–15*. Oxford: National Perinatal Epidemiology Unit, University of Oxford; 2017.

Office for National Statistics. (2016). Statistical bulletin: Birth characteristics in England and Wales: 2015 https://www.ons.gov .uk/peoplepopulationandcommunity/birthsdeathsandmarriages/livebirths/bulletins/birthcharacteristicsinenglandandwales /2015#women-aged-between-35-and-39-are-most-likely-to-have-a-home-birth Accessed 18 June, 2018.

Pilbery R. Meningococcal Disease. *Standby CPD*. 2011;1(7).

Resuscitation Council (UK) Resuscitation and support of transition of babies at birth. (2015). https://www.resus.org.uk /resuscitation-guidelines/resuscitation-and-support-of-transition-of-babies-at-birth/. Accessed 18 June, 2018.

World Health Organization (2017). *WHO Recommendations on Prevention and Treatment of Postpartum Haemorrhage and the WOMAN Trial*. http://www.who.int/reproductivehealth/topics/maternal_perinatal/pph-woman-trial/en/. Accessed 19 January, 2018.

World Health Organization. *WHO Recommendation on Tranexamic Acid for the Treatment of Postpartum Haemorrhage*. Geneva: WHO; 2017.

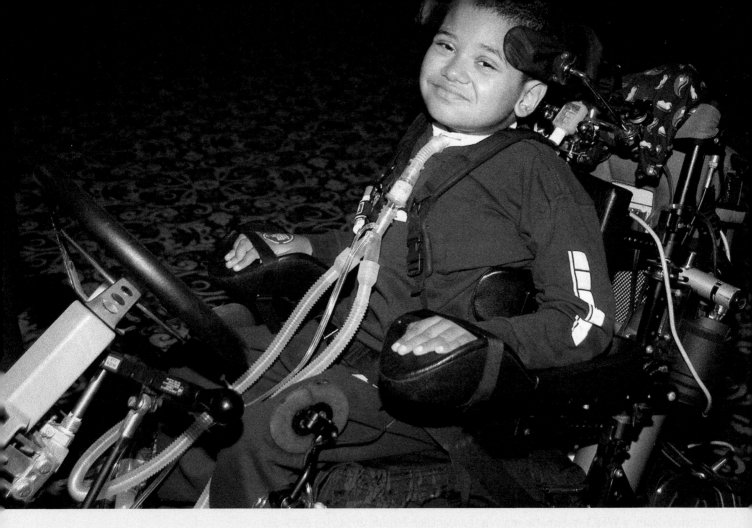

Learning Objectives

1. Define and describe two examples of cognitive disabilities, physical disabilities, and chronic conditions seen in children.

2. List important modifications of field assessment techniques for children with special health care needs (CSHCN).

3. Outline common transport considerations for CSHCN.

4. Describe the most common complications associated with assistive devices (tracheostomy tubes, central venous lines, gastrostomy tubes or gastric feeding tubes, cerebrospinal fluid (CSF) shunts, ostomies, implantable pacemakers and defibrillators) and the emergency management of those complications.

5. Discuss the management of behavioural emergencies in children.

6. Describe the use of health information technology (HIT) including an interoperable emergency information form (EIF) or Emergency Health Care Plan for CSHCN.

Children With Special Health Care Needs

Chapter 11

Introduction

According to an article by McPherson in *Pediatrics*, children with special health care needs (CSHCN) are defined as "those who have or are at an increased risk for a chronic physical, developmental, or emotional condition and who also require health and related services of a type or amount beyond that required by children generally".

The conditions can be either acquired or congenital. These children are a diverse group of patients who frequently need out-of-hospital emergency assessment and treatment. This high-user group includes but is not limited to children who were born prematurely; have suffered closed head injury and have central nervous system (CNS) injuries; or have chronic problems of the lungs, brain, or kidneys. Examples of acquired conditions include cerebral palsy or bronchopulmonary dysplasia. Examples of congenital problems are cyanotic heart disease or spina bifida.

Children assisted by or dependent on technology are a subgroup of CSHCN who need medical devices for their survival. Common devices include tracheostomy tubes, home ventilators, indwelling central venous lines, feeding tubes, pacemakers, and cerebral spinal fluid (CSF) shunts.

Today CSHCN are surviving longer and often live at home. They need emergency medical care more frequently than children without special health care needs. Because of their unique baseline status, CSHCN pose unique challenges in field assessment and treatment. Therefore, prehospital professionals should recognise common types of CSHCN, incorporate modifications during assessment, and understand management of frequent problems.

Cognitive and Physical Disabilities

The Disability Discrimination Act (DDA) (1995), since replaced by The Equality Act (2010), defines a disabled person as a person with "a physical or mental impairment which has a substantial and long-term adverse effect on his ability to carry out normal day-to-day activities".

Case Study 1

You are called to the scene of a 9-month-old girl with multiple underlying medical problems, including ventilator dependence through a tracheostomy tube.

On your arrival, her caregiver states that the girl has had difficulty breathing all day with fever and increased tracheostomy secretions. The child has cerebral palsy, with spasticity and a seizure disorder. She depends on a ventilator because of chronic lung disease as a result of prematurity at birth and respiratory distress syndrome. The child receives carbamazepine for her seizures and received her morning dose. Currently, she is receiving her feedings through her gastrostomy tube, which is connected to a pump.

Your assessment shows a child who is in bed and connected to a home ventilator. She does not engage visually and has subcostal retractions and nasal flaring. Her skin is pink. She has wheezing and crackles on lung examination. Her heart rate is 130 beats/min, despite a ventilator rate of 20 breaths/minute, she is breathing at an additional rate of 20 breaths/minute, blood pressure is 85 mm Hg/palp, and pulse oximetry is 90%. Her ventilator is set at 20 breaths/min.

1. What are the key principles in assessing this child?

2. Describe treatment and transport approaches.

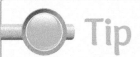 **Tip**

Intellectual disability is less offensive and is the preferred term when referring to those with cognitive disabilities.

Mental processes, such as judgment, reasoning, memory, and comprehension, are cognitive in nature and develop as the child acquires knowledge. Cognitive impairments are present when there is an alteration in the child's ability to think, reason, learn, and abstract. Several examples are outlined in **Table 11-1**.

Physical disabilities may alter the child's ability to be mobile or to accomplish activities of daily living independently. Medical and traumatic emergencies may occur that have nothing to do with the actual physical impairment. Several examples of physical conditions are outlined in **Table 11-2**.

Chronic conditions are present when the child receives ongoing treatment for an injury or illness. Even if the child seems to be healthy, he or she may be on maintenance medications or treatments to prevent complications. Examples of chronic conditions are listed in **Table 11-3**.

Assessment of CSHCN
Modifications

The most important resource for the prehospital provider is the child's caregiver. He or she usually knows how to care for the child's particular condition and understands the child's equipment. Often caregivers have forms or cards that outline the child's medical history, medications, and **baseline** general appearance, oxygen saturation, and vital signs.

Begin evaluation of CSHCN with emergency paediatric assessment techniques adjusted to the child's developmental level, rather than his or her chronologic age. Caregivers can usually provide the child's developmental age, weight, and baseline vital signs. *With children assisted by technology, do not become distracted by their specialised equipment.* Care for the child, not the machinery. Caregivers are often extremely helpful in figuring out the baseline status of CSHCN or in operating or troubleshooting the equipment. *Ask for assistance from the caregiver!*

The assessment of CSHCN has the following important modifications:

1. Baseline status: Ask the caregivers what is usual for the child. Most likely, they will know the child's baseline better than anyone.

2. Rely on the caregivers' opinions: What do they think is wrong? In what ways is the child "acting differently"?

3. If the child is physiologically stable, take a full history on scene. Caregivers usually know the child's medical history, health problems, medications, medical devices, and current complaints. They are also aware of what approaches work best.

4. The child may be slow to answer questions or may be unable to talk. Use a patient approach to the stable child and begin by talking directly to the child, rather than to their caregiver.

5. Seemingly minor illnesses can be life-threatening in some CSHCN. An example is a cold in a child with chronic lung

Table 11-1 Examples of Cognitive Disabilities

Disability	Definition	Behaviours
Attention-deficit/ hyperactivity disorder (ADHD)	Hyperactivity, impulsivity, or periods of inattention	• Usually present before 7 years of age • Occur for at least 6 months • No identifiable cause • Children experience difficulty with impulse control, motor activity, and sustained attention
Autism	Pervasive, developmental disorder characterised by a lack of social interaction and a lack of communication skills	• Speech is affected. May repeat words spoken by others. May not speak at all. • Inability to maintain eye contact • Decreased number of play interests and activities • May exhibit repetitive behaviours (e.g., hand flapping, rocking, flipping a light switch, spinning in circles)
Intellectual disability	Limited mental function in two or more of the following areas: • Self-care • Social skills • Communication • Home living • Health and safety • Self-direction • Leisure • Functional academics • Community use	• Causes are many, and include disease, toxin exposure, genetic causes, metabolic disorders, and psychiatric conditions • Support and therapy are required to participate in activities of daily living

Adapted from: Wertz, E. (2002). *Emergency Care for Children*. Albany, NY: Delmar.

Table 11-2 Examples of Physical Disabilities

Disability	Definition	Characteristics
Cleft lip	The presence of one or more openings in the upper lip, caused by a genetic anomaly; openings may be an indent in one or both sides of the upper lip, or a deep, wide opening up to the nose.	• Infants may have difficulty sucking; creates difficulty feeding and therefore difficulty in receiving adequate nutrition • May affect the teeth, which may be absent or deformed
Cleft palate	An opening in the middle of the upper palate of the mouth, caused by a genetic anomaly; often exists concurrently with cleft lip. May occur in soft palate alone, or may extend through the hard palate into the nose.	• Creates difficulty feeding and therefore difficulty in receiving adequate nutrition • May cause choking, aspiration, vomiting • Ear infections and speech impairments are common

Hearing impairment	A condition in which the ear has a reduced response to pitch and loudness.	• Types:
		  - Hard of hearing: person has impaired hearing ability
		  - Deaf: person is born with inability to hear
		• Speaking ability can be affected
		• Potential solutions: hearing aid, cochlear implant, sign language, lip reading, or separate communication device

Visual impairment	A condition in which the eye has a reduced ability to see.	• Can be caused by obstruction that prevents light from reaching the retina
		• Degrees of visual impairment:
		  - Partial sight: some visual impairment
		  - Low vision: inability to read at usual viewing distance, even with eyeglasses or contact lenses
		  - Legally blind: less than 20/200 vision in at least one eye or a very limited field of vision
		  - Totally blind: no vision
		• Total blindness requires use of nonvisual media or reading by Braille

Adapted from: Wertz, E. (2002). *Emergency Care for Children*. Albany, NY: Delmar.

Table 11-3 Examples of Chronic Conditions

Condition	Definition	Characteristics
Asthma (reactive airway disease)	A disease caused by increased responsiveness of the tracheobronchial tree to various stimuli, resulting in inflammation, bronchoconstriction, mucosal oedema, profuse secretions, and ultimately severe airflow obstruction	• Most common chronic disease of childhood; affects 1.1 million children (1 in 11 children) in the UK (https://www.asthma.org.uk/about/media/facts-and-statistics/) • Possible causes of an asthma attack include upper respiratory infection, exercise, exposure to cold air, emotional stress, and passive exposure to smoke • Patient experiences tachypnoea, tachycardia, increased work of breathing, and wheezing on exhalation

Bronchopulmonary dysplasia (BPD)	Chronic lung disease that develops in premature infants	• Potential causes: pneumonia, cyanotic heart disease, meconium aspiration, persistent pulmonary hypertension; also can occur in response to oxygen and positive pressure ventilation given after birth
		• Patient usually has respiratory distress
		• Long-term complications:
		  - Hyperexpansion of lungs
		  - Airway hyperreactivity
		  - Infections
		  - Gastroesophageal reflux
		  - Cardiac conditions
		  - Seizures
		  - Poor growth and nutrition, failure to grow
		  - Neurodevelopmental conditions
		  - Visual problems
		  - Overall decreased pulmonary function

Cancer	A pathological lack of regulation of production of cells, leading to a neoplasm or tumour	• There are multiple types, determined by location, signs, and symptoms • Chemotherapy and radiation treatments are used; these can produce nausea, vomiting, hair loss, decreased appetite, fatigue, and burns to the skin
Cerebral palsy	A disorder of movement and posture that results from brain injury during foetal development or during delivery	• Symptoms: abnormal muscle tone, poor coordination, fixation and flexion of a joint, "scissoring" of the legs, exaggerated arching of the back, perceptual problems, intellectual involvement, language deficits • Patient may wear ankle-foot orthosis or braces to help prevent contractures • Patient may use a specialised wheelchair controlled by hand or head movements
Congenital heart disease (CHD)	Functional or structural defect of heart or great vessels formed in utero	• Major cause of death during first year of life • Cause unknown, suspected to be mother who is older than 40, has type I diabetes, is an active alcoholic, or who contracts rubella (measles) during pregnancy • Can be cyanotic or acyanotic • Signs and symptoms: tachycardia, tachypnoea, dyspnoea, costal retractions, oedema, diaphoresis with exertion, distended neck and peripheral veins, mottled skin caused by poor perfusion, cold extremities, hypotension, slow capillary refill, clubbed toes and fingers
Cystic fibrosis	A condition in which mucus-producing or exocrine glands do not function properly	• Involves sweat and sebaceous glands • Progressive • Symptoms: thick mucous gland secretions, autonomic nervous system abnormalities, high sodium and chloride concentrations in sweat • Complications: pulmonary complications, drug-resistant infections, impaired digestion or absorption of nutrients
Down syndrome	A congenital disorder in which a person is born with three copies of chromosome 21; also called trisomy 21	• Patients have varying levels of cognitive delay • 50% have some form of congenital heart defect • Increased risk of medical complications: cardiovascular, endocrine, orthopaedic, haematological, neurological, gastrointestinal

Condition	Definition	Characteristics
Haemophilia	A congenital condition in which the patient lacks one or more of the blood's normal clotting factors	• Prolonged bleeding can occur anywhere inside the body or from the body • Bleeding into joint cavities is most frequent, affecting range of motion • Children may receive in-home transfusions of the missing clotting factor
Human immuno-deficiency virus (HIV) / Acquired immunodeficiency syndrome (AIDS)	HIV: a virus that is transmitted through direct contact with bodily fluids, and which causes AIDS AIDS: disease causing decreased immunity, which leads to opportunistic infections; debilitating with poor prognosis	• Present in children whose mothers were HIV positive • Symptoms include poor weight gain, opportunistic infections
Muscular dystrophy	Genetic, progressive, disabling muscle disorder in which muscle fibres gradually degenerate	• Multiple types occur • Symptoms: muscle weakness, muscle wasting, deformity, loss of strength, contractures • Psychologically, many children understand that they will eventually be completely dependent on someone else for their care and then die from the disease

Spina bifida	A congenital anomaly where the posterior elements of the vertebrae have failed to fuse together; the spinal cord and meninges may protrude	• Forms:
		  - Myelomeningocele or meningomyelocele: sac on outside of body contains portion of spinal cord with nerves, spinal fluid, and meninges
		  - Meningocele: sac-like cyst contains CSF and meninges
		  - Encephalocele: meninges and brain herniate through defect in skull; sac present on back of neck
		  - Most children have an Arnold-Chiari malformation (ACM) in which a portion of the brain herniates through an enlarged foramen magnum
		• Leads to neurological impairment in the lower extremities
		• Surgery to repair the defect usually occurs soon after birth
		• Most children have hydrocephalus and have a shunt implanted to drain the extra CSF
		• Symptoms: decrease in skin sensation leading to pressure sores, loss of bladder or bowel control, and loss of voluntary muscle movement
		• Latex allergies are VERY common

Transplants	Performed in children because of defects in organ structure, organ failure, or disease	• Kidney, liver, and heart transplants are most common in children • Medications are given to lessen the potential for rejection of the transplanted organ • Complications: immunosuppression (most frequent), infections, organ rejection

Adapted from: Wertz, E. (2002). *Emergency Care for Children*. Albany, NY: Delmar.

disease who is dependent on a ventilator. The child may have little reserve and may easily become hypoxic.

6. Communicate with the child using developmentally appropriate language, gestures, and techniques, as discussed in the *Using a Developmental Approach* chapter.

7. If a caregiver is not present, find out if the child has a form or card with information about his or her medical problem, normal vital signs, medications, and other important medical data. There are several versions of this medical information card depending on location. Northern England Network has developed an Emergency Health Care Plan in their region. The Council for Disabled Children outline core principles for Emergency Health Care Plans, and have also developed a generic NHS template. ReSPECT: Recommended Summary Plan for Emergency Care and Treatment offers further information.

8. Look for a bracelet or necklace that might describe the child's condition.

9. The usual baseline vital signs for a CSHCN may be "out of the normal range" compared to a child of the same age who does not have special health care needs. Standard vital signs may have limited value in assessment of these children. Pay more attention to the Paediatric Assessment Triangle (PAT) and observations from the caregiver.

10. Do not assume that a child with a physical disability is cognitively impaired. Many children with cerebral palsy, for example, have **spasticity** but do not have cognitive limitations. Discreetly ask the caregiver about the child's typical level of functioning, understanding, and interactions.

11. Be polite and professional. Listen to the caregiver and take his or her concerns seriously. Families of CSHCN often have had a lot of experience with the medical system. If

most of their experience has been positive, they view the prehospital professional as an ally. However, if they have had bad experiences with the medical system, they may be suspicious or aggressive.

12. Keep in mind the amount of stress caregivers of a CSHCN may be experiencing.

13. Ask the caregivers what therapies or interventions have been already undertaken in response to their child's emergency.

14. If possible, try to transport CSHCN to their "medical home" facility. Always follow local protocol.

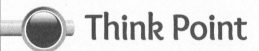

Think Point

Do not become distracted by the specialised equipment used by children assisted by technology. Care for the child, not the machinery.

Paediatric Assessment Triangle

The PAT is a good way to look and listen for signs that help determine the type of physiological problem and the urgency for treatment of a CSHCN. However, because CSHCN often have altered baseline physiology, there are several limitations and modifications to the PAT.

Appearance

Although the child's overall appearance reflects the adequacy of oxygenation, ventilation, and perfusion, as well as CNS status, appearance is the part of the PAT that may differ the most in CSHCN. The underlying medical problem may cause abnormal muscle tone, such as the increased tone and spasticity in a child with cerebral palsy or the decreased tone seen in children with Down syndrome. There may be decreased interactiveness, a common behavioural state in a child with brain damage or an intellectual disability. Look or gaze is helpful because many CSHCN can recognise their caregiver by looking or by hearing their voice. A CSHCN may be unable to speak, but the strength and quality of his or her cry or facial expressions may be a useful sign of health or distress. For example, a high-pitched cry in a child with a CSF shunt may mean obstruction.

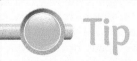

Tip

Approach the child with an intellectual disability using techniques appropriate to his or her developmental level, not age in years.

Work of Breathing

Many CSHCN have respiratory problems. Children with chronic pulmonary disease, such as bronchopulmonary dysplasia (BPD), have rapid respiratory rates and increased work of breathing. When such children have a fever or experience an added respiratory illness or injury, such as pneumonia or chest trauma, they have less reserve. Therefore, work of breathing in these patients increases rapidly with any acute illness or injury.

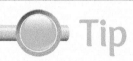

Tip

Assess appearance by asking the caregiver about the child's baseline.

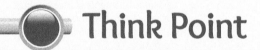

Think Point

Do not assume that a child with a physical disability is mentally impaired. Many children with cerebral palsy, for example, have spasticity but not cognitive limitations.

Assess abnormal breath sounds (stridor, wheezing, or grunting) from across the room. Some "abnormal" airway sounds may be usual for a CSHCN. For example, a child with a tracheostomy tube usually has noisy breathing, and an infant with BPD may have slight expiratory wheezing. Children with BPD or congenital heart disease are much more likely to develop respiratory infections, especially from respiratory syncytial virus (RSV), in the winter. They can decompensate quickly. CSHCN who have an intellectual disability and neurological problems are at high risk for aspiration, pneumonia, and respiratory failure.

Unusual positioning, such as tripoding and head bobbing, are important visual signs of increased work of breathing and hypoxia, and usually indicate serious breathing problems. For the child who usually has mild retractions, the degree or location of retractions provides clues to increased work of breathing. For example, the baseline retractions may be mild and only subcostal, but are now severe and also suprasternal. Nasal flaring is an indication of increased work of breathing, especially when associated with tachypnoea, grunting, or retractions.

Circulation to Skin

The skin colour may appear different in CSHCN, such as in infants with cyanotic congenital heart disease, chronic lung disease, cancer, or liver failure. A child with cyanotic congenital heart disease or chronic lung disease may have bluish

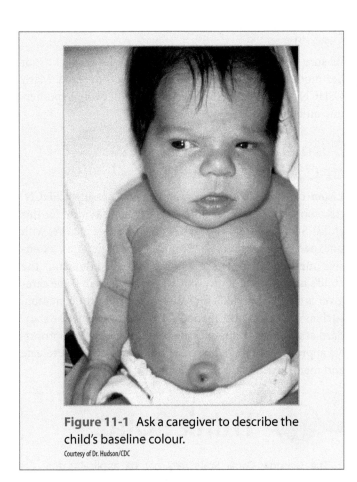

Figure 11-1 Ask a caregiver to describe the child's baseline colour.
Courtesy of Dr. Hudson/CDC

lips and mucous membranes, nail beds, and extremities at baseline. A child with cancer may appear pale, whereas the skin of a child with liver disease may appear yellow. Ask a caregiver to describe the child's baseline colour (**Figure 11-1**).

Adaptations in the Hands-on <C>ABCDEs

After performing the PAT, complete the primary assessment by adjusting the evaluation of the <C>ABCDEs to the child's baseline.

Airway

Open and maintain the airway. Keeping an open airway may be more difficult with the CSHCN. The child may have poor muscle tone and head control, or copious secretions. In children with Down syndrome, the large, protruding tongue may make airway procedures difficult. Getting, and then keeping, the right head position may require several manoeuvres: a shoulder roll to correctly position the head in a neutral axis with the airway, and a chin lift or jaw thrust to open the airway. Always have suction available.

Many children with spina bifida have an Arnold-Chiari malformation (ACM) in which the base of the brain pushes down through a large foramen magnum. Do NOT hyper-extend the neck of a child with spina bifida because any pressure on the herniated brain may cause the child to stop breathing. For these children, use in-line stabilisation for any airway manoeuvres even if no trauma is suspected.

Special Management in CSHCN: Tracheostomy Care. A child with a tracheostomy has an artificial airway that is easily blocked by secretions or by dislodgment of the device. The tracheostomy section of this chapter addresses specific management techniques for these children.

Breathing

Count the respiratory rate. Listen to the lungs for bilateral air movement and abnormal chest sounds. Listening may not give accurate results in the CSHCN who cannot sit still or who has noisy breathing. Also, obtain pulse oximetry and compare to baseline. Keep the child in a position of comfort. Give supplemental oxygen to any CSHCN with increased work of breathing or increased respiratory rate by blow-by, face mask, or bag-valve-mask device. If the caregiver knows the usual baseline oxygen saturation, only give oxygen to achieve baseline levels. Children with chronic lung disease or some forms of congenital heart disease can get worse if too much oxygen is given. For CSHCN, the caregiver may know the best way to give oxygen to the child. For infants or children already on home oxygen, increase the flow rate. For a patient with a tracheostomy tube, place the oxygen directly over the tube or stoma.

Special Management in CSHCN: Bronchodilator Administration. If a CSHCN has a history of breathing problems or uses bronchodilators at home, give a nebulised bronchodilator when wheezing is present.

Circulation

Assess heart rate, pulse quality, skin temperature, and capillary refill time. These are not usually different in CSHCN and require no modifications in clinical interpretation. If the child's age is 3 years or less, consider obtaining a blood pressure. However, the value may be difficult to obtain and interpret in this age group. Attempt to measure blood pressure at least once in all children older than 3 years of age. Tachycardia is a common baseline finding in some CSHCN, and by itself does not indicate shock. This is diagnosis-dependent, so asking the child's caregiver about the child's usual heart rate can be helpful. To evaluate heart rate and blood pressure, assess with the other key characteristics of circulation, as outlined in the *Respiratory Emergencies* chapter.

In some CSHCN, management of shock may be no different than for children without disabilities. Standard management includes oxygen, positioning, and bag-valve-mask support as needed. Some CSHCN may need volume replacement, unless the child has a congenital heart defect and possible heart failure. The CSHCN has the same fluid requirements as any other child. If the patient is injured, transport immediately and attempt vascular access. Give 20 ml boluses of crystalloid fluid on the way to the emergency department (ED) as per JRCALC guidelines.

If the child is ill and has compensated shock, transport and attempt access and fluid administration on the way. If the ill child has decompensated shock, make one attempt at vascular access on scene, if possible. In extreme cases, intraosseous access may be necessary. When a child has a vertical chest scar or a history of congenital heart disease, consider cardiogenic shock as an explanation for poor perfusion. Because a CSHCN may be more difficult to assess accurately, and because vascular access is often troublesome, always transport a child with suspected shock as soon as possible.

Some children with severe, uncontrolled epilepsy may be on the ketogenic diet. This regimen eliminates foods with glucose and keeps the child in a state of ketosis to control the seizures. For these children, do NOT use any fluids containing <u>dextrose</u>.

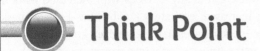

Think Point

Do not give glucose or glucose-containing fluids to children on a ketogenic diet.

Special Management in CSHCN. Bradycardia is not usual for CSHCN. It is a sign of hypoxia or inadequate brain perfusion. Suspect hypoxia in a child with BPD or other chronic cardiopulmonary condition who has a heart rate below normal for chronologic age. Suspect increased intracranial pressure in a child with a CSF shunt.

Disability

Many CSHCN often have a compromised baseline neurological status. Assess neurological status by looking at appearance as part of the PAT, and establish level of consciousness with the Alert, Verbal, Painful, Unresponsive (AVPU) mnemonic. Compare the findings to the child's baseline. In the assessment of motor activity, assess purposeful movement, symmetrical movement of extremities, seizures, posturing, or flaccidity. Treat altered mental status if it is a change from baseline. The Glasgow Coma Scale may not be applicable for assessment of CSHCN because many CSHCN have baseline cognitive and physical challenges that would affect the score. It is better to describe the child as being different from baseline.

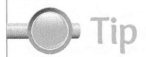

Tip

The usual baseline vital signs for a CSHCN may be different or "out of the normal range" for the child's chronologic age.

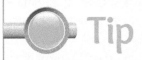

Tip

Bradycardia is not usual for CSHCN.

Exposure

Be sure to inspect the child's entire body, but respect his or her modesty. Do not allow the child to become cold. Many CSHCN have minimal body fat and can become hypothermic quickly.

Summary of Assessment of CSHCN

Listen carefully to the caregiver when assessing CSHCN. Ask about the child's baseline status. What is typical for this child? Such children may present a confusing picture, with unexpected behaviours, communication difficulties, extensive medical histories, and complicated equipment. The child's neurological status is often compromised. If the caregiver is not present, look for sources of baseline information, such as a medical information form or a bracelet. Use standard assessment techniques and developmentally appropriate approaches modified by baseline comparisons to evaluate and manage acute problems. Transport early.

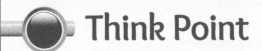

Think Point

The Glasgow Coma Scale may not be applicable for assessment of CSHCN because many CSHCN have baseline cognitive and physical challenges that affect the score.

Transport

Table 11-4 lists key principles of transport of CSHCN. *Always restrain children in the ambulance.* The best type of restraint device and the best method for securing the device in the ambulance are controversial issues. In general, if the child is critically ill or injured, restrain the child on his or her back secured on a stretcher. Try to use a spinal board or paediatric vacuum mattress for spinal stabilisation if the child has suffered an injury to the head or has a spinal injury. Be careful if the child has any contractures or rigid posturing, such as scissoring of the legs or an exaggerated arching of the back seen in children with cerebral palsy. Pad any open areas and do not force the child to conform to the equipment. When immobilising a small child, consider using a vest-type immobilisation device, such as a Kendrick extrication device (KED), which can work very well. Check with the caregiver about positioning and availability of any special car seat. In some children, the supine position may compromise the airway because of an abundance of secretions, poor tone, or anatomical differences. The child's specially designed child restraint system or car seat may be the best option if it can be safely secured in the ambulance.

Many CSHCN have supplemental oxygen and oxygen delivery equipment. It is unsafe to transport liquid oxygen in an

Table 11-4 Principles of Transport of a CSHCN

1. Transport a CSHCN who is on home oxygen with the oxygen (except for liquid oxygen). If the child has no respiratory distress, continue the same rate of oxygen flow.

2. Transport a child on a home ventilator with the ventilator if there are no equipment problems. If there is a concern about the ventilator, provide assisted ventilation by bag-valve-mask. Regardless of the method of ventilation, always secure the child's home ventilator in the ambulance and transport with the child, so that it can be assessed by hospital personnel for potential problems and appropriate settings.

3. If the child has poor muscle control, or increased muscle tone, immobilise the child as needed in a position that is comfortable for him or her. If the child has a special seat, wheelchair, or other equipment (e.g., feeding pump or suctioning device), transport these items to the ED if these items can be safely secured in the ambulance while still allowing enough room to safely care for the child during transport.

4. If the child has any contractures or rigid postures, such as scissoring of the legs or an arched back, pad around any open areas when the child is on the stretcher or during spinal immobilisation. Do NOT force the child to conform to the equipment.

© Jones & Bartlett Learning

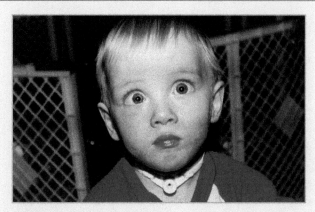

Figure 11-2 A tracheostomy.
Courtesy of Cindy Bissell

Table 11-5 Indications for a Tracheostomy

1. To bypass an obstruction in the upper airway caused by trauma, surgery, or a birth defect

2. To allow clearance of secretions

3. To provide long-term mechanical ventilation of children with chronic respiratory problems, injuries to the lungs, major CNS deficits, or severe muscle weakness

© Jones & Bartlett Learning

ambulance. Consider transporting non-liquid (or gaseous) oxygen and the child's personal devices or equipment to the ED.

Summary of Transport

CSHCN often have special transport considerations. Make sure the child is safely restrained in the ambulance. This may require using a special seat. Address the issue of transport with the caregiver, and consider bringing supportive equipment to the ED if it can be safely secured in the ambulance.

Children Assisted by Technology

Children assisted by technology have devices that may malfunction at home. The most common devices are **tracheostomy tubes**, **cerebral spinal fluid (CSF) shunts**, **indwelling central venous catheters**, and **feeding tubes** (buttons). Equipment malfunction can cause a range of problems. Some malfunctioning may have minor or no immediate effects, such as loss of a feeding tube or clotting of an indwelling central venous catheter. Other malfunctioning may cause serious physiological effects, such as respiratory distress from loss of a tracheostomy tube or intracranial pressure elevation from obstruction of a CSF shunt.

Tracheostomy Tubes

A tracheostomy is a surgical opening (stoma) in the front of the neck into the trachea. A tracheostomy tube is an artificial airway passed through this opening that allows the child to breathe (**Figure 11-2**). Infants and children may have a tracheostomy for several reasons, as noted in **Table 11-5**.

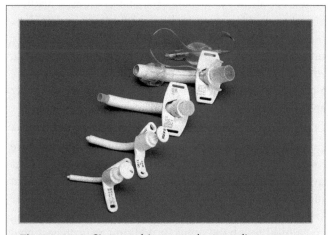

Figure 11-3 Sizes and inner and outer diameters are often written on the wings of tracheostomy tubes.
© Jones & Bartlett Learning

There are several types of tracheostomy tubes, and they come in many sizes. The size is written on the wings or flanges of the tube. The size and name (indicating type of tube) are also on the box. The inner and outer diameters are often on the wings (**Figure 11-3**). The most common paediatric tube sizes are 2.5–10 mm (sizes 000–10). Tracheostomy tubes have a standard outer opening or hub outside the neck so a bag-valve-mask device can be attached. For some tubes, an adapter may be needed to make this connection.

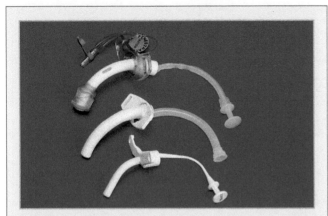

Figure 11-4 Fenestrated, double-lumen, and single-lumen tracheostomy tubes (top to bottom).
© Jones & Bartlett Learning

Types of Tracheostomy Tubes

The main types of tracheostomy tubes are fenestrated, double lumen, and single lumen (**Figure 11-4**). Tubes can also come with or without a cuff. These cuffs can be filled with air or foam. All tubes have an **obturator**, which is a solid plastic guide placed inside the tube to make insertion easier. Use the obturator to clear the tube of secretions in an emergency if a suction catheter is not available.

A single-lumen tracheostomy tube has one hollow tube or cannula for airflow and suctioning of secretions. Uncuffed, single-lumen tubes are usually used for neonates, infants, and young children. A double-lumen tube has a hollow outer cannula and a removable (also hollow) inner cannula. Remove the inner cannula for cleaning, and keep it in place to provide mechanical ventilation. Never remove the outer cannula unless the entire tube must be replaced.

A fenestrated tube has holes (fenestrations) for air to flow upward through the vocal cords and mouth. This structure lets the child talk and breathe naturally. Fenestrated tubes have a decannulation plug attached to the outer cannula that blocks airflow through the stoma. If the child cannot breathe through the nose or mouth, remove this plug so breathing is possible through the stoma. In addition, many fenestrated tubes also have a hollow inner cannula that must be in place for mechanical ventilation.

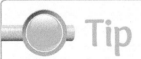 **Tip**

If the inner cannula of a double-lumen tracheostomy tube has been removed, a bag-valve-mask device will not secure to the outer lumen of the tube. To ventilate a tracheostomy tube with the inner cannula removed, secure an infant face mask onto the bag, and then cover the tracheostomy tube's opening and seal the face mask on the neck.

Oxygen Delivery and Assisted Ventilation Through a Tracheostomy Tube

A child with a functioning tracheostomy tube can receive oxygen from the blow-by method, by a face mask or tracheostomy mask placed directly over the tube opening, or by manual ventilation with a bag-valve-mask device.

1. Provide blow-by oxygen. Place a stoma mask or paediatric face mask a short distance above the tracheostomy tube or stoma and give oxygen at 10–15 l/min.

2. Secure a face or tracheostomy mask directly over the tracheostomy tube opening and secure the straps around the neck.

3. Attach a bag-valve-mask device to a tracheostomy tube adapter. Attach a bag-valve-mask device directly to the outer end of the tracheostomy tube (**Figure 11-5**).

For a child who has a stoma (surgical opening in the neck) but no tracheostomy tube, or when a tube cannot be reinserted, apply a seal with a mask over the stoma and ventilate through the stoma; or cover the stoma with a **sterile** gauze, and ventilate with a mask to the mouth or mask to the mouth and nose technique. Begin bag-valve-mask ventilation as needed.

Tracheostomy Complications: Obstruction

Obstruction of the tracheostomy tube is a life-threatening emergency. Obstruction can be caused by secretions, incorrect insertion (tube malposition), improper positioning of the child's head, or mechanical problems with the tube. Obstruction causes respiratory distress and failure.

Assessment. When a child has an obstructed tracheostomy tube, the chest is not rising and the child cannot breathe on his or her own. The PAT shows poor appearance, increased work of breathing, and cyanosis in cases of respiratory failure. The <C>ABCDEs further indicate poor air movement and bradycardia.

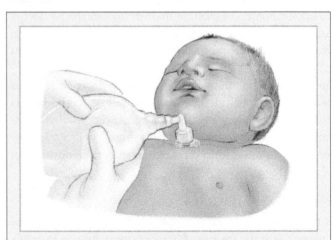

Figure 11-5 Bag-valve-mask device attached directly to the external end of the tracheostomy tube.
© Jones & Bartlett Learning

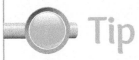

Tip

The most common complication of a child with a tracheostomy tube is respiratory distress caused by obstruction of the tube.

Treatment: Clearing an Obstructed Tube. To clear an obstructed tracheostomy tube, follow these steps:

1. Position the child's head with a towel roll under the shoulders. Ensure that the outer opening of the tube is clear.

2. Check that the tube is in the proper location. The wings or flange should be against the neck, and the obturator should not be in place.

3. If the child has a fenestrated tube, remove the decannulation plug.

4. If the child has a double-lumen tracheostomy tube, remove the inner lumen to clear secretions.

5. If none of these manoeuvres work, suction the tube with a suction catheter.

Treatment: Suctioning a Tracheostomy Tube. If efforts to clear the obstruction are unsuccessful, suction the tracheostomy tube using the following procedure (**Figures 11-6** and **11-7**):

1. Ask the caregiver if he or she has suction catheters, equipment, and supplies. If so, use these. Otherwise, choose a suction catheter small enough to pass through the tube.

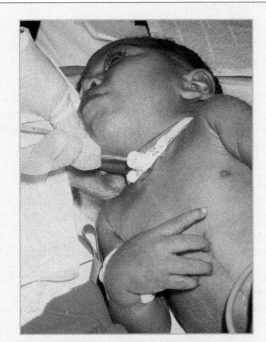

Figure 11-6 Suctioning a tracheostomy tube.
© Jones & Bartlett Learning

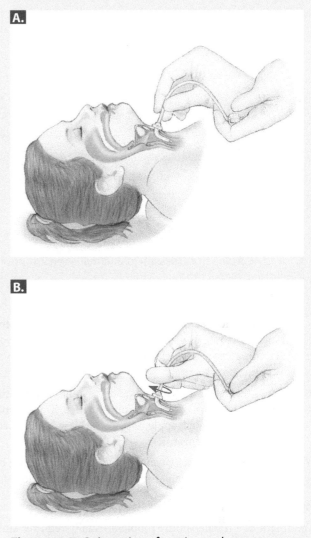

Figure 11-7 A. Insertion of suction catheter to proper depth; suction port remains open. **B.** Suctioning airway in circular motion as catheter is removed; suction port is closed.
© Jones & Bartlett Learning

(A size 1.0 (or 3.0-mm) tube will take a size 6 to 8 French catheter.) The caregiver may know the right size catheter. If equipment is not immediately available, insert the obturator to try to clear the obstruction.

2. If using a portable suction machine, set it to 100 mm Hg or less.

3. Give oxygen via a ventilation bag with a mask, and then loosen secretions by placing up to 1.0 to 2.0 mL of normal saline into the tube.

4. Insert the suction catheter approximately 2 inches (5 cm) into the tube. If the child begins to cough, the catheter is through the tube and into the trachea, and the depth of insertion is too deep. Do not use suction while inserting the catheter, and never force the catheter.

5. Cover the suction port (hole on the tubing) and suction for 3 to 5 seconds, while slowly removing the catheter. Never

Case Study 2

You are called to the home of a 6-year-old boy whose central venous catheter has bleeding around the insertion site. His mother panicked because it is a new catheter and she is not used to taking care of it. She tells you that he has a history of short-gut syndrome caused by an infarcted bowel sustained 6 months ago. He also has a gastrostomy tube through which he receives some medications, but he is totally reliant on his central venous catheter for his nutrition.

On arrival, you note a thin 6-year-old boy sitting quietly on the family's couch. His skin is yellowish. He has no increased work of breathing. His respiratory rate is 22 breaths/min, his heart rate is 95 beats/min, and his blood pressure is 90/50 mm Hg. Pulse oximetry is 98%. There is a tiny ooze of blood from the insertion site of the catheter in the right neck.

1. What are the key historical points?

2. Outline the assessment and management priorities.

suction for longer than 10 seconds. Always monitor the child's heart rate and colour during this procedure. Stop suctioning immediately if the heart rate begins to drop or the child becomes blue.

6. If the obstruction is removed, and the child can breathe on his or her own, do not suction further. If additional suctioning is needed, apply oxygen (by blow-by or direct ventilation) and repeat steps 3–5.

7. Always provide supplemental oxygen after suctioning by using the blow-by method or with manual ventilations.

Replacing a Tracheostomy Tube

Treatment of a tracheostomy problem usually requires simple techniques to establish a patent airway, such as suctioning or removal of the old tracheostomy tube and replacement with a new tube (**Figure 11-8**). Occasionally, it is impossible to ventilate a child through an existing tracheostomy

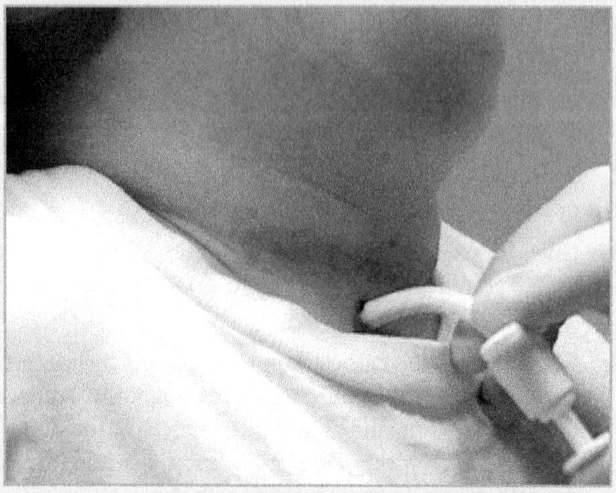

Figure 11-8 Replacing a tracheostomy tube.
© Jones & Bartlett Learning

tube because of decannulation or complete obstruction. Under these conditions, the prehospital professional must place a new tracheostomy tube to save the child's life. For a step-by-step explanation of this procedure, see **Removing and Replacing a Tracheostomy Tube, Procedure 19**.

Central Venous Catheters

Many children receive nutritional support or medications at home through a <u>central venous catheter</u>. This includes children with poor weight gain caused by gastrointestinal or liver problems, children with cancer who require chemotherapy, and children with infections who are receiving antibiotics at home.

Many central venous catheters require a surgical incision, but some can be placed percutaneously or through intact skin (often called PICC lines for percutaneously inserted central catheter). They can enter through the skin of the chest, neck, or arm, and the internal end usually lies in or near the <u>superior vena cava</u> or right <u>atrium</u>. Some are single-lumen lines. Others are double lumen, with two separate external openings, but only one internal opening or port.

Types of Catheters

Central venous catheters may be inserted into the femoral, internal jugular, and subclavian veins (**Figure 11-9**). The skin entry site for the catheter is usually on the chest or arm. This is called a **peripherally implanted central catheter (PICC)**.

<u>Totally implanted devices (mediport)</u> are catheters attached to totally implanted injection ports or reservoirs. The catheter is in a central vein, such as the superior vena cava. Instead of coming out of the skin, as in partially implanted catheters, the end is attached to a reservoir (dome or port) that is in a subcutaneous pocket, usually on the chest. Therefore, there are no external parts visible, just a bulge or bump where the device rests.

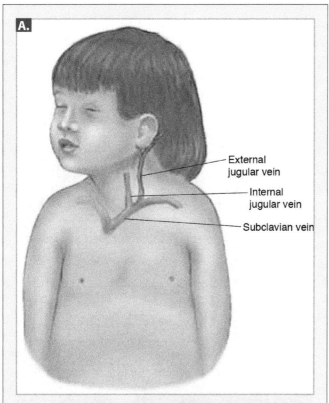

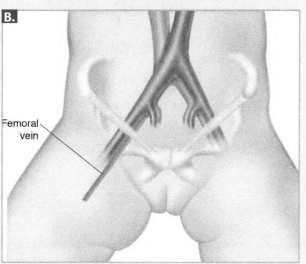

Figure 11-9 Possible insertion sites for a central venous catheter. **A.** Subclavian, internal jugular, and external jugular sites. **B.** Femoral vein locations.
© Jones & Bartlett Learning

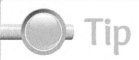

Tip

The most common complication in a child assisted by technology with a partially implanted central venous catheter is a broken or dislodged catheter. If the bleeding is from the catheter and the catheter is in place, inspect the catheter and its end. If a cap is missing, replace the cap, if possible.

Table 11-6 Common Central Venous Catheter Complications
Dislodged or broken catheter
Infection at catheter site
Problems with accessing or flushing the catheter (obstruction)
Air embolism
Medical problems related to **infusion**

© Jones & Bartlett Learning

Complications of Central Venous Catheters

Table 11-6 lists common complications of central venous catheters. The most common problem with partially implanted devices is a broken or dislodged catheter. Check the site for bleeding. If the catheter is in place, but there is bleeding from the entry site, apply direct pressure with sterile gauze. Likewise, if the catheter has been completely pulled out, and there is bleeding, apply direct pressure with sterile gauze.

Clamping a Leaking Central Venous Catheter. If the child is bleeding through a hole or cut in the catheter, clamp the exposed end. The caregiver usually has a clamp available, but if this has been misplaced, wrap the tips of a haemostat with gauze and apply to the catheter. If no haemostat is available, open the emergency delivery kit and use an umbilical clamp. If there has been bleeding, estimate the amount of blood loss.

Provide appropriate fluid therapy if there are signs of poor perfusion or shock. Do not use the central venous catheter.

Infection at Catheter Site. Infection can occur at the site where a partially implanted catheter enters the skin or in the pocket where a totally implanted device is placed. Signs of infection are redness, tenderness, swelling, warmth, or yellow discharge (pus) from the site.

The child can also have a blood infection with fever, chills, and shock. In this case, treat for septic shock, as described in the *Shock* chapter. If the line is possibly infected, do not use it for vascular access.

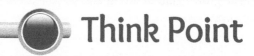

Think Point

If the indwelling central venous catheter seems infected, do not use it for vascular access.

Obstruction. A problem with accessing or flushing the catheter usually means obstruction. This complication can occur with all types of catheters. All that is required is patient assessment and transport. The major concern is a child who depends on **hyperalimentation** (intravenous (IV) nutrition) for calories and glucose. If the line is malfunctioning, and the child has not received any nutrition, their blood glucose may be low.

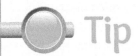

> **Tip**
>
> In a child who depends on hyperalimentation for calories and glucose, if the line is malfunctioning and the child has not received any nutrition, their blood glucose may be low.

Treatment of Hypoglycaemia. Perform a quick finger-stick check of the blood sugar if there are signs or symptoms of hypoglycaemia. For low blood sugar, basic life support (BLS) providers can give oral glucose per local protocol or advanced life support (ALS) providers can treat with IV Glucose 10% or intramuscular (IM) glucagon as described in the *Medical Emergencies* chapter.

Air Embolism. This complication can occur if air accidentally gets into a central venous catheter when the line is being flushed or if the catheter breaks. Symptoms of air embolism include shortness of breath, chest pain, and coughing. Sometimes there is cardiovascular collapse and cardiopulmonary arrest.

Treatment of Suspected Air Embolism. Clamp the catheter or ask the caregiver to clamp the catheter, provide the child with oxygen, place the child on his or her left side in the head-down position, and transport to the ED.

Medical Problems Related to Infusion. Because of the various fluids and medications delivered through central venous catheters, several medical problems can develop, such as allergic reactions, abnormal heart rate or rhythms, or respiratory problems. Treat the appropriate problem, and bring the fluids that were being infused to the ED for analysis.

Feeding Devices

A feeding device provides an avenue for nutrition and medications to CSHCN who are unable to take food or fluids by mouth. This device allows the child to take in enough calories for adequate growth and nutrition and may be used to administer medications.

Types of Feeding Tubes

Some feeding tubes go through the nose (nasogastric (NG)) or, occasionally, through the mouth (orogastric (OG)) and into the stomach or small intestine (nasojejunal (NJ), orojejunal) (**Figure 11-10**). These tubes are usually long catheters that are taped in place on the child's face. Another type of feeding tube goes directly into the stomach from an external site on the abdomen (gastrostomy tube or G-tube).

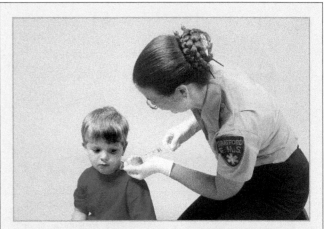

Figure 11-10 Nasojejunal catheter taped in place on the child's face.
© Jones & Bartlett Learning. Courtesy of Glen Ellman.

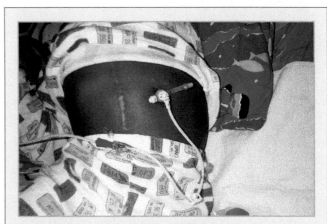

Figure 11-11 A percutaneous endoscopic gastrostomy, with connector attached.
Courtesy of Cindy Bissell

Another example is a device called a percutaneous endoscopic gastrostomy (PEG) or button that is inserted into an opening in the stomach (**Figure 11-11**). It has a balloon on the end inserted into the stomach that is similar to the balloon on an intubation tube. It is inflated to keep the button in place. There is also a small cap with a valve on the outside to allow access. It can be replaced by the child's caregivers. Many caregivers prefer a button because there is no tube hanging from the abdomen that could be dislodged during physical activity.

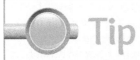

> **Tip**
>
> The main complication of feeding tubes is dislodgment.

Complications of Feeding Tubes

The main complication of a feeding tube is dislodgment. The child may have aspirated fluid if a nasal or oral feeding tube has come out. For tubes inserted into the abdomen, there may be bleeding or leakage of fluid. For a button, a replacement button may not fit into the stoma on the abdomen if it is the wrong size or there was a delay in replacing it. Perform an assessment, paying special attention to the work of breathing, chest auscultation, and pulse oximetry.

Treatment

If an implanted tube (G-tube) comes out, check the site for bleeding and apply direct pressure with a sterile dressing. If the insertion site around the implanted tube seems irritated or infected (the skin seems red, warm, or swollen), apply a sterile dressing to the site.

Whenever a tube dislodges or there is evidence of infection, transport the child to the ED. Ask the caregiver to bring the tube that fell out with the child to the hospital for sizing purposes. If the child was on an infusion of fluid or medication, ask the caregiver to disconnect the pump (infusion device) and transport it with the child. If the child has received fluid through a feeding catheter within 30 minutes of ambulance service arrival, consider transporting the child in a sitting position to prevent reflux, vomiting, and possible aspiration.

Removing a Feeding Tube. If the NG or OG tube seems to be in place but the child is having respiratory difficulty, ask the caregiver to check its position. If position cannot be confirmed, remove the tube.

CSF Shunts

A CSF shunt is a device that drains excess CSF from the brain. It is usually inserted from a ventricle (in the brain) under the skin, then down the neck into the peritoneum of the abdomen (ventriculoperitoneal or VP shunt), the pleura of the chest (ventriculopleural or V-Pleural shunt or VPS, VPL or VPLS) or the heart (ventriculoatrial or VA shunt) (**Figure 11-12**). Its path (or track) can usually be felt on one side of the head and down the neck until the track reaches a scar on the chest wall or abdomen. A CSF shunt helps a child with hydrocephalus maintain normal brain pressure. The hydrocephalus may be caused by a congenital problem or by an acquired condition, such as bleeding, trauma, or infection.

Complications of CSF Shunts

The major complications with a CSF shunt are obstruction and infection. The most common complication is a shunt obstruction and malfunction. **Table 11-7** lists key questions to ask during assessment to evaluate the severity of the complaint and the urgency for treatment.

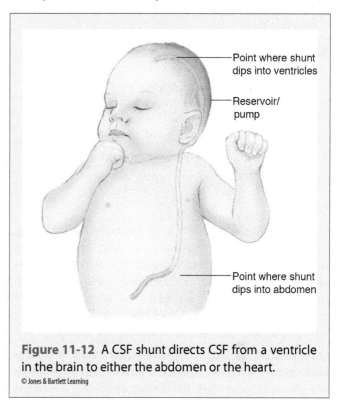

Point where shunt dips into ventricles

Reservoir/ pump

Point where shunt dips into abdomen

Figure 11-12 A CSF shunt directs CSF from a ventricle in the brain to either the abdomen or the heart.
© Jones & Bartlett Learning

Table 11-7 Key Questions for Suspected CSF Shunt Malfunction

When was the CSF shunt placed?
Is the child acting the same as the last time there was a shunt problem (obstruction)?
Has the child had a fever?
Has the child complained of a headache, vomiting, or nausea?

© Jones & Bartlett Learning

Assessment of a Child With a Possible CSF Shunt Obstruction or Infection

Symptoms of a CSF shunt obstruction are the same as those of increased intracranial pressure and include headache, lethargy, sleepiness, irritability, nausea or vomiting, or trouble walking. Fever is usually a sign of a shunt infection or an intercurrent illness, but can occur with a shunt malfunction alone. Signs of a shunt obstruction are abnormal appearance, high-pitched cry, seizures, or altered mental status. A very worrisome finding is Cushing triad (bradycardia, elevated blood pressure, and irregular respirations), which indicates increased intracranial pressure caused by an obstructed shunt.

A child with a shunt infection may have a fever, headache, feeding difficulty, or altered behaviour. Signs of a shunt infection include abnormal appearance, altered mental status, and shock.

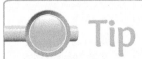

> **Tip**
>
> Many CSHCN, especially those with spina bifida, have a sensitivity or allergy to latex. Always use latex precautions with these patients. Reactions to latex can range from a localised skin reaction to anaphylaxis

Treatment

Make sure the child has a clear airway and effective breathing. Supply supplemental oxygen and transport the patient. Keep the head in midline position and elevate 30° to 45° whenever possible. If the child has bradycardia, irregular respirations, and elevated blood pressure (Cushing triad), there is increased intracranial pressure and herniation is imminent. Begin bag-valve-mask ventilation and rapidly transport.

Hyperventilation for Suspected Increased Intracranial Pressure. Hyperventilation is a treatment for children with impending or frank herniation. However, the effects of hyperventilation in treating out-of-hospital intracranial pressure elevation from hydrocephalus are complex. Hyperventilation, through carbon dioxide reduction and cerebral vasoconstriction, reduces brain perfusion. However, overly aggressive ventilation may dangerously decrease perfusion and cause brain ischaemia. If a child with a CSF shunt has signs of impending or frank herniation, treat with mild hyperventilation using capnography to keep $ETCO_2$ at 35 mm Hg. This is the same treatment as outlined for traumatic brain injury in the *Trauma* chapter.

Ostomies

Some conditions, such as Crohn's disease, spinal cord injury, cancer, distal ureter or bladder defects, and necrotising enterocolitis in an infant, interfere with regular elimination of urine and faeces. Several types of ostomies are created to accomplish this bodily function. With a colostomy or ileostomy, an opening in the abdomen is formed when the small or large intestine is surgically brought out to the surface and sutured in place, creating a stoma. This procedure allows the digestive system to continue functioning while bypassing any inflamed or damaged bowel. An external pouch is placed over the stoma to collect digestive waste matter. The intestines below the colostomy site may not have been removed if there is a possibility of reconnecting the bowel at a later time. Colostomies can be temporary or permanent. With a urostomy, a stoma is surgically created to allow the elimination of urine.

Complications of Ostomies

Complications of ostomies include dehydration, infection, and pouch displacement. Because of an increased risk for dehydration, a child with a colostomy needs to be assessed carefully for clinical signs and symptoms of dehydration and shock, particularly if there is a history of diarrhoea or decreased oral intake.

Signs of infection at the ostomy site include red, warm, tender skin spreading away from the stoma site. Ask the child or caregiver if the area is more tender than usual. If the child has signs of infection, transport the child for further evaluation.

Replacing a Pouch

Ask the caregiver to empty the pouch before transport, especially if the pouch is full. Before the pouch is emptied, document the amount of fluid in the pouch. Be sure the pouch is resealed after emptying to prevent leakage. In some instances, the pouch breaks or is torn off. If another pouch is not available, circle the stoma with moist gauze and then attach anything available that can serve as a substitute collection device. If no pouch is available, place several thicknesses of moist gauze over the stoma until a proper replacement is found. Another option is to secure a non-rebreather face mask over the stoma. The reservoir in the mask collects the excreted stool or urine.

Lastly, be respectful of the child's privacy. Keep the site, and pouch if in place, covered in public.

Internal Pacemakers and Defibrillators

Pacemakers are implanted medical devices that regulate the heart rate. Indications include bradycardia that does not maintain adequate perfusion, a previous cardiac arrest, and heart block especially after open heart surgery. They usually include a generator and leads. The generator houses the software and battery and supplies the electrical impulse. The leads are insulated wires that carry the electrical impulse to the heart and carry information about the heart's natural rhythm back to the pulse generator.

Complications of Internal Pacemakers

Several complications can occur for children with pacemakers. Some devices do not allow the child's heart rhythm to go above a certain rate. If that child is in shock or shock is impending, the body cannot compensate by increasing the heart rate. Begin treatment and transport immediately. Another complication is pacemaker failure. The child's heart rate drops and becomes too slow to maintain perfusion. Again, begin treatment and transport immediately. A third complication is pacemaker malfunction. The child may experience bradycardia if the pacemaker is not firing. In another instance, the leads may become dislodged and cause the child's diaphragm to contract instead of the heart muscle every time the pacemaker fires. The respiratory rate will equal the preset pacemaker rate. One unusual problem may be dislodgement of the leads after some type of chest trauma. Monitor the heart rate closely and transport.

Internal Cardiac Defibrillators

An **automatic implantable cardioverter-defibrillator (AICD)** or internal cardiac defibrillator (ICD) is an electronic device implanted under the skin. Its purpose is to monitor the heart rhythm and slow down or stop excessively fast heart rates that originate in the ventricles. Such rhythms include ventricular tachycardia and ventricular fibrillation.

The mechanical parts of an AICD include a generator and a lead. This generator is a tiny battery-operated electronic device located inside a case that monitors and records the heart rhythm. It sends out shocks to convert excessively fast heart rates when needed. The computer also records any shocks that it sends to the heart. A lead (or wire) is attached to the generator and is connected to the heart muscle to monitor the heart rhythm and carry shocks to the heart.

For any child with a pacemaker, ICD, or AICD, prehospital professionals should ask the caregivers the following questions:

- What type of heart problem does the child have?
- What rate is the child's underlying rhythm?
- What type of pacemaker, ICD, or AICD does the child have?
  - If a pacemaker, is the child dependent on the pacemaker? What are the settings?
  - If an ICD or AICD, what are the settings, at what heart rate does the ICD fire, and how many shocks has the child felt? In addition, has the child experienced any of the following:
    - More than three shocks in a row?
    - Continuation of unusual symptoms after experiencing a shock?
    - Sensations of dizziness, light-headedness, palpitations, and so forth for a period of time yet has felt no shock?

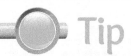

Tip

The internal pacemaker can easily be felt near the clavicle or in small children in the abdomen. Never place defibrillator paddles, "hands off" defibrillating-pacing patches, or automated external defibrillator (AED) patches directly over the internal pacemaker or defibrillator generator. The battery life for implanted pacemakers and defibrillators is 3–5 years.

Vagal Nerve Stimulator

The **vagal nerve stimulator (VNS)** was approved by the Federal Drug Administration (FDA) in 1997 for those patients with intractable epilepsy. Some children continue to have seizures despite conventional medication, surgical procedures, and diet. The VNS provides hope for better seizure control.

The VNS is an implantable device that looks like a pacemaker and is surgically placed by a neurosurgeon just under the skin in the left upper chest. It is programmed to provide baseline intermittent stimulation of the left vagus nerve, which leads directly to the brain. The patient or caretaker activates the device by placing over it a handheld magnet.

When responding to a call involving a CSHCN with an implanted VNS who is seizing, first assist the caregiver with activation of the VNS. Alternatively, contact medical control for guidance. Children with VNS devices should otherwise be treated as any other patient who is seizing with attention to airway, breathing, and circulation.

Dialysis Shunts

Chronic renal failure is a progressive and irreversible inadequate kidney function caused by permanent loss of nephrons. This disease develops over months or years and causes scarring in the kidneys, leading to diminished kidney function and the build-up of waste products and fluid in the blood. **Renal dialysis** is a technique for filtering toxic wastes from the blood, removing excess fluid, and restoring the normal balance of electrolytes. There are two types: **peritoneal dialysis** and **haemodialysis**.

In peritoneal dialysis, large amounts of specially formulated dialysis fluid are infused into and back out of the abdominal cavity. This fluid stays in the cavity for 1–2 hours, allowing equilibrium to occur. It is very effective yet carries a high risk of peritonitis. Many patients undergo peritoneal dialysis at home after the caregivers have received appropriate training. Prehospital professionals are not usually involved in this process.

In haemodialysis, the patient's blood circulates through a machine that functions much like a kidney and requires the use of some type of shunt or surgically created connection between a vein and an artery. External shunts may be located near the wrist, in the upper arm, or on the proximal anterior thigh. Some patients have an internal shunt also known as an arteriovenous (AV) fistula that is usually located in the forearm or upper arm (**Figure 11-13**).

When moving and transporting the patient, make sure the external shunt is protected and is not compromised by any straps. For all blood pressure measurements, use the arm without the device. If the patient has an internal shunt or AV fistula, do NOT attempt to access the fistula to draw blood or to infuse any fluids.

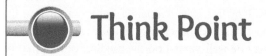

Think Point

Never use an AV fistula for vascular access.

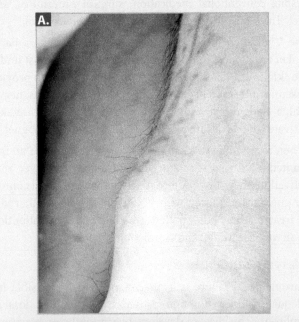

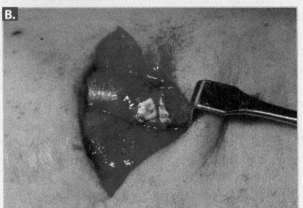

Figure 11-13 A. With an AV fistula, a bulge is created by arterial pressure. **B.** An AV graft creates a raised area that looks like a large vessel (operative photo).

A: © Visuals Unlimited, Inc; **B:** © Michael English, MD /Custom Medical Stock Photo

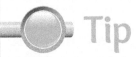

Tip

The best method of hyperventilation for out-of-hospital intracranial pressure elevation from hydrocephalus is guided by capnography. Aggressive ventilation may dangerously decrease perfusion and cause brain ischaemia.

Behavioural Emergencies in Children

There has been an increase in the number of children suffering from behavioural and psychiatric conditions and a concomitant rise in the number of children presenting to EDs with these complaints. These children are a subset of CSHCN. There are many barriers to effective treatment, including few resources for inpatient and outpatient treatment of mental health problems, a lack of tools for screening in the ED setting, and a lack of education of health care providers. Many hospitals do not have psychiatrists or other mental health workers on staff to perform emergency evaluations. Psychiatric conditions are sometimes present in children with cognitive impairments and in children with normal intelligence. Sometimes the behaviour of these children is "out of control" or violent. The child may be at school or at home at the time of the crisis.

Assessment and Transport of the Child With a Behavioural Emergency

First, consider provider safety. Attempt to establish a rapport with the child while assessing the likelihood for violence (**Figure 11-14**). If the child seems cooperative and gives permission to be touched for examination purposes, take a thorough history and perform a physical examination. Next, assess mental status. Is this child a risk to himself or others?

Summary of Children Assisted by Technology

Children assisted by technology may encounter many challenging problems with their equipment. The prehospital professional must be familiar with the basic purpose, design, and common complications of tracheostomy tubes, central venous catheters, feeding tubes, CSF shunts, and pacemakers and implantable defibrillators. Always ask the caregiver about the equipment, and transport all devices and infusions with the child to the ED. Ask whether the current problem has ever happened before, and how the situation was handled previously. Finally, remember that the child may be well-versed on the medical device that he or she uses. Consider asking the child your questions about the device; in doing so, you may gain his or her trust, which ultimately leads to better patient care.

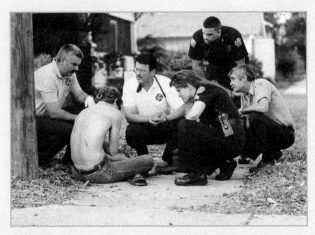

Figure 11-14 Establish a rapport with the child while assessing for the likelihood of violence.

© Craig Jackson/In the Dark Photography

Lastly, determine the need to transport the child. Consider restraints if the patient is a danger to himself or herself, or others. Always bring or ask the caregiver to follow the ambulance to the hospital.

Using Restraints for Assessment and Transport

Explain to the child's caregivers what you are doing and why you are restraining their child. Enlist their assistance. Talk to the child. Explain what you are doing and why, but do not negotiate. Do not attempt restraint placement alone. Often, securing the child in his or her car seat provides sufficient restraint, and may be preferable to the child, since he or she is already familiar with the seat. Before restraining a child, consider calling the police to provide assistance. Do not allow the child to become positioned near an escape route. Should this happen, the child can escape or attempt to injure the clinician who has lost the ability to quickly escape. Apply restraint humanely, allowing the child as much dignity as possible. Document carefully the reasons for and the types of restraints in the medical record. Perform periodic assessments. Keep restraints as loose as possible to avoid injury.

The use of midazolam as a chemical restraint is generally not supported in UK practice for adults or children. However, it may be considered in specific circumstances if local protocols exist and under the direction of the clinical advice team or an appropriate medical provider.

There may be conflict between parental wishes and the needs of the child. If the child is in immediate danger of self-harm or is an immediate danger to others, notify the police to provide assistance with restraining the patient if necessary and with transport to the closest appropriate facility.

Care in the Home Environment for CSHCN

Care coordination for CSHCN who often have involvement of multiple organ systems is quite complex. CSHCN usually see multiple physicians, therapists, home care personnel, and other health care providers to manage their chronic conditions. To co-ordinate that care, these clinicians need to communicate with the medical home and one another in an effective manner. Traditionally, communication has occurred on paper with hospitals and offices faxing reports or sending copies to one another. This system is flawed in that some of these paper reports are lost, are misfiled, or do not arrive at the office or hospital in time for additional visits or procedures. For example, if the child sees the paediatric neurologist and is prescribed different medications to manage seizures, the GP may not know about this change and prescribe another medication for an illness, which may cause a dangerous interaction that could be detrimental to the child. In addition to adverse drug reactions, the poor coordination of care may result in unnecessary hospitalisations, duplicate testing, advice from one clinician that contradicts that of another, and poor clinical outcomes.

The Institute of Medicine (IOM) identified ineffective care coordination as a cause of poor clinical outcomes and recommended electronic health records (EHRs) as one way to improve the quality of care for patients with chronic conditions. By documenting care and treatment in an EHR, the child's past medical and surgical histories, medications, allergies, contact information for multiple providers, schedule of preventive services, baseline neurological status, and other information can be immediately available. Electronic documentation can be beneficial, but sharing that information across systems of care presents yet another challenge. The UK utilises electronic records systems however not all areas use the same system. Access to electronic records can be limited and in many areas, these records are not readily available for paramedics to view. Parents are always encouraged to keep copies of discharge notes and consultant letters to take with their child whenever seeking medical help to ensure there is no delay in accessing vital information. If a caregiver is not present, find out if the child has a form or card with information about his or her medical problem, normal vital signs, medications, and other important medical data. There are several versions of this medical information card depending on location. The Council for Disabled Children outline core principles for Emergency Health Care Plans, and have also developed a generic NHS template.

Additional Considerations for CSHCN

1. Many CSHCN, especially those with spina bifida, have a sensitivity or allergy to latex. Always use latex precautions with these patients. Reactions to latex can range from a localised skin reaction to anaphylaxis.

2. Speak quietly and calmly to the child, and explain what he or she can expect by using words appropriate for that child's developmental level. This approach decreases the child's anxiety and increases cooperation. Recognise that most CSHCN respond best with slower movements and firm, secure contact.

3. Children with musculoskeletal conditions, such as cerebral palsy or muscular dystrophy, need special care during preparation for transport. Children with cerebral palsy are often stiff and may have contractures. Do not force movements. Secure these children in their natural position, and pad any open areas. Children with paralysis or muscular dystrophy may not have regular sensation, so special care should be taken to ensure that their limbs are secured on the stretcher and do not hang off the edges.

4. Assess pain in CSHCN. If the child cannot communicate, then ask the caregiver if the child is in pain or use an appropriate pain assessment tool, such as FLACC, **Table 11-8**. FLACC, the Face, Legs, Activity, Cry, Consolability scale is suitable for use with young children (less than 7 years of age) or children who are unable to verbally express pain (JRCALC, 2016).

Table 11-8 The FLACC Scale

Face	0	1	2
	No particular expression or smile	Occasional grimace or frown, withdrawn, disinterested	Frequent to constant frown, clenched jaw, quivering chin
Legs	**0**	**1**	**2**
	Normal position or relaxed	Uneasy, restless, tense	Kicking, or legs drawn up
Activity	**0**	**1**	**2**
	Lying quietly, normal position, moves easily	Squirming, shifting back and forth, tense	Arched, rigid, or jerking
Cry	**0**	**1**	**2**
	No cry (awake or asleep)	Moans or whimpers, occasional complaint ·	Cries steadily, screams or sobs, frequent complaints
Consolability	**0**	**1**	**2**
	Content, relaxed	Reassured by occasional touching, hugging, or talking to; distractible	Difficult to console or comfort

Position the child for comfort. Use blankets under vulnerable areas of the body. If local protocols allow, administer medications for pain control after ensuring the caregivers did not give the child any pain medication before ambulance service arrival.

5. When leaving the home of a CSHCN:

- Ask the parents or caregivers for the child's "go bag". This bag contains all of the supplies necessary (and that are not routinely stocked on ambulances) to manage the child's tracheostomy tube, feeding catheter, or central venous line.

- Ask the parents for the child's daily medical information form, which contains pertinent medical information regarding the child's medical condition, baseline vital signs, allergies, doctors' names and numbers, medications,

therapies, and necessary home support equipment. Ask how you can make the patient most comfortable.

- Ensure any compressed air or oxygen in the home is turned off before departure.

6. Request that the child's direct caregiver accompany the child to the hospital to continue assisting with the child's care. The caregiver not only becomes a valuable resource for repeated assessments and interventions, but also provides familiarity and reassurance to the child in the midst of an unfamiliar and potentially chaotic environment.

7. Recognise when the caregiver is overwhelmed with emotion or exhaustion. In these circumstances, it may be best to offer the caregiver a more passive role in the child's care while allowing him or her to continue to be with the child.

Case Study 3

A distraught mother calls 999 because her infant son is having difficulty feeding and appears more blue than usual. She tells you that the child is a 2-month-old boy with Down syndrome and a heart defect. He has been home for a few weeks and is being allowed to grow before surgery to repair his heart. His mother confirms that he usually has a pulse oximetry reading in the 80s. She hands you a card with the child's medical history, medications, and hospital information, and states that he has been vomiting since the day before and has not kept down any of his medications.

You approach the child and note that he is cyanotic and poorly interactive. There are retractions and nasal flaring. The chest has crackles, and the pulse oximetry is 75%. His heart rate is 130 beats/min, respiratory rate is 70 breaths/min, and blood pressure is 86 mm Hg/palp.

1. What is the likely physiological problem?

2. What are your primary interventions?

CASE STUDY ANSWERS

Case Study 1 — page 218

Assessment of the airway, breathing, and circulation suggests respiratory distress. Ask the child's caregiver about her baseline vital signs and activity level. Ask if there have been any changes and, if so, what is different.

Take the child off the ventilator and manually ventilate with a bag-valve-mask device. Determine the ease of air entry through the tracheostomy tube and determine if aided respirations help the child's respiratory distress. Ask the caregiver when was the last tracheostomy tube change and the frequency of suctioning. Suction the tracheostomy to determine if this helps the child's breathing. Consider a tracheostomy tube change if there are copious secretions or there is difficulty with air entry during manual ventilations.

Consider an albuterol nebuliser treatment. Albuterol may help clear secretions and can open the child's airways to alleviate distress. In this case, the parent states that he has had to suction more frequently than usual and that he has already changed the tracheostomy tube that day. He states further that he thinks the child is getting sick and that her older sister has had a cold for the last few days. This history makes an exacerbation of the child's chronic lung disease more likely, and a mucous plug obstructing the tube less likely.

You decide to transport this child to her medical home hospital and continue the albuterol nebuliser treatment through her tracheostomy tube en route. You ask the caregiver to disconnect the feed through the gastrostomy tube to prepare for transport.

This patient has bronchopulmonary dysplasia (BPD), a chronic lung disease occurring in infants characterised by stiff lungs and chronic lung disease. BPD is a worldwide problem, affecting one of every three low-birth-weight (LBW) newborns, and ranking with cystic fibrosis and asthma as one of the most common chronic lung diseases in infants. BPD develops primarily in infants with a birth weight of less than 2 pounds or 1,000 grams who have respiratory distress syndrome (RDS), a lung disease common in premature babies. BPD occurs in 97% of all infants weighing less than 1,250 grams. Babies born before 32 weeks gestation may not have enough surfactant to keep these air sacs open. However, BPD development is not limited to RDS survivors; BPD may result from alveolar damage caused by lung disease, exposure to prolonged high oxygen concentrations, or mechanical ventilation after birth (caused by such conditions as neonatal pulmonary hypertension, pneumonia, or other infections or trauma to the lungs), all of which can cause harmful chemical reactions in the lungs.

A combination of fewer alveoli with a lack of surfactant can result in abnormally stiff lungs. This increases the work of breathing for affected infants, who can quickly tire out. As they progressively weaken, carbon dioxide builds up in the lungs and blood. Respiratory infections can also worsen the inflammatory response in the lungs, leading to more fluid in the lungs or bronchospasm. Wheezing results when tiny muscles in the bronchial tubes become narrower and spasm. Other emergencies directly related to BPD include pulmonary oedema, aspiration of food or stomach contents into the lungs, and apnoea. Signs and symptoms of BPD can vary in severity depending on the infant's lung maturity. They may include tachypnoea, retractions, paradoxical respirations, abnormal posturing, and wheezing.

BPD causes the most difficulties during the first year of life. Most deaths from BPD also occur during this first year. Problems after the first year become increasingly uncommon. The most common long-term lung complication of BPD is asthma. Approximately one half of the children with BPD will have asthma. Other less common complications resulting from BPD include apnoea during infancy, gastroesophageal reflux, pulmonary hypertension, high blood pressure, pulmonary oedema, aspiration, subglottic stenosis, and tracheomalacia. Infants who have BPD are at risk for frequent hospitalisations because of their borderline respiratory reserve, hyperactive airway, and increased susceptibility to respiratory infection. A useful resource for identifying risk of serious illness is the NICE guidelines traffic light system. It is used widely by both pre-hospital and in-hospital healthcare professionals.

Case Study 2 — page 228

This boy is in no distress. The PAT is normal. His vital signs are stable. He is totally dependent on this central venous catheter for his nutrition and hydration. Ask the caregiver how long the catheter site has been bleeding. Check the catheter for dislodgement or breakage. Apply direct pressure to the site to stop the bleeding. Ask the caregiver to disconnect the catheter if it is still connected. Prepare the child for transport so that the catheter can be repaired or replaced.

Another very common problem is dislodgement of a feeding catheter. This is especially true if the child is totally dependent on the gastrostomy tube (G-tube) for all nutrition and hydration. Also, the longer the tube is out, the more difficult it is to replace. Ask the family to bring the dislodged tube to the hospital, and if they have a replacement tube, bring that as well. Not all hospitals have the proper size tubes for children, so either call ahead to the local ED if the community children's nursing team are not able to manage the patient safely within the community.

Short gut syndrome results when a large section of the bowel has become necrotic and dies as a result of poor perfusion of the blood vessels. This phenomenon is more likely to occur in premature children, but can also occur in children who experience shock or hypoxaemia to the bowel from infections, obstruction of the intestines, or trauma. These children often receive their nutrition through feeding catheters as this child did; however, if they have lost a significant amount of their bowel, they may need their nutrition (hyperalimentation and lipids) delivered through a central venous line. This boy no longer could receive all of his feeds through the gastrostomy tube and needed supplementation through his central venous catheter.

A young child who misses many hours of fluids may be tachycardic and have signs of dehydration, such as sticky mucous membranes and no tears, in the early stages of hypoperfusion. Interventions include oxygen supplementation, keeping the child warm, covering the stoma site with a dry gauze, and transporting the G-tube that fell out (along with any special adaptors) for sizing purposes. In addition, check fingerstick glucose level as it may be low.

ALS interventions include a 20 ml/kg crystalloid fluid by peripheral IV bolus in a child who seems dehydrated with a G-tube out or dislodged or a broken central venous line as per NICE guidelines.

If the glucose is low, provide IV Glucose 10% or IM Glucagon.

Case Study 3 — page 236

Assess airway, breathing, and circulation. You decide that this child needs assisted ventilations and begin to manually ventilate with a bag-valve-mask device. As your partner is looking for an appropriate IV site, she notes that the child has peripheral oedema. You then consider that this child is in congestive heart failure and opt not to start this child on IV fluids without further medical advice. Because blood pressure and perfusion are adequate, do not start a pressor drug. Transport immediately to the ED.

Down syndrome affects 1 in 800 births. This is lower than in the 1970s as a result of prenatal diagnosis and termination. Children with Down syndrome are at increased risk of medical complications. Some of the organ systems affected include cardiovascular, sensory, endocrine, orthopaedic, dental, gastrointestinal, neurological developmental, and haematologic systems. People with Down syndrome are developmentally delayed.

Cardiovascular defects are the leading cause of neonatal death caused by congenital abnormalities. When an infant is born with a severe cardiac anomaly, interventions are primarily directed toward home health care until definitive surgery can be performed or toward supportive treatment in the home of a child whose defect cannot be surgically repaired.

SUGGESTED READINGS

Textbooks

Adirim T, Smith E. *Special Children's Outreach and Prehospital Education (SCOPE)*. Burlington, MA: Jones & Bartlett Learning; 2006.

American Academy of Pediatrics and the American College of Emergency Physicians. *APLS: The Pediatric Emergency Medicine Resource*. 5th ed. Burlington, MA: Jones & Bartlett Learning; 2012.

Joint Royal Colleges Ambulance Liaison Committee. *UK Ambulance Services Clinical Practice Supplementary Guidelines 2016*. Bridgwater: Class Professional Publishing; 2016.

Articles

American Academy of Pediatrics, Committee on Children with Disabilities. Care coordination: integrating health and related systems of care for children with special health care needs. *Pediatrics*. 2005;116:1238–1244.

National Task Force on Children with Special Health Care Needs. EMS for children: recommendations for coordinating care for children with special health care needs. *Ann Emerg Med*. 1997;30:274–280.

Spaite DW, Conroy C, Karriker KJ, et al. Improving emergency medical services for children with special health care needs: does training make a difference? *Am J Emerg Med*. 2001;19:474–478.

Spaite DW, Conroy C, Tibbitts M, et al. Use of emergency medical services by children with special health care needs. *Prehosp Emerg Care*. 2000;4:19–23.

Spaite DW, Karriker KJ, Seng M, et al. Training paramedics: emergency care for children with special health care needs. *Prehosp Emerg Care*. 2000;4:178–185.

References

Bhandari A, Bhandari V. Pitfalls, problems, and progress in bronchopulmonary dysplasia. *Pediatrics*. 2009;123:1562–1573. doi:10.1542/peds.2008-1962.

Burton LC, Anderson GF, Kues IW. Using electronic health records to help coordinate care. *Milbank Quarterly*. 2004;82:457–481. doi: 10.1111/j.0887-378X.2004.00318.x.

Council for Disabled Children. Emergency Health Care Plan. https://councilfordisabledchildren.org.uk/sites/default/files/field/attachemnt/ehcp_e-form_may_2012_0.pdf. Accessed 20th June 2018.

Council for Disabled Children. Emergency Health Care Plans: Core Principles. https://councilfordisabledchildren.org.uk/sites/default/files/field/attachemnt/ehcp.core_.linksfinal.pdf. Accessed 20th June 2018.

Institute of Medicine. Committee on Identifying Priority Areas for Quality Improvement. In: Adams K, Corrigan J, eds. *Priority Areas for National Action: Transforming Health Care Quality*. Washington, DC: National Academies Press; 2003:1–13.

McPherson M. A new definition of children with special health care needs. *Pediatrics*. 1998;102:137–139.

National Center for Medical Home Implementation. www.medicalhomeinfo.org. Accessed September 24, 2012.

National Down Syndrome Society. (2011). Down syndrome fact sheet. National Down Syndrome web site. http://www.ndss.org/Documents/NDSS%20Down%20Syndrome%20Fact%20Sheet%20English.ppt%20%5BCompatibility%20Mode%5D.pdf. Accessed September 12, 2012.

National Heart Lung and Blood Institute. (2011). Who is at risk for bronchopulmonary dysplasia. http://www.nhlbi.nih.gov/health/dci/Diseases/Bpd/Bpd_WhoIsAtRisk.html. Accessed March 26, 2011.

National Institute for Health and Care Excellence. Diarrhoea and vomiting caused by gastroenteritis in under 5s: diagnosis and management. https://www.nice.org.uk/guidance/cg84/chapter/1-guidance#assessing-dehydration-and-shock. Accessed June 20, 2018.

National Institute for Health and Care Excellence. Intravenous fluid therapy in children and young people in hospital. https://www.nice.org.uk/guidance/ng29/resources/intravenous-fluid-therapy-in-children-and-young-people-in-hospital-pdf-1837340295109. Accessed June 20, 2018.

National Institute for Health and Care Excellence. Traffic light system for identifying risk of serious illness. https://www.nice.org.uk/guidance/cg160/resources/support-for-education-and-learning-educational-resource-traffic-light-table-189985789. Accessed June 20, 2018.

Northern England Clinical Networks. Emergency Health Care Plan. http://www.necn.nhs.uk/wp-content/uploads/2014/06/EHCP-NHS-Print-form-v14-April-2013.pdf. Accessed June 20, 2018.

ReSPECT. Information for Patients and Carers. https://www.respectprocess.org.uk/patientsandcarers.php. Accessed June 20, 2018.

Wertz E. *Emergency Care for Children*. Albany, NY: Delmar; 2002.

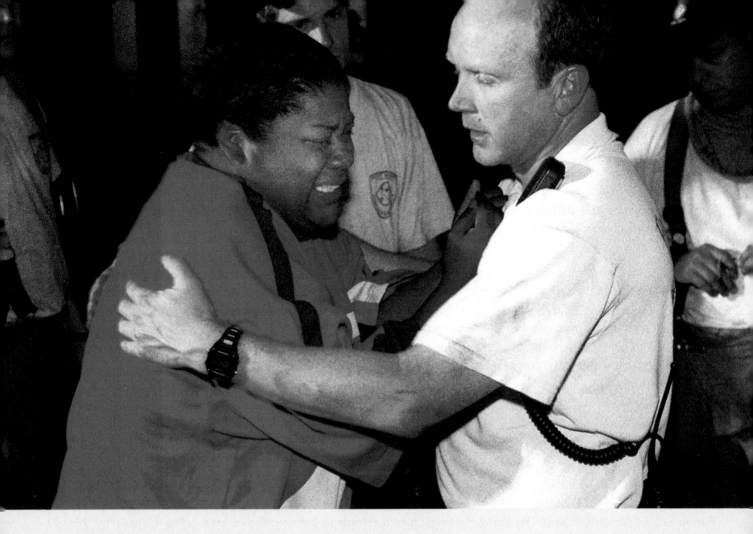

Learning Objectives

1. Describe the common clinical presentations and risk factors for sudden unexpected death in infancy (SUDI).
2. Understand the differences between SUDI and the critically ill child.
3. Discuss the actions of the clinician in the setting of suspected SUDI.
4. Define a critically ill child and discuss assessment, management, and transport considerations.
5. Recognise responses of the family to the death of an infant or child.
6. Recognise emotional responses of clinician to the death of an infant or child.
7. List community resources for support after the unexpected death of an infant or child.

Sudden Unexpected Death in Infancy (SUDI) and Death of a Child

Chapter **12**

Introduction

Sudden unexpected death in infancy (SUDI) and the death of a child are extremely difficult, emotional experiences for the clinician.

The death of a child is an unparalleled family crisis and creates difficult emotional issues for caregivers and clinicians. The infant may be in the care of a parent, child care provider, or babysitter at the time of death and may not be at home. Absence of one or both parents may complicate on-scene management and interactions.

Definition of SUDI

SUDI is the death of a baby less than one year of age that occurs suddenly and unexpectedly and whose cause of death is not immediately obvious before investigation. On the other hand, sudden infant death syndrome (SIDS) is defined as the sudden and unexpected death of an infant under one year of age that remains unexplained after a thorough post-mortem examination, examination of the place of death, and review of the clinical history. SUDI is a broader term, because it encompasses SIDS, unknown causes of death, and accidental suffocation and strangulation in bed. Hence, SUDI cannot be diagnosed at the scene or in the emergency department.

The term "cot death" was commonly used in the past to describe the sudden death of a baby; however, the term is no longer used because it gives the misleading impression that the infant must be present in their cot for the death to occur. This is untrue, because death may occur in a variety of settings.

SUDI Epidemiology

Sometimes a sudden, unexpected infant death is not caused by SUDI, and the coroner identifies a specific illness or injury as the cause. This group includes deaths caused by child maltreatment, as discussed in the *Child Maltreatment* chapter. On scene, the clinician cannot determine the true cause of death of an infant. Treat every caregiver as a grieving parent. *Never discuss child maltreatment as a possible cause of death while on scene.* Be sure, however, to note details of the death scene and record observations on your patient care record. To help identify deaths that may not be from natural causes, document any observations related to the scene assessment, physical assessment of the infant, or focused history that seem atypical or inconsistent with SUDI. For example, dangerous or unclean home conditions, bruises or burn marks on the child's body, or changing or implausible

Case Study 1

You are dispatched for an infant not breathing. On your arrival you find a 6-month-old boy in his mother's arms, with dark purplish bruising on his face and chest. He has pink frothy sputum around his mouth and nose. He is cold, pulseless, and apnoeic. His arms and jaw are stiff. His mother is weeping, "I think he is dead."

1. Is this a SUDI death?

2. What can you do to assist the family with the death of their child?

stories are possible red flags for child maltreatment that require explicit documentation, as discussed in the *Child Maltreatment* chapter. Twins and multiples have approximately twice the risk of SUDI compared with singletons. Components of risk vary in different studies and include pre-term gestation, low birth weight, and zygosity (whether identical or non-identical).

Sudden Infant Death Syndrome (SIDS) is the sudden and unexplained death of an infant where no cause is found after detailed post mortem (**Figure 12-1**). Data from the Office for National Statistics shows that:

- 212 unexplained infant deaths occurred in England and Wales in 2014, a rate of 0.30 deaths per 1,000 live births. This follows the decreasing trend that has generally been seen over the last decade from 0.5 in 2005.

- 60% of these deaths were recorded as sudden infant deaths with the remaining 40% recorded as unascertained (where no other cause of death is recorded).

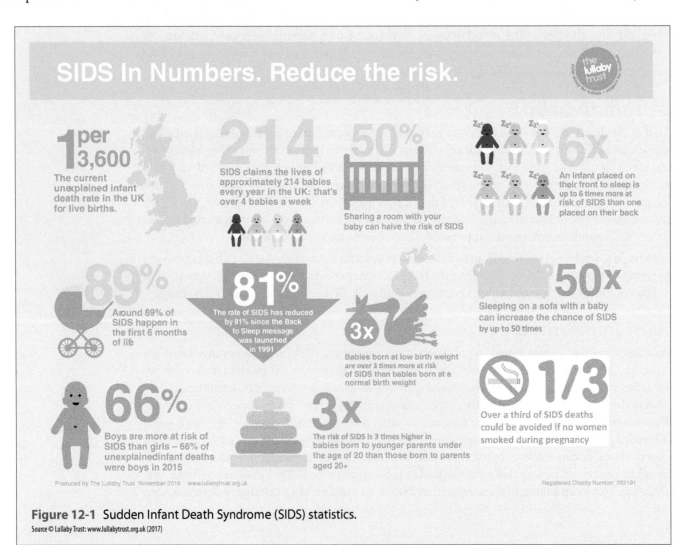

Figure 12-1 Sudden Infant Death Syndrome (SIDS) statistics.
Source © Lullaby Trust: www.lullabytrust.org.uk (2017)

- Just over half (55%) of all unexplained infant deaths were boys in 2014 (117 deaths).

- The rate of infant deaths rose for mothers aged 20 to 24 and 25 to 29 in 2014 while the rate fell for all other age groups.

Source: Office of National Statistics, National Records of Scotland and Northern Ireland Statistics and Research Agency 2016

Key information about mechanism for suffocation includes adults sharing a bed with the infant, soft bedding, and wedging and entrapment of the infant between two objects. Information provided by prehospital clinicians can assist in the later determination of the cause of death, so the scene survey is very important. **Figure 12-2** provides more data on SIDS.

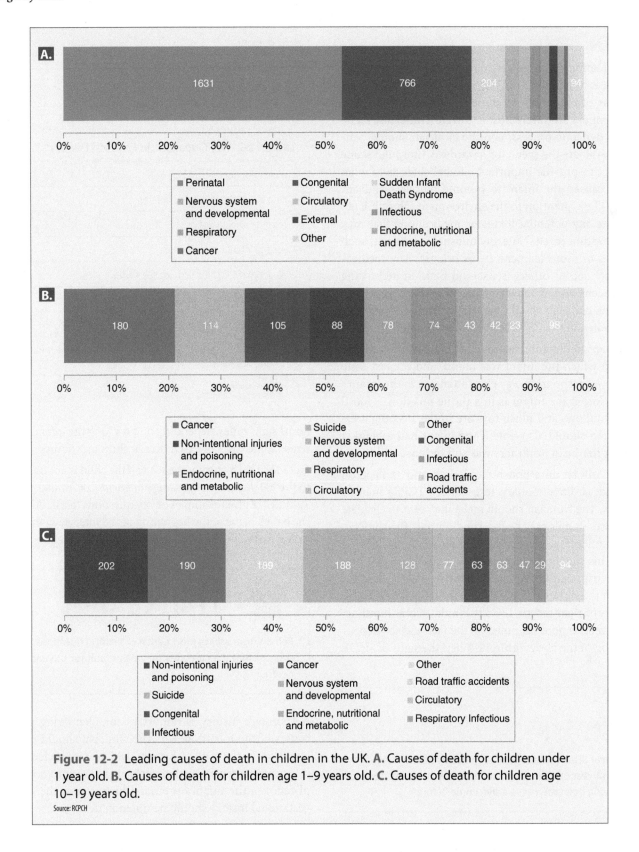

Figure 12-2 Leading causes of death in children in the UK. **A.** Causes of death for children under 1 year old. **B.** Causes of death for children age 1–9 years old. **C.** Causes of death for children age 10–19 years old.

Source: RCPCH

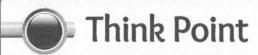

Think Point

Never discuss possible causes of death on the scene with the parents/caregiver.

Common Clinical Presentation of SUDI

When evaluating an unresponsive infant, a thorough scene assessment is imperative. The scene may be potentially hostile because of the emotions present. Although emotional family members are rarely hostile toward clinicians, scene safety is a dynamic process, and the clinician should constantly re-evaluate the scene for hazards. A thorough scene evaluation can provide important clinical clues as to what may have caused the infant to become pulseless and apnoeic. Pay close attention to the environment. The clinician should note any potential toxins or medications that may have been within reach. Note any unusual conditions, such as extremes of room temperature or odours. Any medications, prescribed or otherwise, should be indicated to the police on scene and, if conveying, taken with the patient to the ED. The clinician should also pay attention to signs of abuse, as noted in the *Child Maltreatment* chapter.

The clinician should note the time the infant was found, the position in which the infant was found, and the last time the infant was responsive. Pay close attention to the infant's position. Note if the infant is in a prone position. Record how many pillows and plush toys are in the sleeping area. The clinician should also note if the infant had a blanket over his or her head or if there was soft or loose bedding.

The infant will be unresponsive, pulseless, and apnoeic on arrival, and cardiopulmonary resuscitation (CPR) may be in progress. The clinician should make it a point to evaluate central pulses. Pupils may be fixed and dilated. The clinician will also notice asystole on the electrocardiogram (ECG) monitor. This should be confirmed as per local policy, and additional strips may be required to hand over to the coroner. Along with the signs listed previously, the clinician may also note lividity or rigor mortis. Lividity is reddish blue mottling, caused by venous pooling, noted on the face and the dependent portion of the body. **Table 12-1** lists the signs of SUDI.

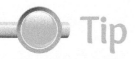

Tip

The typical SUDI scenario is an apparently healthy baby, less than 1 year of age, who is found dead in his or her bed after having been seen alive a short time before.

Table 12-1 External Appearance of SUDI Victims
Cold skin
Frothy or blood-tinged fluid in the mouth and nose
Lividity or dark, reddish blue mottling on the dependent side of the body
Normal hydration and nutrition
Rigor mortis
Vomitus (uncommon)

© Jones & Bartlett Learning

Table 12-2 Key Questions in Focused History*
What happened?
Who found the infant and where?
What did the parent or caregiver do?
Has the infant been moved?
What time was the infant last seen alive?
Had the infant been sick?
Was the infant receiving any medications?
*When asking these questions, use the infant's name rather than "the infant."

© Jones & Bartlett Learning

Some signs differ, depending on how long the infant has been dead. Some cases of SUDI do not show any of these signs.

Get a focused history at the scene if the child is not transported to the ED. *Refrain from asking judgmental or leading questions.* **Table 12-2** gives examples of key questions to ask. Always ask the baby's name at the beginning of the interview, and use his or her first name in all discussions with the caregiver.

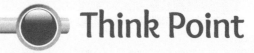

Think Point

Refrain from asking judgmental or leading questions that suggest that the caregiver may be at fault for the infant's death.

A thorough history is important for identifying potential causes of the infant's death. The clinician should pay close attention to the patient history, which may include recent infections, potential birth defects, or a variety of other complications. The infant's pre-natal history and the maternal gestational history should be noted in detail.

Actions in Suspected SUDI

The clinician's first actions when SUDI is suspected must always be to assess and treat the baby. Immediately begin resuscitation, according to the current Resuscitation Council Guidelines, JRCALC, and local ambulance protocols, unless the infant meets the JRCALC criteria for situations unequivocally associated with death, or recognition of life extinct (ROLE). In many SUDI cases, the baby has easily recognisable signs of death, and interventions or resuscitation are not indicated. If resuscitation is indicated, encourage the family to remain present during the resuscitative attempt, whenever possible.

After assessing the child's cardiopulmonary status, unless the patient meets ROLE criteria, begin CPR if there is no detectable heart rate or other signs of life. If resuscitation is started and the child responds, transport as soon as medically appropriate, as discussed in the *Transport Considerations* chapter.

Table 12-3 Pros and Cons of Transporting Suspected SUDI Infants

Pros	Cons
ALS capability in ED	Caregiver concern about infant's body
Facilitation of post-mortem	Disruption of scene
More medical personnel to manage infant	High costs
Physician involvement in management	Possible violation of family's culture
Religious services	Removal of family from familiar setting
Social services for grief counselling	Transport liabilities, especially ambulance crashes and adverse bystander reactions

© Jones & Bartlett Learning

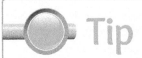

Tip

In all cases of cardiopulmonary arrest, immediately begin resuscitation using standard treatment protocol, unless the infant meets ROLE criteria.

If resuscitation is considered to be futile on the clinician's arrival at the scene or if the initial response to CPR is unsuccessful, it may be appropriate to leave the scene and allow the coroner or police forensic examiner to facilitate the death investigation. *The clinician must not leave the scene after a child has died until the appropriate authorities have arrived.* **Table 12-3** lists the pros and cons of transporting suspected SUDI infants. Because the clinician cannot distinguish a child with SIDS or SUDI from any other child in cardiopulmonary arrest, use standard principles of treatment and transport for children in cardiopulmonary arrest, as discussed in the *Resuscitation and Dysrhythmias* chapter.

Value of Transport After Failed ALS Treatment in Cardiopulmonary Arrest. The value of immediate or delayed hospital transport when a child does not respond to resuscitation is controversial. The chances of neurological survival of a child in the ED, after failed ALS on scene, are almost zero, unless rare extenuating circumstances (e.g., profound hypothermia, barbiturate overdose) are present.

Sometimes, local policy will state that the infant must be conveyed to the local ED regardless of the situation; this will depend upon local ambulance service and police joint protocols. In this situation, transport the baby to the hospital in a controlled transport mode (no lights or siren) with the parents or caregiver, if possible. Risks generally far outweigh the benefits of lights and siren transport. Allow the parents or caregiver a chance to touch or hold the child before transport. This may be the last time the parents or caregiver have to be with the child. This may not be possible if the scene is related to a crime but is an important step in the grieving process.

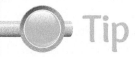

Tip

Encourage family presence during the attempted resuscitation.

The clinician's emotional support of the parents or caregivers is extremely important. When possible, have one person stay with the parents to provide information and support. Let family or caregivers stay with the child and do not separate them even during attempted resuscitation and transport. If family chooses to ride with the patient, ensure that they remain restrained with a seat belt according to manufacturer's recommendations and local protocols. *Be clear that the child is dead.* Do not use euphemisms, such as "your child has left us" or "she has gone to a better place." Avoid well-intentioned but inappropriate remarks, such as, "You can always have other children," "I know how you feel," or "You will get over this in time." **Table 12-4** suggests specific ways to communicate with caregivers when there is an unexpected death of a child.

Table 12-4 Communicating About an Unexpected Death of a Child

Use the child's name.
Show **empathy** and express condolences.
Ask questions in a non-judgmental manner. Never become hostile or angry.
Use a calm and directive voice.
Be clear with instructions and answers to questions.
Provide explanations to the caregivers about treatment and transport.
Repeat statements when necessary.
Reassure parents or caregivers that there was nothing they could have done.
Allow the parent or caregiver to accompany the baby if possible.

© Jones & Bartlett Learning

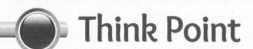

Think Point

In discussion with the family, do not obscure the fact that the child is dead by using ambiguous language.

It is vital that clinicians create a clear picture of the events that occurred through their documentation, which should be objective in nature. Any statements that are pertinent to the documentation should be captured with quotation marks. This patient-care report should be extremely detailed and include dispatch information, a scene evaluation, thorough head-to-toe assessment, interventions, response to interventions, transport decision and reasoning, and transfer of care. Also note any communication that occurs with the family, coroner, police, emergency operations control (EOC), or any other entity involved. Failure to adequately document can cause a significant amount of stress on the clinician and parents.

Summary of SUDI

SUDI is one of the common causes of infant death seen by the ambulance service. It is unpredictable and silent. The clinician cannot "diagnose" SUDI on scene, and the emergency physician cannot diagnose SUDI in the ED. Determining the cause of death requires a post-mortem. There are, however, common clinical signs and important risk factors that may be helpful in identifying probable SUDI cases.

When faced with an infant in cardiopulmonary arrest, begin or continue CPR according to the local and national

ambulance service policies on death at scene. **Figure 12-3** provides a typical sequence of events when there is a suspected SUDI case.

Responses to an Infant Death
Parent or Caregiver's Response

The clinician is often the first person on scene following the discovery of the dead infant. Responses of parents or caregivers to the sudden and unexpected death of an infant are not predictable and may vary from numb silence to rage. Common reactions include denial, anger, hysteria, withdrawal, intense guilt, or no visible response. The parent or caregiver may or may not accept that the infant is dead and that resuscitation is not possible. The parent or caregiver may cling to the hope that the clinician can do something to save the infant, even though the child is obviously dead.

The death of a child is likely the most stressful and tragic moment in the life of a parent or caregiver. It is not uncommon for parents in this situation to express strong preferences or make "demands" of the clinician. Remember, this is the individual's last chance to fulfil their role of protecting and caring for their infant. Respond to the parents gently and professionally. The parent or caregiver may:

- Ask repeated questions
- Request that you not start care or that you stop resuscitation efforts
- Request to be alone with the infant
- Want to know the cause of death
- Physically interfere with care
- Insist on continuation of care or that resuscitation efforts begin

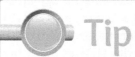

Tip

Responses of the parent or caregiver to the sudden and unexpected death of an infant are not predictable and may vary from numb silence to rage.

When the parents or family expresses their preferences or asks difficult questions, use a calm and professional approach. Keep explanations simple. Be honest and direct with family members. Follow local and national guidance on resuscitation and ROLE and maintain an empathetic and nonjudgmental attitude. Allow room for the family to grieve. Be respectful of the family's religious beliefs, customs, or traditions.

If there is no indication to attempt to resuscitate the infant, while awaiting the police or coroner at the scene ask the family member or caregiver if someone can be called

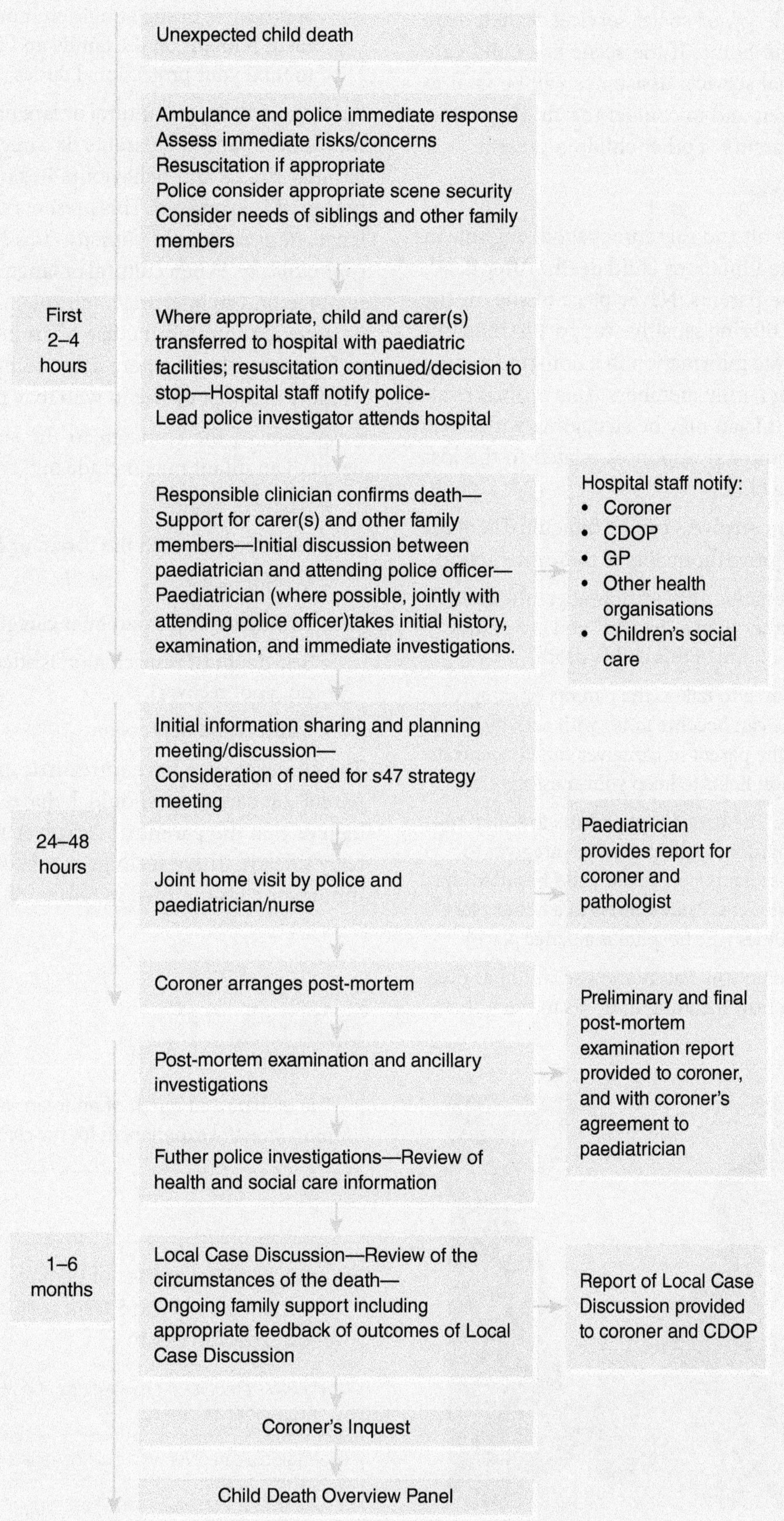

Figure 12-3 The joint agency response to an unexpected infant death.
© Crown copyright

to give them support (**Figure 12-4**). This may involve calling friends, relatives, clergy, or social services to help care for other children at the home. If the scene is a child care setting, police and social services assistance will be vital to assist with other children and to contact the child's parents or caregivers and the parents of other children present.

Clinician's Response

The clinician has a difficult and sometimes agonising role in the setting of unexpected infant or child death. After death is declared, comfort the parents. Never place blame on the parents or caregivers. Offering sensitive support to the family and gathering accurate information in a non-threatening manner helps surviving family members. This is often challenging, because the clinician may be struggling with overwhelming personal emotional responses related to the loss of a patient, especially a child.

Talking to the family or caregivers can be difficult. There are techniques that may improve the quality of these interactions:

- Use the child's first name. This acknowledges the child as an individual rather than a "patient" and the unique, intensely personal nature of this child's death.

- Try to find a quiet area to talk to the parents or caregivers. Often the scene can become noisy with activity. Finding an area where the parent or caregiver can concentrate on your conversation helps to keep your message clear.

- Use concrete terms. The use of euphemisms to soften the news can make it harder for the parent or caregiver to understand what has happened. "Your child has died" has a finite meaning, whereas "Your child is in a better place" has infinite possibilities (the hospital is a better place).

- It is okay to show emotion. Parents whose child has died often comment on how meaningful it was to them that

the clinician clearly cared. Expressing your emotions is appropriate in such tragic circumstances, so long as the focus remains on the family and child and you are able to fulfil your professional duties at the scene.

Sometimes there are cultural or language differences between the clinician and the parents or caregiver. There may be unfamiliar rituals and behaviours in how death is regarded or how grief is expressed. This presents another important challenge. *Respect cultural diversity. This is necessary to effectively communicate.* When cultural or language differences arise, attempt to find an interpreter to explain and translate. This may be accessed through the use of an interpreting service such as "Language Line" where calls are more reliable than using a family member or friend who may not interpret correctly.

Responses of the clinician to the sudden and unexpected death of an infant may include one or more of the following:

- Anger or blame
- Identification with the parent or caregiver
- Withdrawal
- Avoidance of the parent or caregiver
- Self-doubt (if resuscitation is attempted and the child does not recover)
- Sadness and depression

The clinician may have unrealistic expectations of how the parent or caregiver should behave and respond, or may believe that the parent or caregiver was responsible for the baby's death. These feelings can become obstacles to communication, as outlined in **Table 12-5**.

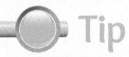

Tip

The unexpected death of an infant or child is one of the most stressful experiences for the clinician.

Figure 12-4 Caregivers can react to the death of a child in many ways, but all need support. Attempt to contact identified individuals who might give comfort.

Table 12-5 Responses of Clinician That Hinder Communication With Parents or Caregivers After an Unexpected Death

Having stereotyped expectations of how the caregiver should respond to the event
Judging a caregiver who did not initiate CPR
Distrusting a caregiver who has recognised the infant is dead and does not want resuscitation
Misunderstanding the mourning and grief behaviors of persons of different cultures or religious beliefs

Case Study 2

You are called to a family home. On arrival, there is a large, concerned, group congregated at the doorway, speaking in a language that you do not recognise. You enter the house to find a mother and father sitting on a couch, quietly weeping. They gesture toward a cot, where a cold 3-month-old infant with lividity lies covered in a pile of blankets. Through a neighbour who speaks English, you explain that the baby is dead and ask if they would like to hold her. They decline, and seem offended by the proposal.

1. How should you react?

2. What steps do you take from this point?

Common Clinical Presentation of the Critically Ill Child

Similar to SUDI, critical illness generally presents with a stressful scene. A thorough scene assessment should be used when evaluating scene safety, while ascertaining clinical clues that may have caused the event. Primary assessment should include evaluating the patient's airway for patency. The clinician should evaluate the patient's breathing rate, depth, and quality. Breathing patterns may be slow, shallow, or have some other disruption in minute volume causing breathing to be inadequate. Circulation should be assessed by palpating pulses for rate, regularity, and quality; assessing capillary refills; and assessing skin colour, temperature, and condition. Pulses may be bradycardic and weak, capillary refills may be greater than 4 seconds, and skin may show signs of hypoperfusion or hypoxia.

A thorough history should be obtained. Onset should be noted so a timeline can be developed. The clinician should note if anything makes the patient's symptoms better or worse. Pain is generally difficult to assess, especially in children who are non-verbal or not able to communicate. History should be obtained from the child's caregiver. If any long term conditions are present, listen to the caregiver on how to manage these; they have probably dealt with the condition for years and are the ones who can manage equipment and machines best.

Identify the patient's signs and attempt to identify symptoms. If any allergies are known at this age, they should be noted. Any medications that the patient is taking should be evaluated for potential side effects and cross-referenced with any potential treatment plans. The patient's entire medical history is pertinent at this age. Identifying the patient's last oral intake and events leading up to it may help point toward a potential diagnosis.

Vital signs should be assessed on all critically ill patients. This should include pulse rate, respiratory rate, blood pressure, pulse oximetry, and blood glucose analysis. A thorough, hands-on, head-to-toe assessment should be performed, noting any abnormalities. Auscultation of lungs and bowel should occur. Reassessments should be done every 5–15 minutes depending on severity and interventions.

Actions

Clinical Interventions

If the child appears unstable or needs urgent treatment, complete the secondary assessment en route to the chosen appropriate hospital. The clinician must pay close attention to and protect the patient's airway as necessary. It is imperative that supplemental oxygen be given as early as possible if indicated. Always transport the child, even if the complete assessment reveals no abnormalities. Serious illnesses in newly born and young infants are sometimes subtle and difficult to detect, and congenital abnormalities often improve before worsening again.

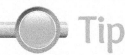

Tip

In the child with underlying health issues, listen to the parents—they have often been dealing with the condition for many years and understand the child's needs.

Summary

The critically ill child may be an indicator of serious occult illness or injury that may not be identified on scene. Perform a standard assessment and treat if there is a demonstrable physiological or anatomical problem. In most cases, transport alone is the most important intervention.

Stress Management

Stress is an unavoidable part of the clinician's job. The death of a child may be the most stressful situation in the clinician's career. Acknowledging emotions is a key element in

Table 12-6 Signs and Symptoms of Critical Incident Stress

Anger and irritability
Changes in eating habits
Changes in sleeping patterns
Depression
Excessive alcohol consumption
Inability to concentrate
Mood changes and emotional instability
Physical illness
Recurring dreams or frightening images
Withdrawal

© Jones & Bartlett Learning

successfully coping with stress and maintaining a healthy mental attitude. **Table 12-6** lists the frequent signs and symptoms of stress.

There are many ways to decrease the impact of stress related to the death of an infant or child. TRiM: Trauma Risk Management may be an important technique for helping cope with the emotional toll of SUDI. TRiM has been developed in the UK to support organisations that operate in high-risk or high-threat locations and staff who in the course of day-to-day work are likely to face traumatic or potentially traumatic situations. Other techniques to help decrease stress include the following:

- Talk to line managers and experienced clinicians to share feelings.
- Maintain a well-balanced lifestyle outside of work. Exercise, plan leisure time, and limit overtime hours.
- Get adequate rest and eat a balanced diet.
- Avoid excessive alcohol or drugs.
- Write a personal diary.
- Obtain religious or peer counselling.
- Request professional psychological assistance.

Community Resources

Community resources available to parents or caregivers and clinicians to help them cope with the unexpected death of a child include the following (dependent on local availability):

Local support groups include:

- 2 Wish Upon A Star: Immediate support, counselling and support groups for suddenly bereaved parents in Wales.
- Cardiac Risk in the Young: Counselling for those affected by young sudden cardiac death.

- Care For The Family Enquiries: Provide parenting, relationship, and bereavement support through events, resources, courses, training, and volunteer networks.
- Child Bereavement UK Support and Information: Support for bereaved parents on helpline. Face-to-face support groups in Bucks, Milton Keynes, West London, Newham, Cheshire, Carlisle & Eden and South Lakeland.
- Child Death Helpline: A free helpline started by volunteer bereaved parents for all those affected by the death of a child.
- Child Funeral Charity Enquiries: Assists families financially in England and Wales for funeral expenses for under 16s (excluding headstones or funeral plots).
- Cruse Bereavement Care Helpline: Helpline and face-to-face support for bereaved people.
- SANDS (Stillbirth and Neonatal Death Charity): Stillbirth and neonatal death charity, providing a helpline and support groups.
- Scottish Cot Death Trust Enquiries: Scottish charity supporting families and providing professionals with education and information on sudden unexpected death in infants and pre-school children.
- TAMBA (Twins and Multiple Births Association): Helpline, support groups and advice on raising multiples.
- The Compassionate Friends Helpline: Supporting bereaved parents and their families after a child dies.
- The Coroners' Courts Support Service Helpline: A registered charity whose volunteers give emotional and practical support to families and other witnesses attending inquests at 30 coroners' courts around England.
- The Lullaby Trust Helpline: Specialist support for bereaved families and anyone affected by a sudden infant death.
- Winston's Wish Helpline: A childhood bereavement charity in the UK offering practical support and guidance to bereaved children, their families and professionals.
- Professional counselling.
- Emergency Services Chaplain.

For contact details see the list of resources at the end of the chapter.

Parental Education

Due to the uniqueness of the clinician's role, you can also play a key role in educating parents in your care on ways to decrease the risk of SUDI. This includes the promotion of the Lullaby Trust's "Back to Sleep" campaign and active support of their recommendation to place babies on their backs to sleep. A "Back to Sleep" fact sheet is available on the Lullaby Trust's website, as well as a guide for clinicians;

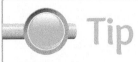

Tip

TRiM may be an important technique for coping with the emotional toll of SUDI.

Controversy

The value and appropriate timing of TRiM is not known. Although the clinician suffers predictable stress after the death of a child in his or her care, how and when such intervention should occur has not been studied.

Controversy

Risk reduction and risk counselling are important community prevention activities. Further research must help define the appropriate educational role of the clinician at the scene of an injury or death.

Tip

Clinicians can play a key role in educating parents in the community on ways to decrease the risk of SUDI.

these are listed in the further reading at the end of the chapter. Although side-sleeping is several times safer than prone sleeping, the risk of SUDI for the side-sleeping position is still double the risk of the supine position. Clinicians can participate in community risk reduction by advocating for firm, flat mattresses in safety-approved cribs, and avoidance of soft or bulky blankets or comforters and overheating in the infant's sleeping area.

Recommendations for reducing the risk of SUDI are:

- Place your baby to sleep on his or her back for every sleep.
- Place your baby to sleep on a firm sleep surface.
- Keep soft objects, loose bedding, or any objects that could increase the risk of entrapment, suffocation, or strangulation out of the crib. This includes pillows, blankets, and bumper pads.
- Place your baby to sleep in the same room where you sleep but not the same bed.
- Breastfeed as much and for as long as you can.
- Schedule and go to all baby checks and see the health visitor regularly.
- Keep your baby away from smokers and places where people smoke.
- Do not let your baby get too hot.
- Offer a dummy at nap time and bedtime.
- Do not use products that claim to reduce the risk of SUDI, such as wedges and positioners.

Support of anti-smoking campaigns is also important. Recent research shows that the risk of SUDI doubles among babies exposed to cigarette smoke after birth, and triples for those exposed both during pregnancy and after birth. As for all infants, encouragement of breastfeeding is a useful action.

Case Study 3

You are dispatched to a co-worker's home where a grandmother is weeping and largely incoherent. She leads you to a bedroom where a 3-month-old boy lies motionless in his crib, face down on a sheepskin. He is apnoeic and pulseless, has lividity on his chest and face, and is stiff. In between sobs, the grandmother tells you she put the baby to sleep 4 hours ago and found him this way when she checked on him 10 minutes ago. She asks you if he is dead.

1. What are your key medical actions?

2. How should you deal with the grandmother? The co-worker?

CASE STUDY ANSWERS

Case Study 1 — page 242

The infant has many findings commonly associated with a SUDI death. Sleeping prone (indicated by the lividity on the chest and face), the pink frothy sputum, and the absence of traumatic injuries are the initial clues to a SUDI death. However, remember that SUDI is a diagnosis of exclusion made by a medical examiner or coroner at post-mortem and cannot be made on scene.

In this setting, provide a direct and calm explanation to the parent that the child is dead. Find out the child's name and use it. Do not ask questions in a way that suggests blame. Use controlled and supportive dialogue with the parent. If the child is not transported, try to get grief counselling for the parent, by contacting the family GP, contact the coroner from the scene, and consider critical incident stress management for yourself and your partner. Signpost to further support resources.

Case Study 2 — page 249

Different cultures have different beliefs about death, afterlife, and the proper handling of a dead body. There may be rituals or taboos with which you are unfamiliar and different ways of coping with loss. Because there is no medical intervention that will help this child, your focus must be on providing support to the survivors. Obtaining a professional interpreter, where available, is an important part of the scene management and death investigation. Through an English-speaking neighbour, you can inquire about family needs, who they might want you to contact, and any way that you might assist them at the scene. Remember that even with an interpreter present, concepts may be difficult to translate and the family may have a very different belief system than do you with regard to illness, health care, and cause of death. If you cannot communicate the rationale for your treatment or non-treatment to the family, transport (this will depend on local policy and procedures).

Case Study 3 — page 251

In most ambulance services, this child would meet ROLE criteria and would not require any resuscitation attempt. If you are uncertain about whether resuscitation is indicated, begin CPR and call senior support to clarify treatment options.

The grandmother may need to be medically evaluated if she cannot be calmed down. Provide a calm and controlled environment. Do not place blame.

Try to minimise radio communications if your co-worker may be listening. If the employee is at work, have a supervisor contact the co-worker and provide safe transportation to the scene. Contact other family, friends, or clergy if the situation warrants. Watch for symptoms consistent with that of critical incident stress and initiate TRiM if indicated.

SUGGESTED READINGS

References

American Academy of Pediatrics. SIDS and other sleep-related infant deaths: expansion of recommendations for a safe infant sleeping environment. http://pediatrics.aappublications.org/content/128/5/e1341.full. Accessed July 18, 2012.

American Academy of Pediatrics. AAP expands guidelines for infant sleep safety and SIDS risk reduction. http://www.aap.org/en-us/about-the-aap/aap-press-room/pages/AAP-Expands-Guidelines-for-Infant-Sleep-Safety-and-SIDS-Risk-Reduction.aspx. Accessed July 18, 2012.

Centers for Disease Control and Prevention. Sudden unexpected infant death and sudden infant death syndrome. Centers for Disease Control and Prevention web site. http://www.cdc.gov/sids/index.htm. Accessed November 17, 2015.

Garstang J, Griffiths F, Sidebotham P. What do bereaved parents want from professionals after the sudden death of their child: a systematic review of the literature. *BMC Pediatr* 2014;14:269.

HM Government. 2015. Working Together to Safeguard Children: A guide to inter-agency working to safeguard and promote the welfare of children. Department for Education.www.gov.uk/government/publications/working-together-to-safeguard - children—2. Accessed June 21, 2018.

The Lullaby Trust. 2013. When a Baby Dies Suddenly and Unexpectedly. London: The Lullaby Trust website. https://www .lullabytrust.org.uk. Accessed June 21, 2018.

Mathews TJ, MacDorman MF, Thoma ME. Infant mortality statistics from the 2013 period linked birth/death data set. http:// cdc.gov/nchs/linked.htm. Accessed November 18, 2015.

National Institutes of Health. Infantile apnea and home monitoring. NIH Consensus Statement Online 1986;6(6):1–10. National Institutes of Health web site. http://consensus.nih.gov/1986/1986InfantApneaMonitoring058html.htm. Accessed September 12, 2012.

Office for National Statistics. 2014. Unexplained Deaths in Infancy, England and Wales. https://cy.ons.gov.uk/people populationandcommunity/birthsdeathsandmarriages/deaths/bulletins/unexplaineddeathsininfancyenglandandwales /2014?:uri=peoplepopulationandcommunity/birthsdeathsandmarriages/deaths/bulletins/unexplaineddeathsininfancyenglan dandwales/2014. Accessed June 21, 2018.

Royal College of Pathologists. Sudden Unexpected Death in Infancy: A multi-agency protocol for care and investigation. The report of a working group convened by The Royal College of Pathologists and The Royal College of Paediatrics and Child Health. London: RCPath and RCPH. Chaired by The Baroness Helena Kennedy QC. 2004. https://www.rcpath.org/resource Library/sudden-unexpected-death-in-infancy-and-childhood-report.html. Accessed June 21, 2018.

Shapiro-Mendoza CK, Camperiengo L, Ludvigsen R, et al. Classification system for the sudden unexpected infant death case registry and its application. *Pediatrics.* 2014;134:e210–e219.

Sidebotham P, Fleming PJ. *Unexpected Death in Childhood: A Handbook for Professionals.* Chichester, UK: Wiley; 2007.

Resources

The Lullaby Trust. Safer Sleep for Babies Fact sheet 1. Back to Sleep. https://www.lullabytrust.org.uk/wp-content/uploads /fact-sheet-back-to-sleep.pdf. Accessed July 16, 2018.

The Lullaby Trust. Sudden Infant Death Syndrome: A guide for professionals. https://www.lullabytrust.org.uk/wp-content /uploads/sids-guide-professionals.pdf. Accessed July 16, 2018.

March on Stress. 2017. Trauma Risk Management (TRiM). http://www.marchonstress.com/page/p/trim. Accessed July 16, 2018.

Local Support Groups

2 Wish Upon A Star Tel: 01443 853125 Support@2wishuponastar.org

Cardiac Risk in the Young (CRY) Tel: 01737 363222 cry@c-r-y.org.uk

Care For The Family Enquiries: 029 2081 0800 mail@c.org.uk

Child Bereavement UK Support and Information: 0800 02 888 40 support@childbereavementuk.org

Child Death Helpline: 0800 282 986; from a mobile: 0808 800 6019

contact@childdeathhelpline.org

Child Funeral Charity Enquiries: 01480 276088 enquiries@childfuneralcharity.org.uk

The Compassionate Friends Helpline: 0345 123 2304

Northern Ireland helpline: 028 8778 8016 helpline@tcf.org.uk

Cruse Bereavement Care Helpline: 0808 808 1677 www.cruse.org.uk

Language Line: Available at: https://www.languageline.com/uk

SANDS (Stillbirth and Neonatal Death Charity) Helpline: 020 7436 5881 helpline@uk-sands.org

Scottish Cot Death Trust Enquiries: 0141 357 3946 contact@scottishcotdeathtrust.org

TAMBA (Twins and Multiple Births Association) Twin-line: 0800 138 0509 asktwinline@tamba.org.uk

The Coroners' Courts Support Service Helpline: 0300 111 2141 (o ce hours) or 020 3667 7884 (answerphone) info@ccsupport.org.uk

The Lullaby Trust Helpline: 0808 802 6868 support@lullabytrust.org.uk

Winston's Wish Helpline: 08452 03 04 05 info@winstonswish.org.uk

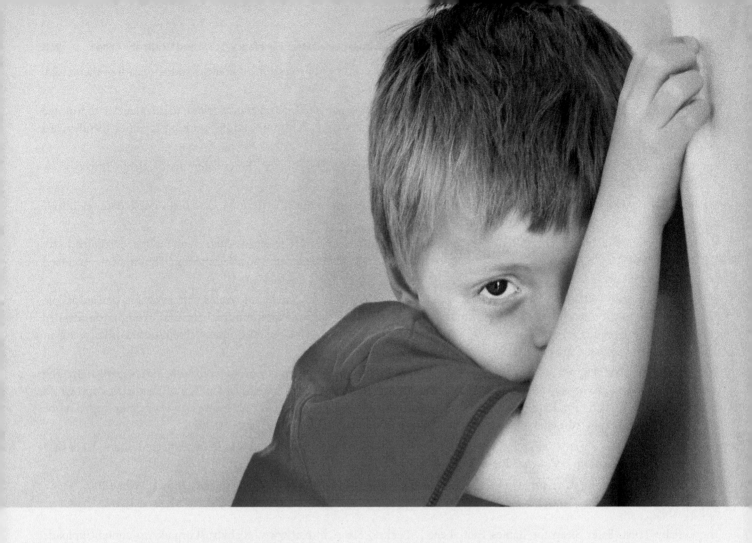

Learning Objectives

1. Discuss the known signs, causes, and complications of child maltreatment.
2. Define the terms physical abuse, emotional abuse, sexual abuse, and child neglect.
3. Explain the role of local authority social services in the management of suspected child maltreatment.
4. Distinguish features in the scene assessment, in the history and physical assessment, and in the caregiver's behaviours that suggest child maltreatment.
5. Describe appropriate communication with caregivers of suspected victims of maltreatment.
6. Outline the prehospital professional's legal responsibility to document and report suspected child maltreatment.

Child Maltreatment

Introduction

Prehospital professionals must know when to suspect child maltreatment. Although providing emergency medical care is always the top priority, prehospital professionals have a legal duty to report safeguarding concerns and are often the first step in the reporting process of suspected cases of maltreatment. Likewise, they provide valuable scene assessment documentation. All of these actions are critical to protect vulnerable children and to break the cycle. When caring for a paediatric patient who has suffered obvious trauma, prehospital clinicians need to remain vigilant in looking for potential signs of abuse.

Unfortunately, child maltreatment is common. It is one of the leading causes of death in infants less than 12 months of age. Physical abuse and neglect are often detectable, but sexual abuse, emotional abuse, and child neglect may not be so obvious. Some children who die from maltreatment are known to the local authority who are one of the legal organisations in the community who monitor, manage, and prevent child maltreatment. These deaths are sometimes preventable. Abused or neglected children have a high probability of being maltreated again. Early recognition is important to prevent future injury or death.

Background, Cost, and Definition

In 2015–2016 there were 621,470 requests for services to be provided by children's social care in the UK. Survivors of child maltreatment or neglect can suffer from lifelong consequences, either physical and or emotional. Survivors may themselves become abusive or neglectful to children, thus perpetuating the cycle of abuse. The number of children who suffer long-term effects from neglect is not as well documented, but it is believed to be substantial. **Table 13-1** lists some of these long-term complications.

It is estimated that 199 children die from abuse and neglect in the UK each year, a little under 4 children per week. Males are slightly more likely to be maltreated than females (52.7% vs 45.3%). A small percentage occurs prenatally and the gender is unknown. The largest age group are those aged 10–15 years, accounting for 30.6% of abused or neglected children; 23.6% are under 5 years. It has been estimated that the annual cost of child sexual abuse in the UK was £3.2 billion in 2012–2013.

Definition of Child Maltreatment

Child maltreatment is a general term that includes all types of abuse and neglect. Yearly, approximately 43.8% of substantiated maltreatment is classified as neglect, 8.7% is physical, 4.6% is sexual abuse, and 37.8% is emotional. The remaining percentage is a combination of these different types of maltreatment.

Factors identified at the end of "child in need" assessments found that of all cases domestic violence was a factor in 49.6%, emotional abuse in 19.3%, neglect in 17.5%, physical abuse in 14%, sexual abuse in 6.45%, child sexual exploitation (CSE) in 3.9%, self-harm in 4.35%, gangs in 1.2%, and trafficking in 0.3%.

Case Study 1

999 is called for an unresponsive infant. On arrival, you find a 10-month-old male infant who is unresponsive and has irregular respirations. The mother's boyfriend (mum is at work) tells you that he found the baby in this condition when he went to get him up from his nap. You note that it is 7 PM. The boyfriend is not holding the infant and when you pick the baby up from the cot, you also note that there is no muscle tone and the infant is flaccid. During your assessment and treatment, you note bruises on both upper arms. What are your initial patient management priorities?

1. What concerns you about the history reported by the boyfriend and the infant's injuries?

2. What do you suspect is the primary injury?

Table 13-1 Potential Complications of Maltreatment

Low self-esteem and underachievement
Psychological disorders or psychiatric symptoms
Abnormal growth and development
Permanent physical or neurological damage
Poor school performance
Teen promiscuity and pregnancy
Social withdrawal
Eating disorders
Substance abuse
Negative learned behaviour
Criminal behaviour beginning in young adulthood
Vulnerability to further abuse
Suicidal tendencies
Increased survivor health care costs to family and society
Death

© Jones & Bartlett Learning

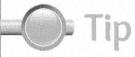 **Tip**

When adults with poor coping skills are faced with stressful situations, a cycle of child maltreatment may result.

Physical Abuse

Physical abuse occurs when a person intentionally inflicts injury, or allows injury to be inflicted, on a child younger than 18 years of age, which causes or results in risk of death, disfigurement, or distress.

Emotional Abuse

Emotional abuse occurs when there is an ongoing and consistent pattern of behaviour that interferes with the normal psychological and social development of a child. This includes unreasonable, excessive, or aggressive demands on the child that are not age-appropriate; setting tasks that are beyond the physical ability of the child; or the caregiver not providing the nurturing, guidance, and psychological support critical for the growth and development of a healthy child. Verbal attacks, such as belittling, insults, rejection, and constant criticism, are a few patterns of emotional abuse.

Sexual Abuse

Sexual abuse occurs when an older child or adult engages in sexual activities with a dependent, developmentally immature child or adolescent for the older person's own sexual excitement or for the enjoyment of other persons (e.g., child pornography or prostitution).

In most cases of sexual abuse, the perpetrator is an adult who knows the child and is often living under the same roof. A common misconception is that child sexual abuse is perpetrated by strangers. According to the National Society for the Prevention of Cruelty to Children (NSPCC), an estimated 90% of sexual abuse perpetrators are known by the child, and approximately a third of sexual abuse is committed by other children or young people. 1 in 3 children who are being sexually assaulted do not disclose the abuse during the time frame in which it is occurring.

Sexual abuse usually does not occur as a single incident. It does not always involve violence and physical force, and commonly leaves no visible sign. The perpetrator may use the power of adult–child authority or the parent–child bond instead of force or violence. The child may be manipulated into thinking that "it's OK" and a normal behaviour or that the child is "special" for making the perpetrator feel good. The child may also be made to feel deeply ashamed and powerless or may even be kept silent by threats from the perpetrator. The insidious nature of this abuse makes it difficult to detect, unless the child discloses the information to a confidant or the prehospital professional.

Child Neglect

Child neglect occurs when a child's physical, mental, or emotional condition is harmed or endangered because the caregiver has failed to supply basic necessities or engages in child-rearing practices that are inadequate or dangerous. Child neglect may involve a caregiver's misuse of drugs or alcohol, or child abandonment. Neglect is the failure to act on behalf of a child and is an act of omission. Neglect may not have visible signs, and it usually occurs over a period of time rather than as a discrete episode.

Neglect may be physical or emotional. Physical neglect is a failure to meet the requirements basic to a child's physical development and safety, such as supervision, housing, clothing, medical attention, and nutrition. Some social service agencies subdivide this category into more specific acts of omission, such as medical neglect, lack of proper supervision, or educational neglect. Emotional neglect is failure to provide the support or affection necessary to a child's psychological and social development.

Abuse Versus Neglect

The difference between abuse and neglect is that abuse represents an action against a child, whereas neglect represents a lack of action for the child. *Abuse is an act of commission; neglect is an act of omission.* In abuse, a physical or mental injury is inflicted on a child. In neglect, there is a failure to meet the basic needs of the child for adequate food, supervision, shelter, guidance, education, clothing, or medical care.

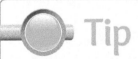

Tip

Abuse represents an action against a child (commission). Neglect represents a lack of action for the child (omission).

High-Risk Groups

Younger aged children are more vulnerable and at risk for maltreatment than older children who have more resources available to them and can better take care of themselves. Child maltreatment involves risk factors and lapses in child protection at the individual, family, community, and societal levels. No geographic, ethnic, or economic setting is free of child maltreatment. Abuse is present in all communities. The data from 2016 in **Table 13-2** shows that most children in need are from the white ethnicity group and the highest referrals per age group are from the 5–9 years age group.

Table 13-2 Characteristics of Children in Need: 2015 to 2016

Breakdown by age at 31 March:	
Unborn	1,020
Under 1	5,080
1–4	13,720
5–9	14,810
10–15	13,810
16 and over	1,870
Breakdown by ethnicity:	
Total known ethnicity	48,750
White	38,120
Mixed	4,360
Asian or Asian British	2,980
Black or black British	2,500
Other ethnic group	800

Source: Department of Education © Crown copyright

The prehospital clinician must consider maltreatment whenever circumstances suggest it, regardless of the family's socioeconomic status. Other risk factors for child maltreatment, besides nonverbal toddlers and infants, include factors where additional stressors and insufficient resources are available to the parents or caregivers, such as children with special needs (mental and physical disabilities and developmental issues) and children with chronic medical conditions—all conditions in which there are increased responsibilities to care for the child and a financial impact that may also affect the level of stress in the home.

A perpetrator of child maltreatment can be any person who has care, custody, or control of the child. This can include the child's parents, relative, teacher, babysitter, or child care staff person, institution staff person, bus driver, playground attendant, coach, religious leader, caregiver, or boyfriend or girlfriend of the caregiver.

Maltreatment happens for many different reasons. Often the perpetrators genuinely care for the child, but lack the resources or the parenting skills to deal with frustration and cope with anger. Likewise the person calling for help should not be assumed to be the perpetrator. For example, non-accidental head injury (formerly known as shaken baby syndrome) can present with seizures and apnoea, but the caregiver with the child at the time of the 999 call or ambulance services arrival may not be the individual who injured

Table 13-3 Assessment Factors Associated With Maltreatment

Does the history change over time?
Was there a delay in seeking care, or was the closest treatment centre bypassed?
Are there injuries of multiple ages?
Does the history fit the child's developmental ability?
Do the injuries fit the history?
Does the patient not seek comfort from the caregiver?
Does the caregiver inappropriately respond to the patient's needs?
What are the other sibling's involvements with the patient and caregiver?

© Jones & Bartlett Learning

Table 13-4 Duties of the Prehospital Professional in Suspected Maltreatment

Recognition of suspicious circumstances at the scene
Physical assessment of the child
Assessment of the history given by the caregiver
Communication with the caregiver and family
Careful documentation
Notation of other children living at the scene
Reporting of maltreatment concerns to the proper authority

© Jones & Bartlett Learning

the child. This individual may be unaware of the abuse, or in denial, and unable to believe that the child has been harmed. He or she may also be a victim of abuse or afraid of the abuser.

Rarely does the prehospital professional have sufficient information to determine with certainty that maltreatment has occurred. Information gathered in the field, however, can be critical in the eventual confirmation of maltreatment. **Table 13-3** lists assessment factors that are suggestive of maltreatment. Particularly important is the documentation of the exact history given by the caregiver in cases of presumed injury. A changing story is one of the most common hallmarks of maltreatment. Recognising and reporting suspected child maltreatment is one of the most important ways the prehospital professional can prevent childhood injury.

Duties and Communication by the Prehospital Professional

The prehospital professional has an extremely important role at the scene and a legal duty to ensure that they consider the need to safeguard and promote the welfare of children when carrying out their functions. Health professionals in the emergency department (ED) rely on the scene assessment, verbal handover, and documentation of suspected child maltreatment. **Table 13-4** lists the prehospital professional's duties in suspected maltreatment cases.

Mandatory Obligation to Report

All healthcare professionals, including prehospital professionals, have a legal obligation (mandate) to report suspected child maltreatment and other situations where a crime may have been committed or a vulnerable population is harmed. UK law places a responsibility on all professionals to report any child maltreatment. Not only do prehospital clinicians have a responsibility to report during handover, they also have a duty to provide an individual report to social services. In addition, there is a duty to report suspected maltreatment to the police urgently to protect the child and so that evidence can be protected and obtained. Clinicians also have an individual duty to report directly to the police any witnessed or direct disclosure from a child of female genital mutilation (FGM). *Failure to report suspicion of child maltreatment may result in legal action against the mandated reporter.*

Remember that a report of suspected child maltreatment is not an attempt to harm or punish a family, but an attempt to help the child. All prehospital personnel should become familiar with the particular obligation to report and the local child protection policy and procedures in the region in which they practice.

Assessing the Caregiver's Behaviour

Common characteristics among caregivers of maltreated children are drug use, poor self-concept, immaturity, lack of parenting knowledge, and lack of interpersonal skills. Although none of these factors in and of themselves mean that an individual has abused the child, be alert for these "red flag" behaviours, as noted in **Table 13-5**. Conversely, an "appropriate" caregiver who does not show any of these characteristics may still be maltreating a child. In some cases a caregiver may appear to be overreacting to the child's condition, such as in cases of fabricated illness or non-accidental injury, in which a caregiver may intentionally inflict illness or injury on a child to obtain attention for herself or himself.

Never confront a caregiver with suspicions of maltreatment. Such an approach at the scene may delay care, endanger the child, and create a hostile and dangerous situation for

Table 13-5 "Red Flag" Caregiver Behaviours

Apathy
Bizarre or strange conduct
Little or no concern about the child
Overreaction to child misbehaviour
Not forthcoming with events surrounding injury
Intoxication
Overreaction to child's condition

the prehospital professional. Instead, note the presence of alcohol or drugs in the prehospital report and document any statements from the caregiver that reflect apparent misinformation, inconsistency, or evasiveness. Watch interactions among the caregivers and document them if they seem noteworthy. Be careful, however, to keep the tone of the report objective and neutral. Report what you see and hear, but avoid making judgments or interpreting intent in the written documentation. Particularly note any comments made by the child about how he or she was hurt. However, be aware that young children may attribute injury to an abstract perpetrator, such as a monster or "bad man", rather than identifying the caregivers on whom they depend.

Documentation

There is no difference between basic and advanced level documentation of suspected child maltreatment. Be sure to document your findings of the scene assessment related to possible child maltreatment (e.g., whether there is child-appropriate food and bedding available, heat or air-conditioning, appropriate clothing, toys, supervision, and any safety concerns). Make a note of the child's position and location when you first encountered him or her. It is also recommended to document who else is at the scene (e.g., caretakers) and their relationship to the child. When documenting the history and physical assessment, be thorough but objective. Interjecting feelings or interpreting the facts may make the documentation inadmissible in court. For example, write, "palms show a 1-cm circular burn" instead of "cigarette burn to hand". Use objective, clear, specific terminology. Place in quotation marks and note in the records any statements from caregivers (e.g., father states that "child climbed into hot bathtub").

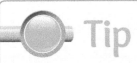

Document physical findings objectively. The facts speak for themselves in court.

Communicating With the Child and Caregivers

Communicate with the child in an age-appropriate manner. When assessing a stable child for whom there is concern of maltreatment, transport the child to the safe environment of the ED for full evaluation as soon as possible.

Communication with the caregiver in suspected maltreatment is a challenging task for the prehospital professional. Resist the impulse to "find out what really happened" or express anger at the caregiver. Do not make accusations or assume a judgmental tone. When confronted with suspicions of abuse, caregivers often respond defensively or angrily, whether or not they were the ones who inflicted the injuries.

Sometimes a caregiver may refuse to cooperate in further assessment, decline transport, or attempt to leave the scene with the child. If you believe the child to be in danger, immediately contact the police for assistance. Never attempt to physically restrain a caregiver or to forcibly take possession of a child, because this may put everyone in danger. If the scene is chaotic but not dangerous, consider contacting your control/clinical advisors, who may be able to convince the caregiver to permit treatment and transport. Never leave a suspected victim of child maltreatment at home.

Patient Assessment
Scene Assessment

First, ensure that the scene is safe for the child and for the prehospital professionals. If you suspect maltreatment, make a mental note of any conditions at the scene, because you need to document the conditions in the patient care report (**Figure 13-1**). Record remarks or specific conversations with the caregiver and document specifics about the environment where injuries were reported to occur. For example, note the approximate height of furniture an infant

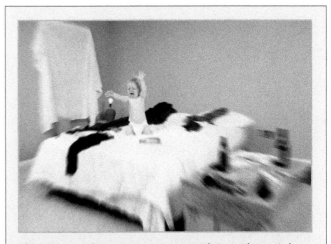

Figure 13-1 Document scene conditions that might support suspicion of maltreatment.

rolled off, the floor surface, or the location and condition of the sink or room where a child was burned.

Consider child maltreatment in every paediatric trauma call and every paediatric cardiac arrest situation in children less than 1 year of age. Suspicious circumstances in the environment, behaviour of the child or caregiver, history, or physical examination may also raise concerns of abuse in responding to calls for unrelated complaints. Look for unsanitary or dangerous home conditions, such as drugs, needles, or other unsafe care situations.

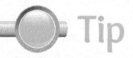

Tip

Consider child abuse in every injury case, as well as in illness cases with suspicious circumstances in the environment, behaviour of the child or caregiver, history, or physical examination.

If the scene is safe, assess the child and provide appropriate medical care. If an infant with suspected maltreatment has an abnormal appearance (e.g., listlessness, inconsolability, weak cry) or altered mental status (abnormal response to verbal or painful stimuli), assess for a traumatic brain injury.

One cause of traumatic brain injury is non-accidental head injury, formerly called shaken baby syndrome. Non-accidental head injury involves diffuse intracranial haemorrhage, usually from violent shaking of the child with or without impact with another object. The signs, symptoms, and physical findings in non-accidental head injury vary depending on the amount of trauma to the brain. These range from lethargy and irritability to seizures, coma, or death. Petechiae or hand grip patterns on the arms or chest (**Figure 13-2**) may also be found in non-accidental head

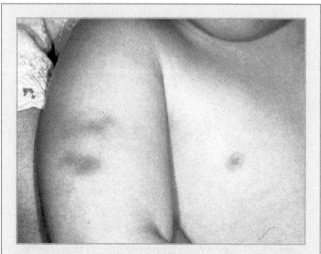

Figure 13-2 Human hand and fingertip marks can appear as oval bruises.

injury. The incidence of permanent neurological damage from non-accidental head injury is high. Seizures, learning disabilities, blindness, and other handicaps are common. The fatality rate in non-accidental head injury is 20%–30%.

If the child with suspected maltreatment is physiologically unstable or has significant injuries, begin transport after the primary assessment. If the scene is unsafe for the child or prehospital professional, call for police back-up and move to the ambulance to complete the assessment and initiate treatment. Transport every child with suspected maltreatment, even if the injuries are trivial.

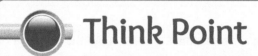

Think Point

Never leave a suspected victim of child maltreatment. Transport every child, even if the injuries are trivial.

Additional Assessment

Stay on scene for additional assessment only if the child is stable and the scene is safe. Take a careful history, using the questions suggested in **Table 13-6**. *The history may be more important than the physical assessment.* Ask questions in a non-judgmental way to maximise the quality of information and to avoid escalating the situation. Pay close attention to and document in detail the caregiver's description of the

Table 13-6 Focused History: Questions and Considerations in Evaluating Suspected Child Maltreatment

Question	Considerations
How did the injury occur?	• Is the caregiver's explanation plausible? • Do the physical conditions at the scene support the alleged mechanism of injury?
When did it happen?	• Was there a long delay before 999 was notified? • Does the injury appearance match the time frame?
Who witnessed the event?	• Do all of the caregivers' or witnesses' stories match? • Was there adequate supervision?
What is the child's medical history?	• Are there pre-existing psychosocial, developmental, or chronic problems?
Does the child have a GP?	• When was the last visit? • Does the GP know the child?

Jones & Bartlett Learning

events leading to the call, noting inconsistencies or evasiveness. Consider the developmental capabilities of the child. Be concerned about inflicted trauma when the history does not account for the observed injuries (**Figure 13-3**), the caregiver's history changes over the course of the interview, or the mechanism of injury described is not plausible given the developmental level of the child. Note any unusual interactions between child and caregiver or other possible perpetrators. Although a child may seem wary or frightened of the perpetrator, at times a child may cling to or try to appease an abusive caregiver to avoid further abusive behaviour.

If the injury is described as an "accident", determine the mechanism. For example, if the caregiver reports that the child fell, determine the distance, the stopping surface, and the initial reactions of the child (**Table 13-7**). The information obtained at the scene may be more accurate than that obtained by the ED staff, social services, and the police.

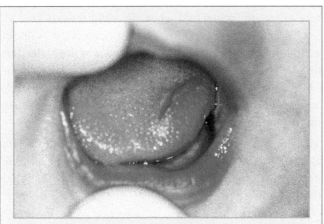

Figure 13-3 A caregiver's history of a child biting his or her tongue is not believable in an infant who has no teeth. This discrepant history suggests an inflicted injury.
Courtesy of Ron Deickmann, MD

Table 13-7 Distinguishing Fact From Common Fiction

History	Fact
"He fell off the couch, and then had a seizure".	Fewer than 1 in 1,000 falls of 4 feet (1.2 m) or less result in serious injury.
"My 1-month-old rolled off the bed".	Most infants cannot roll over until 3–4 months of age.
"He must have bruised himself".	Bruises are rare in infants who are not yet pulling to a stand.
"I found him with his leg stuck in the cot slat",	Without an external force, either intentional or accidental, infants do not sustain fractures.

© Jones & Bartlett Learning

Physical Examination

The prehospital professional may note suspicious findings in the physical examination of the child. Up to 90% of physical maltreatment victims have some kind of skin injury. The physical examination may reveal the suspicious patterns and physical findings of child abuse. In cases of suspected sexual abuse, defer a genital examination to providers with specialised training.

Bruises

Physical findings that suggest inflicted injury include the following:

- Bruises located on soft tissues, such as neck, back, thighs, genitalia, or buttocks
- Bruises on or behind ears
- Bruises in a child less than 4 months of age
- Facial bruises from slapping (**Figure 13-4**)

Any bruising of the torso, ears or neck in any child of 4 years or younger, or any bruising in an infant younger than 4 months, are significant indicators of abuse.

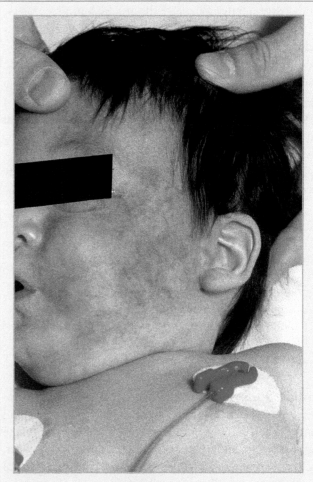

Figure 13-4 The face is a common target for physical abuse.
Courtesy of Ron Deickmann, MD

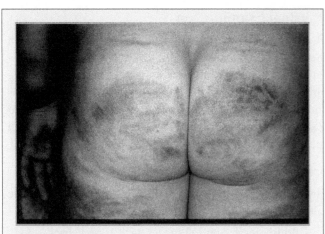

Figure 13-5 Bruises on the buttocks are usually inflicted injuries.
Courtesy of Ron Deickmann, MD

Differentiating bruises resulting from maltreatment versus normal wear and tear depends on appearance, location, and developmental age of the child. Bruises over bony prominences, such as the elbow, forehead, or below the knees, are the common result of play injuries in children. However, bruises over soft tissues, such as the thighs, buttocks, cheeks, ears, or on the back, are less common and should raise suspicions of inflicted injury (**Figure 13-5**).

ANY bruising in an infant who is not yet mobile may suggest inflicted injury. Most children are able to roll over by 4 months of age and able to pull to stand and toddle (cruise) by 9 months of age. A child who is not yet cruising should not have unexplained bruises or fractures—*no cruising means no bruising.* As children become older and increasingly mobile, bruises and lacerations from normal activity become more common.

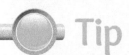

Tip

"Those who don't toddle rarely bruise". In a child who cannot yet pull up to stand and walk while holding onto furniture (toddle), bruising or injury is rare. Most infants do not start "cruising" until they are about 9 months of age.

Any bruise with an identifiable pattern is almost certain to have been inflicted. Common items include belts, cords, and hands. When an object hits the skin with high velocity, the edges leave an outline of petechiae. If a very thin object, such as a switch or a cord, hits the skin, parallel **petechial** lines form as an outline of the object.

It was previously thought that the time that a bruise was inflicted could be determined based on its appearance. This is now known to be inaccurate. Bruises resolve at differing rates based on their location and the mechanism of injury, and bruises of different colours can result from injuries sustained in one event. Nevertheless, document the location and colours of all bruises to provide a complete description of the injuries sustained.

Burns

Inflicted burns are usually from immersion in hot water (scalds) or from forced contact between the child and a hot object. Adult skin can develop a full-thickness burn from 2 seconds of exposure to 65°C water; children may burn even faster. Accidental scald burns typically have varying depths and irregular borders, with a "flow" pattern evident. They are rarely symmetric (i.e., both hands or both feet), and occur infrequently in the pre-ambulatory child. In contrast, scalds from deliberately dipping a child in hot water are clearly **demarcated**, sparing **flexural creases** (e.g., the creases behind the knees or inside the elbows), because these areas are "protected" when the child reflexively tries to withdraw. "Doughnut burns" with sparing of the buttocks occur in children who have been dipped into hot water, but whose buttocks are pushed firmly down against the relatively cooler surface of the tub or sink (**Figure 13-6**). Children with inflicted burns may also have arm or leg bruises where they were restrained.

Pattern burns that are an even thickness throughout or are repeated are red flags for maltreatment. Remember that any **acute** burn can be extremely painful. ALS clinicians should consider the administration of an analgesic as the local protocol allows.

Fractures

Fractures in children who are not yet ambulatory are also suspicious for maltreatment. Although an infant who is being carried and is unintentionally dropped may sustain a fracture, it is not plausible that an infant who is only

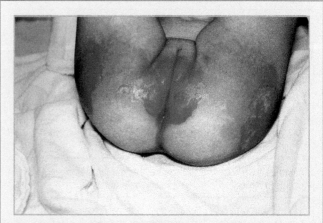

Figure 13-6 Doughnut burn.
Courtesy of Ron Deickmann, MD

crawling or cruising could develop sufficient energy on their own to fracture a bone. Infant fractures of abuse have typical patterns on hospital radiographs. A history of <u>osteogenesis imperfecta</u> or problems causing decreased bone calcification may increase fracture occurrence in some children. Include these conditions in the documentation of the child's history.

Deceptive Skin Signs Masquerading as Abuse

Sometimes, normal physical findings suggest an inflicted injury. For example, "<u>Mongolian spots</u>" are birthmarks frequently seen in children of colour (e.g., African American, Asian, Latino) that can be easily mistaken for bruises (**Figure 13-7**). These birthmarks often take the form of large, flat patches of hyperpigmented skin, most commonly found on the low back or buttocks. Mongolian spots will blanch; bruises will not.

Certain disease states, such as <u>leukaemia</u>, <u>vasculitis</u>, <u>meningococcemia</u>, or bleeding disorders (i.e., <u>haemophilia</u>), can rarely produce skin findings that appear to be bruises. Infectious processes, such as impetigo, can appear to be burns, but are much less painful. Insect bites in some children can cause redness and blistering. Distinguishing intentional injuries with certainty is sometimes impossible in the field.

Another benign skin finding that masquerades as abuse is the pattern of lesions produced by cultural rituals intended to treat illness. The most common of these patterns are associated with Asian practices called <u>cupping</u> (**Figure 13-8**) and <u>coin rubbing</u> (**Figure 13-9**). These superficial lesions have distinctive rounded edges. Caregivers of these children can explain the purpose for such practices—information that can help distinguish inflicted injuries that are intended to help from inflicted injuries that are intended to harm.

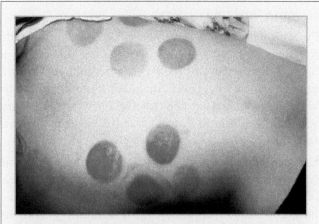

Figure 13-8 Cupping is the cultural practice of placing warm cups on the skin to pull out illness from the body. The red, flat, rounded skin lesions are often more intensely red at the borders.
Courtesy of the American Academy of Pediatrics

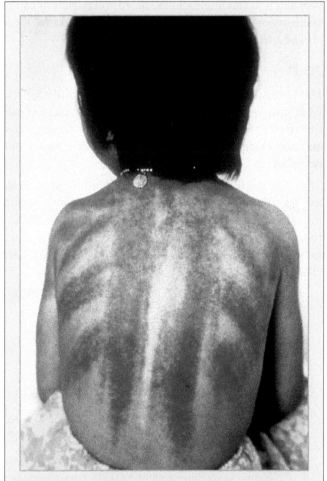

Figure 13-9 Rubbing hot coins, often on the back, produces rounded and oblong red, patchy, flat skin lesions.
Courtesy of the American Academy of Pediatrics

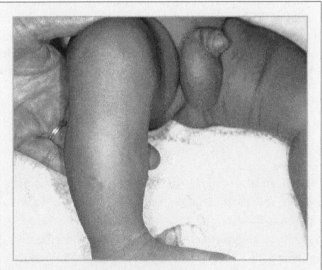

Figure 13-7 Mongolian spots appear on the buttocks, back, and extremities of many infants.

Harmful Cutural Practices

Professionals have a duty to promote and protect the welfare of children living in circumstances that appear to be complex because of their faith and culture. Harmful practices including FGM, so called honour-based violence, forced marriage, and belief in spirit possession and witchcraft are considered child abuse. FGM is illegal in the UK.

So called "honour crime", "honour-based violence", or "izzat" (mainly a South Asian term) embrace a variety of crimes of violence mainly perpetrated towards girls and women, including assault, imprisonment and murder where the person is being punished by their family or their community. The family or communities are punishing them for undermining what they believe to be the correct code of behaviour. Failure to adhere to the correct code of behaviour is an indicator to the family that the person cannot be controlled and made to conform and this brings "shame" to the family. "Honour-based violence" usually occurs with some degree of approval by family and community members and it has an international dimension as victims can be taken overseas where the violence is then perpetrated. It can also be a trigger for a forced marriage.

FGM

FGM is an illegal, extremely harmful practice and a form of child abuse and violence against women and girls. It should therefore should be dealt with as part of existing child and adult safeguarding/protection structures, policies, and procedures.

The World Health Organisation (WHO) defines FGM as: "all procedures (not operations) which involve partial or total removal of the external female genitalia or injury to the female genital organs whether for cultural or other non-therapeutic reasons" (WHO, 1996). FGM has been classified by the WHO into four types:

- Type 1: Circumcision—Excision of the prepuce with or without excision of part or all of the clitoris

- Type 2: Excision (Clitoridectomy)—Excision of the clitoris with partial or total excision of the labia minora. After the healing process has taken place, scar tissue forms to cover the upper part of the vulva region

- Type 3: Infibulation (also called Pharaonic Circumcision)—This is the most severe form of female genital mutilation. Infibulation often (but not always) involves the complete removal of the clitoris, together with the labia minora and at least the anterior two-thirds and often the whole of the medial part of the labia majora

- Type 4: Unclassified—This includes all other procedures on the female genitalia, and any other procedure that falls under the definition of female genital mutilation given above. It includes prickings, genital piercings and tattoos, as well as cosmetic procedures to female genitalia.

Summary of Duties, Communication, and Assessment in Suspected Maltreatment

When child maltreatment is suspected, the prehospital professional faces a challenging and potentially explosive situation. Communication with the child may be difficult or limited, and interactions with the caregiver may be frustrating and sometimes hostile. A professional, nonjudgmental approach is necessary. Document conditions in the environment, the child's and caregiver's behaviours, the history, and relevant physical findings that may suggest maltreatment. The prehospital professional has a moral and legal duty to report suspected cases of maltreatment to the proper authorities.

The prehospital professional is in a unique position to recognise signs of possible child maltreatment. The initial principles of field care are the careful scene assessment, history taking, and careful physical assessment for physiological abnormalities or anatomical patterns of inflicted injuries. Additional assessment and identification of "red flag" child

Case Study 2

You respond to a flat at 3 AM for a baby not breathing. On arrival, an apparently intoxicated female meets you at the door with an unresponsive 6-month-old female in cardiac arrest. Your partner begins treatment, and you are able to determine that the woman is the grandmother who is supposed to be watching her granddaughter while the baby's mother is working a night shift. The grandmother tells you that she and the infant must have fallen asleep on the sofa, and she woke up "next" to the baby and that she found the baby this way. You also notice several beer cans in the room. There are at least three blankets and a pillow piled up on the couch.

1. What are the red flags for maltreatment?

2. What are your medical and legal responsibilities?

and caregiver behaviours are sometimes extremely important to maltreatment investigations. The diagnosis of child maltreatment is rarely possible in the field. All cases require a complete investigation by social services.

Legislation, Principles, and Protocols

Child Protective Services

The local authority has overarching legal responsibility for safeguarding and promoting the welfare of all children and young people in their area and have a number of statutory functions under the 1989 and 2004 Children Acts. The local authority has the legal authority to temporarily remove children at risk of injury or neglect from the home and to secure foster care placement. Local authority social services are responsible for initial investigations of suspected maltreatment. They must make complicated and important decisions about the maltreatment accusations, at times remove children from the home and place them into foster care, and provide services for abusive and neglectful families. **Table 13-8** lists the initial actions of the local authority when a report is filed. The local authority may work in concert with the police to investigate the facts and determine who is responsible for maltreating the child. Local agencies including police and health services have a duty under Section 11 of the Children Act 2004 to ensure that they consider the need to safeguard and promote the welfare of children when carrying out their functions. Most local authorities have a Multi Agency Safeguarding Hub (MASH) where all referrals about child protection are received. Agencies within the MASH include local authority children's safeguarding services, the police, health and other agencies that vary area by area. The benefit of a MASH is that all agencies can review and share the information they have on a child and quickly assess the level of support required.

Ultimately, the judicial system determines if an accused individual is "guilty". Although emotions may run high when the prehospital professional suspects child maltreatment, it is neither appropriate nor safe to confront caregivers with these concerns at the scene.

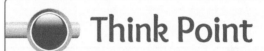

Think Point

Judging or confronting caregivers or attempting to intervene in issues of dysfunctional parenting may interfere with patient care or a subsequent maltreatment investigation. The caregiver may in fact not know how the child was injured or by whom. Your interventions may put you at risk, and a confrontation does not help the child.

The prehospital professional can provide vital scene information that helps social services to determine safe placement of the patient. When maltreatment is suspected, always note the presence of other children in the home. If a determination is made that an environment may be unsafe, contact the police and social services to evaluate the safety of any other children who are present, based on local service guidelines. When a patient is transported to a hospital, communicate any concerns of maltreatment to hospital staff and report to social services. Hospital staff also have a mandatory obligation to report any concerns they have.

The Children Act 1989 & 2004 Section 11, 17, and 47 and 'Working Together to Safeguard Children' 2015 outlines the responsibilities of all agencies to safeguard and promote the welfare of children. Other national resources of note include the NSPCC who provide a range of data and advice on child protection.

Table 13-8 Initial Multi Agency Safeguarding Hub (MASH) Actions

1. When a report of child abuse or neglect is received, either from a health care professional, the police, or another body the protocols of the receiving agency, usually the Multi Agency Safeguarding Hub, (MASH) determine the timing and scope of the initial response.

2. The referral is reviewed with each agency in the MASH checking the information they have on the child to determine best approach to take.

3. The facts having been reviewed determine if a home visit is appropriate and, if so, which members of the team will be involved.

4. The social worker assigned to the case assesses risk to the child, the family's ability to provide safety, and supportive resources available to the family.

5. After the investigation and assessment, a reported incident is determined to be founded, unfounded, or unable to be determined because of lack of information.

6. Appropriate support may be provided to support the child and family following investigation, depending on the outcome of investigations.

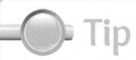

Tip

Note and report the presence of other children in situations suggestive of maltreatment.

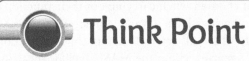

Think Point

Never attempt to physically restrain a caregiver or to forcibly take possession of a child. Call the police if the scene is unsafe.

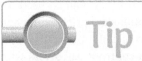

Tip

Even in the face of probable maltreatment, remain non-judgmental with the caregiver and maintain control of the scene and transport.

Controversy

It is the duty of the prehospital professional to ensure that they submit a safeguarding referral when abuse is suspected. This is a legal duty and cannot be passed to another professional. If you witness or suspect child maltreatment you have a duty to act. You should inform the receiving professional of your concerns but you must still make a report to social services, you cannot pass this duty onto another professional, i.e., ED staff.

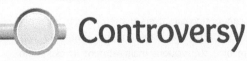

Controversy

The on-scene role of the police in suspected child maltreatment is to ensure the safety of children and other professionals. It is essential to transport a child to the ED. If the scene is not safe or caretakers are refusing transport, the prehospital professional must call the police for protection and assistance.

Case Study 3

999 is called by a babysitter, because a child has been burned. On arrival at the scene, the ambulance crew finds a teenage girl holding a sobbing 2-year-old boy. The teenager states that the child has been fussy and crying for the 2 hours in her care. On changing the child's nappy, the babysitter noted what looked like burns on the buttocks, and on her mother's advice called 999.

The child is alert but upset and is not easily consolable by the babysitter. There are areas of denuded skin on the buttocks covered with nappy rash cream, with one unpopped blister near the sacrum. The centres of both buttocks, and the gluteal cleft, do not appear to be injured. Extremity examination shows no bruises or other abnormalities.

1. Is this injury caused from abuse?

2. What interventions are indicated?

CASE STUDY ANSWERS

Case Study 1 — page 256

Be alert for the signs of non-accidental head injury in any infant or small child with a sudden onset of altered mental status and irregular respirations. Remember that grab bruises and marks may be found on the arms of children that are held and shaken, and their presence should be documented. Carefully document the scene, the comments of the caregiver, and the reported events leading to the injury.

Immediate transportation is critical. One common complication of inflicted head injury is respiratory failure or apnoea as a result of elevated intracranial pressure and compression of the medulla (respiratory centre in the brainstem). Be prepared to provide respiratory support. Ensure that a safeguarding referral is made.

Case Study 2 — page 264

This case may be the result of the grandmother accidently suffocating the infant. Co-sleeping, especially with a caregiver who is under the influence of alcohol or drugs, can have deadly consequences. Adults may roll over on top of infants and not realise it because of their intoxicated state. Infants do not have the strength to push back or to get the adult to notice that they are lying on them. Make a note of the scene and call the police. Your attention needs to be focused on resuscitation efforts for the child.

Case Study 3 — page 266

This child has obvious signs of an inflicted scald injury. The lack of burn in the creases and the centre of the buttocks (doughnut burn) may indicate the child was forcibly held in hot water. There is no way for the prehospital professional to know who inflicted the injury; nor is establishing responsibility part of his or her role.

Provide analgesia if possible. Large burns can lead to significant fluid losses, so ALS providers should start an intravenous (IV) line and begin fluid resuscitation. Document the scene assessment, the child's and caregiver's behaviours, and the history. Transport this child to an ED for burn care as well as an evaluation for inflicted injury. Treatment at a burn centre may ultimately be necessary.

SUGGESTED READINGS

Resources

General Medical Council: Protecting children and young people—The responsibilities of all doctors, 2012: Avilable: https://www.gmc-uk.org/-/media/documents/Protecting_children_and_young_people___English_1015.pdf_48978248.pdf. Accessed June 19, 2018.

NICE. 2009. Guidance on when to suspect child maltreatment; clinical guideline [CG89]. https://www.nice.org.uk/guidance/cg89. Accessed March 3, 2018.

Royal College of General Practitioners. Safeguarding Children and Young People: The RCGP/NSPCC Safeguarding Children Toolkit for General Practice http://www.rcgp.org.uk/clinical-and-research/resources/toolkits/the-rcgp-nspcc-safeguarding-children-toolkit-for-general-practice.aspx. Accessed March 3, 2018.

Royal College of Nursing. 2015. Looked after children—Knowledge, skills and competences of health care staff (Intercollegiate role framework). https://www.rcpch.ac.uk/system/files/protected/page/Looked%20After%20Children%202015_0.pdf. Accessed March 3, 2018.

Royal College of Paediatrics and Child Health. 2014. Safeguarding children and young people: roles and competences for health care staff—Intercollegiate document. https://www.rcpch.ac.uk/sites/default/files/page/Safeguarding%20Children%20-%20Roles%20and%20Competences%20for%20Healthcare%20Staff%20%2002%200%20%20%20%20(3)_0.pdf. Accessed March 3, 2018.

Department for Education, Safeguarding children who may have been trafficked, 2011. Available: https://www.gov.uk/government/publications/safeguarding-children-who-may-have-been-trafficked-practice-guidance Accessed June 19, 2018.

Department for Education, Multi-agency statutory guidance on female genital mutilation, 2016. Available: https://www.gov.uk/government/publications/multi-agency-statutory-guidance-on-female-genital-mutilation Accessed June 19, 2018.

Department for Education, Forced marriage 2013. Available: https://www.gov.uk/guidance/forced-marriage. Accessed June 19, 2018.

Department for Education, Safeguarding children from abuse linked to faith or belief, 2012 https://www.gov.uk/government/publications/national-action-plan-to-tackle-child-abuse-linked-to-faith-or-belief Accessed June 19, 2018.

Department for Education, Radicalisation—Prevent strategy, 2011. Available: https://www.gov.uk/government/publications/prevent-strategy-2011 Accessed June 19, 2018

Department for Education, Radicalisation—Channel guidance, 2012. Available: https://www.gov.uk/government/publications/channel-guidance Accessed June 19, 2018.

Department for Education, Use of reasonable force in schools, 2013. Available: https://www.gov.uk/government/publications/use-of-reasonable-force-in-schools Accessed June 19, 2018.

Department for Education, Child sexual exploitation: definition and guide for practitioners 2017. Available: https://www.gov.uk/government/publications/child-sexual-exploitation-definition-and-guide-for-practitioners Accessed June 19, 2018.

Department for Education, Safeguarding Children in whom illness is fabricated or induced, 2008. Available: https://www.gov.uk/government/publications/safeguarding-children-in-whom-illness-is-fabricated-or-induced Accessed June 19, 2018.

Department for Education, Preventing and tackling bullying, 2013. Available: https://www.gov.uk/government/publications/preventing-and-tackling-bullying. Accessed June 19, 2018.

Articles

Johnson CF. Child maltreatment 2002: recognition, reporting and risk. *Pediatr Int.* 2002;44:554–560.

Kairys S. Distinguishing sudden infant death syndrome from child abuse fatalities. American Academy of Pediatrics. Committee on Child Abuse and Neglect. *Pediatrics.* 2001;107(2):437–441.

Kempe CH. The battered child syndrome. *JAMA.* 1962;181:17–24.

Krug EG, Dahlberg LL, Mercy JA, et al. World report on violence and health. Geneva: World Health Organization; 2002.

Pierce MC, Kaczor K, Aldridge S, et al. Bruising characteristics discriminating physical abuse from accidental trauma. *Pediatrics.* 2010;125:67–74.

Web sites

American Psychological Association. Child sexual abuse: what parents should know. http://www.apa.org/pi/families/resources/child-sexual-abuse.aspx. Accessed September 28, 2012.

References

Child Welfare Information Gateway. 2012. Child maltreatment 2010: summary of key findings. http://www.childwelfare.gov/pubs/factsheets/canstats.cfm. Accessed September 11, 2012.

Saied-Tessier A. NSPCC. 2014. Estimating the Costs of Child Sexual Abuse in the UK. https://www.nspcc.org.uk/globalassets/documents/research-reports/estimating-costs-child-sexual-abuse-uk.pdf. Accessed March 3, 2018.

Department of Education. 2016. Children in need census data. https://www.gov.uk/government/uploads/system/uploads/attachment_data/file/564620/SFR52-2016_Main_Text.pdf. Accessed March 3, 2018.

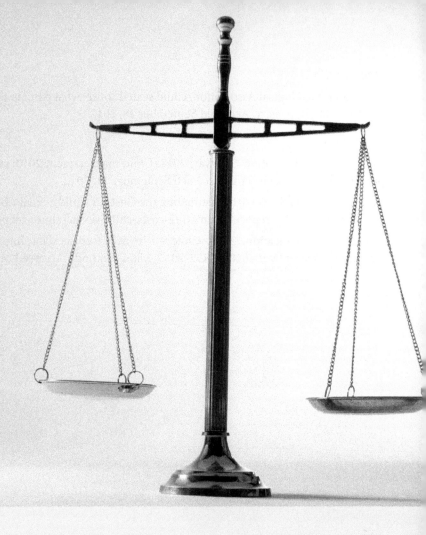

Learning Objectives

1. Identify out-of-hospital ethical and legal issues unique to paediatric emergency care.

2. Discuss the need to act in the best interests of a child or young person when treating them in the out-of-hospital environment.

3. Understand the different ethical and legal challenges when caring for the "young person" and the "child" as opposed to the adult.

4. Outline the prehospital professional's responsibilities when a carer may refuse to give consent to prehospital professionals to treat or transport a child or young person, including the "doctrine of necessity".

5. Review the legal and ethical considerations when faced with a child who has "Do Not Attempt Resuscitation" status.

Medico-legal and Ethical Considerations

Chapter
14

Introduction

The prehospital professional can encounter ethical and legal issues while caring for children and young people. These may include challenges around consent, confidentiality, telling the truth, and the recognition and reporting of possible child protection issues. This chapter discusses these issues and considers the role of prehospital professionals in addressing common paediatric ethical and legal concerns. A number of complex legal situations in relation to the treatment of children are generally avoided in the out-of-hospital setting due to the nature of emergency medicine. Such complex matters will not be addressed in depth in this chapter. If the prehospital clinician is undertaking a more routine, non-emergency role, for example in a doctor's surgery, such legal matters will need to be considered and researched by the individual.

Definitions

The terms "child/children" and "young person/young people" will be used in this chapter to refer to paediatric patients; however, for clinical purposes, the young person is more often treated as an adult. Legally, childhood is the period from birth until the age of 18; however, children acquire some rights and responsibilities before they reach 18 years. For example, in England a child acquires criminal responsibility at age 10, whereas in Scotland the age is 8, with the ability to be prosecuted from age 12. In Scotland, an individual aged between 16 and 18 may get married, whereas a young person of the same age in England and Wales requires parental consent to do the same. In all areas of the United Kingdom, a sixteen-year-old can lawfully join the army and have sexual intercourse. There are two main age ranges for consent in children that out-of-hospital clinicians need to be aware of:

- Under 16 years = child
- 16–17 years = young person

As can be seen in the examples above, the legal systems within the countries that make up the United Kingdom are separate, with legislation differing between England, Wales, Northern Ireland, and Scotland. Although the underlying principles upon which such legislation is formed can be considered to be universal, the resultant laws do differ. Where there are such differences, they will be identified; however, it remains the responsibility of the individual clinician to ensure that they are practicing within the appropriate legal framework of their country of employment.

Case Study 1

You are called to a house where you find a 3-year-old girl in respiratory distress. She is interactive and consolable, but has bilateral wheezes and a pulse oximeter reading of 94%. She is home alone with a 16-year-old babysitter who tells you that the child's parents will not return for several hours and did not leave information about their destination or contact information.

1. Can the babysitter legally withhold consent to treat the child?
2. Can you legally provide care and transport this child?

Consent

The requirement to obtain informed consent from a patient before delivering medical care is a central feature of health care law and ethics. Adults, i.e., people aged 18 or above, are considered to have the capacity to give consent, or withhold consent, for treatment unless they are shown to lack mental capacity (Mental Capacity Act 2005; Adults with Incapacity (Scotland) Act 2000), meaning that they may not be touched, treated, or transported without their consent. Children, however, are not automatically considered to have capacity to consent to, or refuse, treatment, potentially presenting a challenge to out-of-hospital care providers. Only once a person turns 18 are they considered an adult for the purposes of consent.

Consent and the Young Person

Under the Family Law Reform Act 1969 competence is presumed for consenting to medical treatment, meaning that 16- to 17-year-olds are usually treated in the same way as adults and are able to give their consent to treatment, as long as they have capacity to do so. However, there are exceptions, such as solid organ donation and other procedures that are not for the benefit of the young person themselves. Clinicians involved in this type of care must be cognisant of the law in this area for this age group. In Scotland, under the Age of Legal Capacity (Scotland) Act 1991, a person over the age of 16 years has legal capacity and *any* young person may consent to surgical, medical, or dental procedure or treatment where, in the opinion of a qualified attending medical practitioner, the person is capable of understanding the nature and possible consequences of the procedure or treatment.

Refusal of Consent by a Young Person

The legal ability to consent to treatment is not the same as the legal ability to *refuse* consent for medical treatment. A young person who refuses to consent to treatment can have their refusal overridden by a consenting parent or guardian who has parental responsibility (see "Parental Responsibility" below). In the absence of a holder of parental responsibility,

the prehospital clinician should act in the best interests of the young person and, under the doctrine of necessity, can treat the young person in the absence of formal consent.

Such action should only be taken in extreme circumstances where a failure to act would result in serious injury or death to the young person. As with all matters of consent, the patient, and/or their parent/guardian, should be fully informed about the proposed treatment in order for them to make an appropriate decision. Overriding the refusal of a competent young person would normally only be considered in very serious circumstances and is not undertaken lightly. Usually, the Courts are required to arbitrate on such decisions. Due to the emergency nature of prehospital care, such challenges regarding emergency, life-saving treatment in the prehospital setting are rare.

Consent and the Child

Unlike the young person, there are no defined ages where a child can be considered competent to consent to treatment. The nature of the proposed treatment, along with the maturity of the child, are considered and consent is judged on a case-by-case basis. For example, a child of four years of age may be considered competent to consent to treatment for a minor injury, such as a grazed knee, but may not be considered competent to consent to the administration of an intramuscular injection of adrenaline in a case of anaphylaxis. The basis for this position comes from the case of *Gillick v West Norfolk and Wisbech Area Health Authority*, a legal case about a child's access to contraception, with "Gillick competence" referring to the ability of a child to make a decision about their care. This case established that if a child has '*sufficient understanding and intelligence to enable him or her to fully understand what is proposed*' then he or she can consent to that treatment. This position is also reflected in the Age of Legal Capacity (Scotland) Act 1991.

Part of the judgment in the Gillick case is known as the Fraser Guidelines and those guidelines provide specific assistance to health care practitioners in their treatment of children seeking contraception.

Refusal of Consent by a Child

Gillick competence is only related to the ability of a child to consent to treatment, and does not extend to *refusal* of consent. For all children, as with young persons, a refusal can be overridden by a consenting parent or guardian who has parental responsibility (see "Parental Responsibility" below). In cases where the intervention is therapeutic, as opposed to non-therapeutic, e.g., religious or prophylactic treatment, only one parent/guardian needs to consent, addressing situations where there may be a difference of opinion between two parents. This is only the case where treatment is considered to be needed by the child and is in their best interests. When working in non-emergency environments, where the refusal of inoculations and other interventions for religious, cultural or other reasons may be more prevalent, the practitioner must make themselves fully conversant with the legal guidance in respect of this area.

In the rare situations where a holder of parental responsibility refuses to give consent for emergency treatment, the pre-hospital clinician should act in the best interests of the child and, under the doctrine of necessity, can treat the child in the absence of formal consent. Such action should only be taken in extreme circumstances where a failure to act would result in serious injury or death to the child. In such circumstances, it is important to try to understand why a parent/guardian would refuse to consent to treatment. The reasons may be due to a long-term condition of the child, where there are alternative treatment plans in place, or cases of end of life care, where treatment would be against medical advice. In the absence of such reasons, consideration should be given to child protection matters and the general welfare of the child concerned (see Child Maltreatment chapter).

Parental Responsibility

The legislation from which parental responsibility is predominantly derived is the Children Act 1989 and, in Scotland, the Children (Scotland) Act 1995. Different individuals or organisations may have parental responsibility for a child or young person. On occasions, it may be appropriate to identify if a person has parental responsibility for a child. This is less likely to be the case for clinicians working in the emergency, out-of-hospital environment, but may be relevant for those working in GP surgeries or urgent care centres where more routine interventions or inoculations may be undertaken.

Although a child's mother automatically has parental responsibility, not all fathers will have legal parental responsibility for their children. In some situations, the following individuals/ organisations will have parental responsibility for a child:

- Legally appointed guardian
- Person with a residence order for the child
- Local Authority appointed to care for the child
- Local Authority or person with an emergency protection order for the child

Throughout this chapter, the term "carer" will be used to describe individuals who have parental responsibility for the child. As an example, the flowchart in **Figure 14-1** demonstrates who has parental responsibility in England and Wales.

Documentation

As with any patient treatment, the prehospital professional must fully and clearly document on the prehospital record the nature of the medical emergency and any treatment given. In addition, in cases where a carer either refuses to consent to the treatment of a child, or is not available on-scene, the documentation should record any attempts to contact the carer, the reasons the child required immediate treatment or transport, and any discussion that was held between the clinician and the carers.

In situations where a child is at a location such as a youth club, campsite, or sporting facility, there may be members of staff who are acting *'in loco parentis'*, i.e., in the place of the parent, and who are responsible for the welfare of the child in the absence of the child's parents. Such staff may be able to give consent to the treatment of a child, but they cannot refuse consent unless they have formal parental responsibility as described previously. This is also the case for teachers, whose statutory responsibility for children in their care is set out in the Children Act 1989.

Although it might be considered best practice, and sometimes the policy of the club or group, there is no legal requirement for a carer to accompany a child or a young person when they are conveyed to hospital. When considering the best interests of the child, the distress caused by travelling unaccompanied must be balanced against the emergency nature of the clinical presentation; if a short delay would not adversely impact on the health of the child, then it may be in their best interests to await the arrival of a parent, or for an escort to be found.

When conveying an unaccompanied child, it would be advisable to notify the appropriate control/operations centre.

Never confront the carer with accusations, moral judgments, or threats when difficult circumstances develop at the scene. This approach only aggravates the situation and does not help the child. Try to establish whether the carer refuses all care and transport or only certain aspects of care. For example, some carers may prefer that prehospital professionals not initiate therapy, but permit the child to be transported to the hospital. If the child can be safely transported without initiating care, respect the carer's wishes concerning care. It may be appropriate for the carer of a child with a terminal illness or significant disabilities to restrict certain kinds of care for the child.

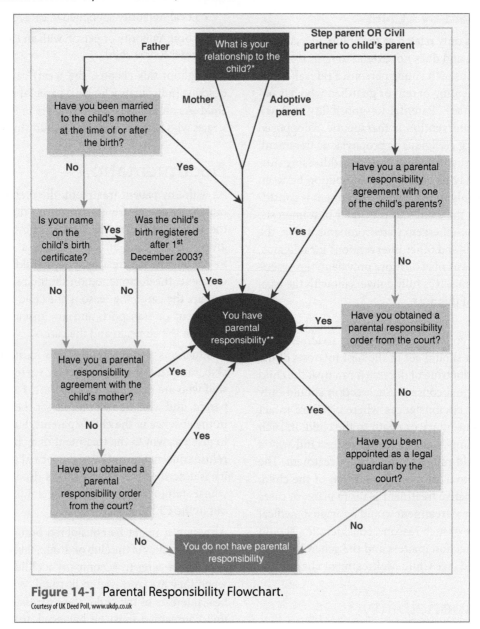

Figure 14-1 Parental Responsibility Flowchart.
Courtesy of UK Deed Poll, www.ukdp.co.uk

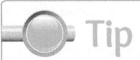

Tip

You may need to gain police assistance when a carer who is impaired or intoxicated refuses care or transport of an ill or injured child. In such cases, consider the safeguarding and child protection matters covered in Chapter 13.

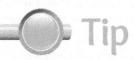

Tip

Never confront the carer with accusations, moral judgments, or threats.

Child Refusal

Children may live in non-traditional families in which they are cared for by grandparents, older siblings, two same-sex parents, or foster parents. It may not be immediately clear who has the responsibility of consenting for the child. In addition, these carers may be the only adults involved with the child on a regular basis despite the fact that they may not have legal responsibility for that child.

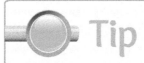

Tip

A child cannot legally refuse care or transport when emergency care is required.

In these situations, determining who has legal parental responsibility for a child may be difficult, however, if the child is acutely ill or injured, it is the responsibility of the prehospital professional to act in the child's best interests and treat appropriately. Legal responsibilities can be explored and determined once initial emergency treatment has taken place.

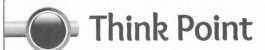

Think Point

Children may live in non-traditional families, and it may be unclear who has parental responsibility for a child.

Summary of Consent

Laws strictly protect the right of adult patients to accept or reject medical care; however, the laws of consent for children can pose special problems. The prehospital professional faces a difficult situation in cases where the carer refuses to consent or where consent to provide care and transport for a child cannot be readily obtained. Every case requires careful scene management and accurate documentation in the prehospital record.

Confidentiality

Medical information is private. Carelessly or inadvertently revealing identifiable information is an ethical and legal risk that prehospital professionals face, because they frequently care for individuals in a public environment. *It is essential to remain aware of the potentially sensitive nature of identifiable information and to take every possible precaution to protect confidentiality.* Conduct all sensitive discussions, when possible, in a setting where bystanders cannot overhear. Avoid using last names, if at all possible, at the scene. Do not share private information with concerned bystanders (other than those legally responsible for the patient).

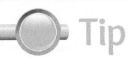

Tip

Prehospital professionals must be aware of the potentially sensitive nature of protected health information and take every possible precaution to protect confidentiality.

Respect for Cultural or Religious Differences

Cultural differences and religious beliefs may present exceptionally difficult situations. Although the care of the patient is always of primary concern, the prehospital professional must attempt to respect requests from the family or patient regarding preferences that may originate from their religious or cultural beliefs, especially when these do not interfere significantly with the provision of treatment to the child. The prehospital professional must always remain non-judgmental about requests that stem from cultural or religious beliefs, acknowledge the importance of these requests to the family, and attempt to accommodate them when possible. When the prehospital professional cannot accommodate requests that are based on cultural or religious beliefs because they would put a child at risk of serious harm, the reasons the requests cannot be accommodated must be respectfully explained.

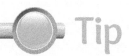

Tip

The prehospital professional must always remain non-judgmental about cultural or religious beliefs, acknowledge their importance to the family, and attempt to accommodate them whenever possible.

Language barriers may also present a challenge as the prehospital professional attempts to communicate with a child's carer. The prehospital professional should be familiar with what resources are available locally to provide translation in a timely manner. Miscommunications can have a significant impact on a child's care, especially if the prehospital professional is unable to obtain information about a child's underlying medical conditions, allergies, current medications, or other factors relevant to clinical care. If professional translation services are available, use these rather than family members or bystanders. If translation services are not available, a family member or neighbour may be asked to assist with translation, with the understanding that the information transferred may be inaccurate or incomplete, especially with regard to medical terminology.

End of Life Issues

The carers of some children who are terminally ill, usually in consultation with their GP, may decide on limitations to treatments and interventions. These decisions usually arise from the child's underlying condition and the desire to avoid futile or burdensome interventions if the child develops a life-threatening condition. Prehospital professionals, in responding to a call about a sick child, may find a **Do Not Attempt Resuscitation (DNAR)** order in place. These orders inform health care providers that cardiopulmonary resuscitation (CPR) or additional resuscitation, such as defibrillation or advanced airway control, should not be initiated in the

Case Study 2

You respond to the scene of a road traffic collision where you find a 10-year-old child with facial bruising; a tense, tender abdomen; and an obviously deformed left thigh. The child is seat belted in the rear passenger seat of the car, which has been struck on the driver's door by a truck. The child seems scared and begins to cry as you begin your assessment. The adult woman who had been driving the car has obvious head injuries and lacks a pulse. Another team begins work on the adult while you tend to the child. As you stabilise the child for transport, she asks you if her mother is okay.

1. Would it be appropriate to tell the child her mother is okay to enable a safe and efficient transport?

2. How should you respond to this child's question?

event of a cardiopulmonary arrest. The DNAR should clearly indicate what treatment is permissible, and what treatment is specifically refused. In some cases, the administration of medication to alleviate distressing symptoms may be permissible, but not treatment that would potentially extend the life of the patient. In cases of children with a DNAR order in place, it is important to understand what action the child's carers are expecting to be undertaken by the prehospital professional. Where a DNAR order has been written, it is done with the involvement of the child's carers as well as the wider medical team responsible for the care of the child and has been produced on the basis that it is in the best interests of the child. The prehospital professional should not presume to overrule such an order and undertake resuscitation based on their own personal beliefs.

Resuscitation

Sometimes resuscitation attempts are ineffective for children in cardiopulmonary arrest, and occasionally such attempts are unnecessary, as discussed in the *Resuscitation and Dysrhythmias chapter*. Clinical guidelines define circumstances when cardiopulmonary resuscitation must be initiated, when it may be withheld, and when it may be stopped.

Clinical guidelines allow prehospital professionals to withhold or stop resuscitation when a child is clearly dead, as defined by specific criteria (e.g., rigor mortis or injuries incompatible with life). This situation may be emotionally difficult for the prehospital provider; however, it is ultimately the decision of the lead clinician on scene, generally a paramedic or a doctor, to stop or to forego a resuscitation attempt, taking into account the views of their colleagues on scene as appropriate. Likewise, it may be difficult emotionally for family members if prehospital professionals do not attempt resuscitation. In cases where resuscitation attempts would clearly be futile, it would not be appropriate to begin resuscitation solely to appease family members on scene.

Being open and honest with the family of the deceased child, while a challenge in the immediate term, supports the grieving process of the family members and does not give them false hope.

Telling the Truth in Difficult Situations

Prehospital professionals should deal as honestly as possible with children and their carers. It is not unusual for carers to ask about the condition of a child or request information about a child's "chances of survival". In such situations, refrain from speculating, but respond instead with honest reassurance. For example, the statements "We'll take the best possible care of your child", or "He is in good hands; everything is being done to help him", provide an honest and reassuring response without speculating about uncertain outcomes.

The prehospital professional may also face situations in which multiple patients have sustained injuries and the parent or child requests information about others involved in the incident. It may be appropriate to deflect such questions, especially when the other party has suffered severe injuries or has died. It may be best to offer an honest statement of reassurance, such as "I need to focus on taking the best care of you right now. My colleagues are doing their best to take care of the others". Although there is an ethical obligation to be honest, it may be appropriate to delay sharing particularly distressing information until a patient has been transported safely and other sources of emotional support are available.

Hospital Destination

The appropriate ED for a sick or injured child may differ from the ED appropriate for an adult with a similar condition. Local service guidelines may identify specialised paediatric centres (e.g., general trauma centres with paediatric capability, paediatric critical care centres, or paediatric trauma centres) as primary receiving facilities for certain paediatric patients. In some cases, a child may meet multiple conflicting triage criteria (e.g., should a severely burned child be transported to a regional children's hospital or a non-paediatric hospital with a regional burn centre). In such circumstances, advice should be sought from the local ambulance control, who will be able to check the admission policies of the local hospitals.

Child Protection

Education of prehospital professionals in identifying possible maltreatment is an essential component of initial education and continuing medical education in paediatrics (see the *Child Maltreatment* chapter). Never confront the carer or others with accusations, moral judgments, threats, or suspicions. Although these situations are emotionally difficult, the immediate goal must always be to provide necessary treatment and ensure the safe transport of the child.

The NHS Constitution for England outlines patients' rights to privacy, confidentiality, security of their medical records, and to be informed about how their information is used. The Statement of NHS Accountability for England, an accompanying document to the NHS Constitution for England, identifies that accountability for the NHS is same across the United Kingdom with the governments of Scotland, Wales, and Northern Ireland all signing up to a set of common principles. The Health and Social Care (Safety and Quality) Act 2015 introduced a duty for health and social care commissioners and providers to share patient information where they consider that the disclosure is likely to facilitate the care provided to the individual and is in their best interest, although this duty to share extends only to England and Wales. Patient information must be securely safeguarded, although individuals also expect that relevant health information is shared amongst their care team.

This legislation requires all health and social care workers, including paramedics, to appropriately report any concerns regarding the safeguarding of any of their patients, including children. Failure to appropriately report such matters may constitute an offence.

CASE STUDY ANSWERS

Case Study 1 — page 272

Although a babysitter, even an adult babysitter, may be acting *in loco parentis*, they cannot withhold consent to treat a child, the doctrine of necessity allows you to treat and transport this child who is in respiratory distress. She suffers from an emergent condition that places her at risk and it would be unsafe to delay treatment. If the babysitter has a telephone number for the parents, call them, apprise them of the situation, and tell them that you will provide necessary treatment and transport. Even if the parents cannot be reached, you should provide treatment for the child's wheezing and respiratory distress with oxygen and a bronchodilator and transport her to an appropriate facility. Finally, make sure this 16-year-old babysitter is safe, and leave information with her to give to the child's carers that explains what happened and where you have transported the child.

Case Study 2 — page 276

Carefully consider your answer to this child's concerned question. On the one hand, avoid being dishonest. Since you do not know whether her mother will survive, you should not assure the child that her mother will be okay. On the other hand, it would be appropriate to withhold your concerns and suspicions about the mother's condition until the child has been transported safely, more is known about the mother's condition, and there are resources (e.g., a social worker) available to assist the child in receiving what may be terrible news. One honest answer might be, "I know you are worried about your mother. My colleagues are taking good care of her. I need to take good care of you, and I'm going to take you to the hospital. Once we get there, we'll try to find out more about your mother".

SUGGESTED READINGS

Textbooks

American Academy of Orthopaedic Surgeons and College of Paramedics. *Nancy Caroline's Emergency Care in the Streets.* Revised 7th ed. Burlington: Jones & Bartlett Learning; 2014.

References

Gillick v West Norfolk and Wisbech Area Health Authority and Another [1985] UKHL 7.

Department of Health and Social Care. NHS Constitution for England. https://www.gov.uk/government/publications/the-nhs-constitution-for-england. Accessed August 7, 2018.

Scottish Government. Adults with Incapacity (Scotland) Act 2000. https://www.legislation.gov.uk/asp/2000/4/contents. Accessed August 7, 2018.

Scottish Government. Age of Legal Capacity (Scotland) Act 1991. https://www.legislation.gov.uk/ukpga/1991/50/contents. August 7, 2018.

Scottish Government. Children (Scotland) Act 1995. https://www.legislation.gov.uk/ukpga/1995/36/contents. Accessed August 7, 2018.

UK Government. Children Act 1989. https://www.legislation.gov.uk/ukpga/1989/41/contents. Accessed August 7, 2018.

UK Government. Family Law Reform Act 1969. https://www.legislation.gov.uk/ukpga/1969/46. Accessed August 7, 2018.

UK Government. Health and Social Care (Safety and Quality) Act 2015. http://www.legislation.gov.uk/ukpga/2015/28/notes. Accessed August 7, 2018.

UK Government. Mental Capacity Act 2005. https://www.legislation.gov.uk/ukpga/2005/9/contents. Accessed August 7, 2018.

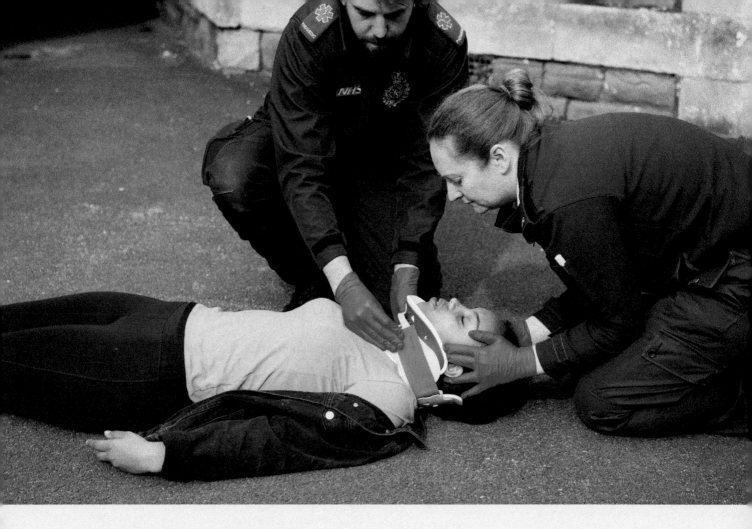

Learning Objectives

1. Explore the decision-making processes required to admit, refer, or discharge a child.
2. Discuss the choice of destination for children who require admission.
3. Outline the process required to refer a child to another healthcare professional.
4. Discuss how to discharge safely, including safety netting and advice to caregivers.
5. Identify when a paediatric patient requires emergency transport.
6. Discuss transport considerations for paediatric encounters in an ambulance, including mode of transport, restraint systems and emergency journeys.

Admission, Referral, and Discharge Considerations

Introduction

All prehospital professionals will make decisions to admit, refer or discharge children. Paediatric patients encounter many of the same presenting complaints as in adults, but because our encounter with this patient group is far less common, the decision-making process is immediately more complex. Age of the child is an important factor, as well as capability of those looking after the child, previous medical history, and duration of illness, to name a few. The decision to admit, refer or discharge a child must always be informed by evidence-based guidelines, as well as the experience of the prehospital professional and the circumstances of the incident.

For children with emergency presentations, the decision is simpler: provide life-saving intervention(s), select the appropriate receiving unit and either transport to that facility or handover care to advanced care teams (i.e., HEMS: Helicopter Emergency Medical Services). For the child with a minor illness, minor injury or other "non-emergency" presentation, the decision is more complex. All of these children will still require a thorough assessment, including a full set of vital signs, but they are less likely to require immediate intervention and transport to an Emergency Department (ED). It is for this group of patients that we must move away from emergency protocols and consider the most appropriate action for each child.

For example, you see a child who has had a fever for 2 days who is well-hydrated with no red flags or abnormal vital signs. You are reassured that the caregivers are sensible and will be capable of monitoring for any deterioration and agree to book an appointment with the GP for review in 48 hours. Now consider the same child, but with worried caregivers who are extremely concerned, and you feel that they would not necessarily detect deterioration, so you may make a different decision. That child may need to see the GP today, or within 24 hours to get additional reassurance. In this short example, the patient presentation is the same; however, the circumstances require a different clinical decision.

This chapter will discuss in detail the considerations required to:

- Admit the child (to ED or other care centre)
- Refer to another healthcare professional
- Discharge at the scene

Decision-Making Process

It is a big decision to admit a child to hospital, refer them to another professional, or discharge them at the scene. Paediatric calls to the ambulance service account for about 10% of all 999 calls received and less than 5% of those will require emergency intervention. Therefore, the majority of our paediatric patients are more likely to have a non-emergency presentation, are less likely to need critical interventions, and should be admitted to Emergency Departments less often.

Case Study 1 – Prolonged Fever

You attend a 5-year-old girl with a fever (38°C). She has been unwell for 5 days and despite regular paracetamol, the fever has persisted and she is now becoming more irritable. In the last 24 hours she has been eating and drinking less and her parents have noticed a rash on her stomach, back, and legs. The rash is red, raised, and is blanching (tumbler-test). Her vital signs are recorded as follows:

RR	26	HR	135	CRT	2s	SpO$_2$	98%

You continue your assessment using the traffic light system provided by NICE (see Chapter 6, *Medical Emergencies*, for details on assessment using the NICE traffic light system).

The child is green (low risk) for colour, activity, respiratory, and circulation/hydration, although the heart rate is towards the limit for amber (intermediate risk) at 135/min. Also, while there is no reported reduction in urine output, the child has had reduced fluid intake in the last 24 hours. The child hits one amber feature "*Fever for ≥5 days*". Using good clinical reasoning, you recognise that the child is at risk of multiple amber features in the next 24–48 hours, and you remember from a lecture that a fever lasting for more than 5 days is a risk factor for Kawasaki disease.

The NICE guideline (CG160) for management by non-paediatric practitioners offers two options for this child:

1. Provide parents or caregivers with a "safety net", which includes one or more of the following:

   a. Including verbal and/or written information;

   b. Follow up appointment at a specified time and place;

   c. Referral to another healthcare professional (e.g., out-of-hours) to ensure direct access should the child require further assessment.

2. Refer to specialist paediatric care.

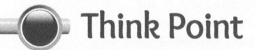

Think Point

1. How do you make this decision currently?
2. Which guidelines, evidence, and resources can you use to help your decision-making process?
3. Do you use all of the tools that are available to you on a regular basis?

Many prehospital professionals will rely on experience to make a decision, as the UK evidence suggests that paediatric education and training is lacking or limited to emergency care. Those professionals who have children often feel more comfortable giving advice to parents than those who do not. But, regardless of personal circumstances, all prehospital clinicians are expected to *be competent in caring*

for sick and injured children (Royal College of Paediatrics and Child Health: 2012).

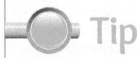

Tip

If the option is available to you, always try to call a GP or paediatric specialist to talk through the case. It is common practice in hospital settings to discuss discharge decisions with senior colleagues.

Summary of Admission, Referral, and Discharge Considerations

- Make use of published guidelines (e.g., NICE) to help to build your decision about the child with a non-emergency presentation.

- When available, speak to the local paediatric team or a GP about your patient—it is good practice to discuss the case with other healthcare professionals. That way you can reach a decision as a team.
- If you aren't sure, or the caregivers seem worried despite your assessment/advice—lower your threshold for admission or referral for a face-to-face assessment.

Admission Destinations

Choosing an appropriate "admission" destination should allow the child to be seen by a clinician with the knowledge and competence to assess and manage their presenting complaint. In order to choose the right destination, we must form a working diagnosis. From this working diagnosis, you can then determine which receiving unit has the capability to manage your patient. In the UK, your choices are limited and dependent on the region in which you work and local pathways that are available. Listed below are common receiving units—the types of patient that they will see will vary region by region, and you should always be familiar with the criteria for your local receiving units:

- Emergency Department/Trauma Centre
- Urgent Care Centre
- Walk-in-Centre
- Minor Illness/Injury Unit
- Paediatric Assessment Unit/Ward
- General Practice

Making a Referral

A referral to another healthcare professional can be defined as *a communication process with the purpose of directing a patient to an appropriate specialist for advice, assessment or admission* (Bradley V, Whitelaw BC, Lindfield D, Phillips RJW, Trim C, Lasoye TA: 2015). As prehospital professionals, the different specialists that we can refer to will vary depending on location and clinical grade. For example, a paramedic will be able to make a referral to the out-of-hours

GP, whereas a specialist paramedic may be able to refer that same patient to the correct ward/department (e.g., urology). The availability of paediatric specific referral pathways is limited across the UK. That said, many of your paediatric patients will be suitable for referral to a GP.

The following numbered points are a suggested format for making a successful referral:

1. Hello, this is _____ and I'm a Paramedic/EMT with _____ Ambulance Service. Can I confirm your name, please? I have a patient and I would like to *refer/ admit/seek advice*.
2. Pause and wait for acknowledgement by specialist.
3. The patient is a ____ year old *male/female* and an ambulance was called for *presenting complaint*.
4. Provide the relevant history and vital signs data.
5. I think the most likely working diagnosis is _____. My clinical impression is that this patient has _____.
6. So far, I have given the following *advice/treatment/ reassurance*.
7. If it is more than just an advice call, state that you "would like the specialist to evaluate this patient". Confirm that you would like a face-to-face appointment, telephone consultation, and admission.
8. The current condition is _____.
9. Thank you. If not already taken, ensure that you document the name of the specialist you are referring to, the time that the referral was accepted OR, if not accepted, the advice that was provided and your next steps.

(Adapted from Go et al. 1998)

Tip

Referrals must be made to another registered clinician. It would not be appropriate to speak to an out-of-hours call taker, receptionist or another non-clinical person.

Case Study 2 — Tonsillitis

You are called to assess a 5-year-old boy with a sore throat, fever and reduced fluid intake. On arrival, the child is alert and interacting well. There is no immediate concern with regard to their appearance, work of breathing or circulation status. The history reveals a 4-day history of fever with a sore throat and in the last 2 hours he has been reluctant to drink water. His vital signs and clinical assessment are as follows:

RR	22	HR	110	Central CRT	2s	SpO$_2$	98%	T	37.9°C

The chest is clear, there is no cough, no rash, and the child is warm peripherally. Cervical lymph nodes are enlarged. If permitted, you may look in the child's ears, and you determine that there is no abnormality.

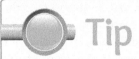

Discharging Safely

Before you make the decision to discharge a child at scene, there are a few things to consider:

- Your own knowledge and experience—is it enough to understand the whole picture and to give the correct advice to caregivers?

- What does your local policy state? Some mandate transport for patients under 2 years of age, some for under 5s, and some for anyone under the age of 18. Policy is difficult to contradict and should be followed, if in place in your place of work.

- Capability of the parent/caregiver—will they be able to retain your advice? Will they be able to recognise the red flags you mention? Do they have the means to access further support?

- What advice are you planning to give and how will you provide it? Ideally, any verbal advice should be complimented with comprehensive written advice. The written advice should include red flags, what support is available, when to access further support and what to do in an emergency.

Once you have taken the above into consideration, you can start to formulate a clinical decision. This should be informed by relevant guidelines, current best evidence and your experience as a clinician.

Emergency Transport

The decision to pre-alert the Emergency Department for a seriously ill or injured child should be straightforward. In the case of major trauma, we have decision tools that support our own clinical judgment to ensure the patient is taken to the most appropriate hospital; see **Figure 15-1**. The seriously ill child may have altered vital signs, a working diagnosis of an emergency condition or the clinical "gut feeling" that something isn't right and this child needs to be seen immediately.

Emergency transport will, more often than not, mean that a patient will arrive at a hospital in less time than driving at normal road speed—however, emergency transport is not a substitute for meaningful intervention on scene. For example, a child with severe/life-threatening asthma must receive standard care (nebulised salbutamol and/or ipratropium

bromide, intravenous steroids and when indicated, intramuscular adrenaline). Some of this may be possible en route to hospital, but you should still consider spending time at the scene to complete these meaningful interventions.

The pre-alert message should prepare the hospital team for what they are about to receive, but that does not mean you will have a team that is prepared on your arrival. For this reason, the information in your pre-alert must be exceptionally clear and you should ask for what is needed on your arrival.

The below example uses SBAR to pre-alert the child with severe asthma:

Situation	I have a 6-year-old female with severe asthma and I am concerned that she is not improving despite treatment at scene.
Background	The child has had frequent admissions and most recently was admitted to PICU (Paediatric Intensive Care Unit) for ventilatory support. No inhaler available while playing sport today.
Assessment/**A**ctions	We have diagnosed severe asthma and treated with nebulised salbutamol and ipratropium bromide and IV steroids, but the child is still deteriorating.
Recommendations	We request a paediatric anaesthetist attend this pre-alert due to failing respiratory effort and will administer IM adrenaline 1:1000, continue supplemental oxygen/nebulisers and will arrive at your ED in 20–25 minutes.

Below is the same patient using the ATMIST mnemonic:

Age	6-year-old female
Time	Onset in last hour
Mechanism	Exacerbation of asthma due to playing sport, no inhaler available
Injuries/**I**llness	Severe asthma attack
Signs	**<C>** – No catastrophic bleeding present **A** – Airway patent, but child exhausted **B** – RR = 34, SpO_2 = 90% on nebuliser (via 100% FiO_2) **C** – HR = 136 **D** – Responding to VOICE **E** – n/a
Treatment	Nebulised salbutamol and ipratropium bromide Preparing to assist ventilations, if necessary IV hydrocortisone Preparing IM adrenaline 1:1000
ETA	15–20 minutes Request PICU attendance

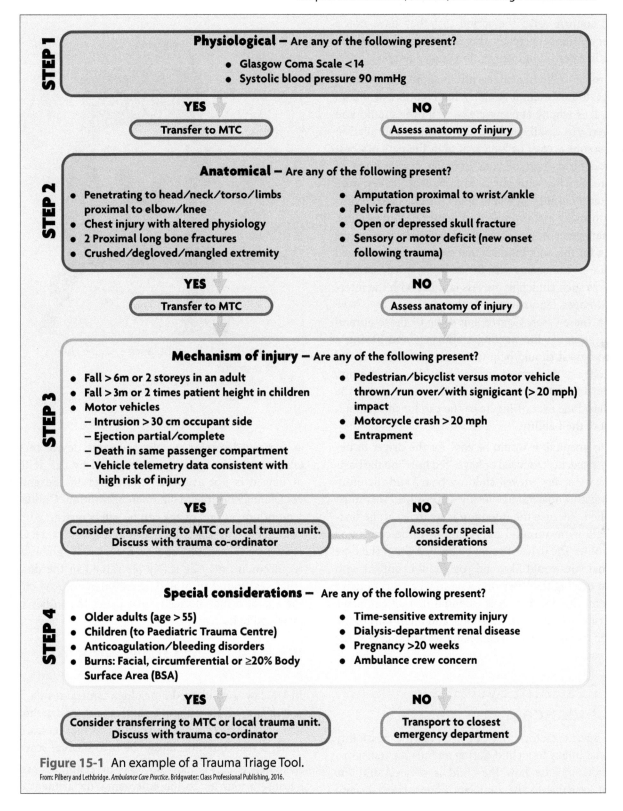

Figure 15-1 An example of a Trauma Triage Tool.
From: Pilbery and Lethbridge. *Ambulance Care Practice*. Bridgwater: Class Professional Publishing, 2016.

SBAR and ATMIST are just two tools; different prehospital systems and clinicians use these and others to pass pre-alert messages. Use one that you are comfortable with and can remember. Use the time during transport (when possible) to prepare/note down your clinical handover and be ready to deliver it confidently, clearly, and succinctly. In the Emergency Department, there will usually be someone appointed to scribe—once you have given your verbal handover, confirm with the scribe that they have noted your interventions correctly, medicine dose/route/time and any other pertinent information (e.g., allergies).

While en route to the ED, interventions should still be continued, but do not attempt complex interventions while on the move. It is wholly appropriate to pull over should you need to perform a skill such as, for example, cannulation or intraossesous access, as long as it is in the patient's best interest and forms part of your ongoing management of that patient. Staying with our asthma patient, if they were to deteriorate en route—it would be reasonable (and recommended) to make a short stop and deliver IM adrenaline, airway management, or commence ventilatory support. The reason for this suggestion is that seriously ill or injured children are a rare occurrence in the prehospital environment, and as such clinicians are less familiar with the interventions, dosages, landmarks and other decisions they have to make in these cases. Controlling some of those human factors, by stopping the moving ambulance and having a colleague to assist should help to ensure that those critical interventions are performed correctly, on the first attempt. The journey to the ED can then continue, knowing that the clinician has done everything he or she can for this patient, to the best of their ability.

En route to hospital, it would be easy for the driver to become distracted, task focused or have "red mist" on the basis that they have a very unwell child on board and therefore they must get to hospital as quickly as possible. This must be controlled, because the intention is to arrive at the hospital and allow meaningful interventions to be continued while en route. The driver should be briefed about the type of drive that you would like, and you should confirm with the person driving that they understand what sort of drive is needed on this journey. It is essential that all clinicians communicate their actions, decisions, and intentions to the whole team to ensure that all clinicians are working towards the same goal.

Child Restraint Systems in Ambulances

There are several factors that can decrease the possibility of additional injury to a child during ambulance transport. These factors include how the child is secured and the equipment available to the ambulance crew. Use age- and weight-appropriate restraints according to the manufacturer's guideline.

UK law requires that all children must normally use a car seat until they are 12 years old or 135 cm tall, whichever comes first. All children over 12 must wear a seatbelt. Newborns and very small babies should be transported in

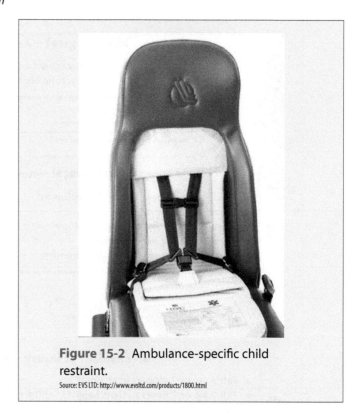

Figure 15-2 Ambulance-specific child restraint.
Source: EVS LTD: http://www.evsltd.com/products/1800.html

an approved carrier, usually the same device that a parent would use to transport the child by car. If this type of device is not available, the driver of the ambulance vehicle may be able to claim an exemption. Children aged 1 month to 5 years of age can be safely restrained using an ambulance-specific child restraint (**Figure 15-2**). Children aged over 12 months, or who meet the height and weight requirement, may be safely restrained in the dual adult/child seat found in most UK ambulances. Any child over the age of 5 may be restrained using the trolley bed and provided belts.

When Can a Child Travel Without a Car Seat?

In UK law, a child aged 3 or older can travel in a the back seat of any vehicle without a child car seat and without a seat belt if that vehicle does not have one. In most cases, children under 3 years old must always be in a child car seat.

Ambulance crews may be able to claim an exemption because a journey to the emergency department or other care centre may be considered an unexpected journey. If the correct child car seat is not available, a child aged 3 or older can use an adult seat belt if the journey is all of the following:

- Unexpected
- Necessary
- Over a short distance.

The law also states that you cannot take children under 3 years old on an unexpected journey in a vehicle without the correct child car seat, unless both of the following apply:

- It is a licensed taxi or minicab
- The child travels on a rear seat without a seat belt.

In this case, ambulance crews will be expected to make a judgment and transport the patient by the safest means possible, using the child restraints and other tools that should be available within the ambulance vehicle.

Summary of Emergency Transport

- Make use of triage tools to support your decision to admit a child under emergency conditions. This will also help to select the most appropriate receiving unit.

- Use pre-alert and handover tools (e.g., SBAR and ATMIST) to send your message and to give a confident, clear and succinct handover to the receiving team.
- Continue and/or provide meaningful interventions en route to hospital, even if that means a short stop to do it correctly—the first time—with support from your colleagues.
- Communicate decisions and intentions to the whole team and brief the driver as to what you expect—a safe, smooth journey that allows interventions to continue and timely arrival at the receiving hospital.

CASE STUDY ANSWERS

Case Study 1 — page 282

In this situation, you would be fully justified in referring directly to specialist paediatric care—which is probably best accessed via admission to an Emergency Department. The child has amber features, altered vital signs, and is at risk of a severe infection, and therefore they require an urgent face-to-face assessment. If we reduced the fever duration down to 3 days (with or without the rash) and with "OK" vital signs, then safety netting and referral may be very appropriate.

Case Study 2 — page 283

On examination of the throat you see what is depicted in **Figure 15-3**.

The working diagnosis is tonsillitis and you now use the "Centor Criteria" (**Table 15-1**) to determine if the child requires a referral +/− antibiotics.

Using the Centor Criteria, this child scores 5 and so is a good candidate for antibiotics. As he is otherwise well but still complaining of pain in his throat, you decide to refer to the GP. This is how the referral conversation might be structured:

1. Hello, this is *Joe Bloggs*—Paramedic with *999 Ambulance Service*. Can I confirm your name and speciality, please? I would like to discuss a patient with you, please.

2. Pause—acknowledged.

3. I have a 5-year-old boy with a sore throat.

4. He has a 4-day history of fever. In the last hour or so he has been reluctant to drink water. He has been treated at home with oral paracetamol but is not improving. His vital signs are:

5.

RR	22	HR	110	Central CRT	2s	SpO$_2$	98%	T	37.9°C

6. Based on inspection of the pharynx, my working diagnosis is tonsillitis.

7. We have given oral ibuprofen as he was in some discomfort on our arrival and had already received oral paracetamol.

8. He has a Centor score of 5, can I arrange an appointment with you to review and consider antibiotics?

9. He is currently alert and interacting well and I have no immediate concern.

10. Thank you (accepted)—I have asked the parents to visit your clinic at 20.00 hrs this evening.

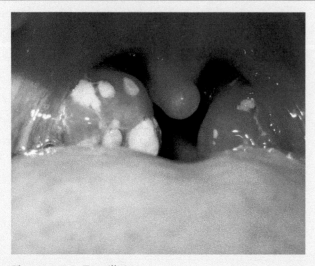

Figure 15-3 Tonsillitis.

Table 15-1 Modified Centor Criteria for Pharyngitis and Tonsillitis

Lack of a cough	1
Tonsillar exudates	1
Tender anterior cervical nodes	1
Fever	1
Age: 3–14 years	1
Age: 15–44 years	0
Age: Older than 45 years	−1

Source: Zoorob R, Sidani MA, Fremont RD and Kihlberg C. Antibiotic Use in Acute Upper Respiratory Tract Infections. *Am Fam Physician.* 2012;86(9):817–822.

REFERENCES AND SUGGESTED READINGS

Bradley V, Whitelaw BC, Lindfield D, Phillips RJW, Trim C, Lasoye TA. Teaching referral skills to medical students. *BMC Research Notes*. 2015;8(1):375. Available at: https://bmcresnotes.biomedcentral.com/articles/10.1186/s13104-015-1369-4. Accessed August 27, 2018.

Department for Transport. 2018. Child car seats: the law. Available at: https://www.gov.uk/child-car-seats-the-rules/when-a-child-can-travel-without-a-car-seat. Accessed July 23, 2018.

Go S, Richards DM, Watson WA. Enhancing medical student consultation request skills in an academic emergency department. *J Emerg Med*. 1998;16(4):659–662.

Houston R, Pearson GA. Ambulance provision for children: a UK national survey. *EMJ*. 2010;27(8):631–636.

Jewkes F. Current topic: Prehospital emergency care for children. *Arch Dis Child*. 2001;84(2):103–105.

Joint Royal Colleges Ambulance Liaison Committee. *UK Ambulance Services Clinical Practice Guidelines 2016*. Bridgwater: Class Professional Publishing; 2016.

Lissauer T, Clayden G. *Illustrated Textbook of Paediatrics*. 4th ed. London: Elsevier Mosby; 2012.

National Institute for Health and Clinical Excellence. *Fever in Under 5s (CG160)*. London: NICE, 2013. Available at: https://www.nice.org.uk/guidance/cg160. Accessed August 27, 2018.

National Institute for Health and Care Excellence. *NICE Clinical Guideline (NG9) Bronchiolitis in Children: Diagnosis and Management*. Manchester: NICE; 2015.

NHS Gloucestershire Hospitals Foundation Trust. Fever advice for children and young people in Gloucestershire. 2018. Available at: www.gloshospitals.nhs.uk. Accessed July 23, 2018.

Pilbery R, Lethbridge K. *Ambulance Care Practice*. Bridgwater: Class Publishing; 2016.

Royal College of Paediatrics and Child Health Standards for Children and Young People in Emergency Care Settings. London; 2012.

Zoorob R, Sidani MA, Fremont RD, Kihlberg C. Antibiotic use in acute upper respiratory tract infections. *Am Fam Physician*. 2012;86:817–822.

Procedure 1: Pre-alert

Introduction

Gathering and organising pertinent information about children to report to other prehospital professionals and the receiving emergency department (ED) requires the use of paediatric terms. Clear, concise communication helps ensure an orderly flow of out-of-hospital tasks: informing the receiving ED personnel about incoming patients; and making an effective transfer of information about the patient's assessment and care. Each ambulance service area will have differences in its procedures for handing over patient information to the receiving ED. Sometimes the pre-alert reporting is made by radio; at other times it may be made by telephone or another form of real-time communication.

In addition to the spoken presentation format for handover, specific documentation is also essential for later review and analysis. Each service has its own patient care record on which the prehospital professional must record clinical information, as well as detailed incident or administrative information.

Indication

Patients who you suspect will require immediate assessment or treatment on arrival at the ED, or will require additional resources to be present, for example, major trauma patients or critically ill children.

Contraindication

Patients that will not require rapid assessment or management on arrival. It may be challenging at times to pre-alert a critically ill or injured child while simultaneously providing necessary interventions; however, it is very important to do so to allow the hospital staff to prepare for their arrival. In such circumstances you should consider asking a colleague or the ambulance control room to pass on a pre-alert message for you.

Equipment

Equipment requirements vary depending on the service. Most UK ambulance services have a digital radio capable of both radio and telephone communications. Other equipment may include mobile telephones, computerised real-time data transmission, or, in the near future, video (telemedicine). The patient care record is essential, as are additional records in some services.

Rationale

A logical and descriptive format for presentation of key information about ill or injured children is essential for effective pre-alerting. Paediatric-specific reporting techniques complement appropriate age-related modifications in assessment, treatment, triage, and transport.

Preparation

1. The prehospital professional should prepare for and practice pre-alerting about children.

2. It is helpful to have a pre-alert format that is agreed on by the ED and the ambulance providers. Some specific pathways may have different pre-agreed formats, e.g., for major trauma patients. The desired format can be printed on small pads as a checklist. This may help in the flow and understanding of patient information during situations when the prehospital professional has multiple tasks and when the environment or equipment makes communicating difficult.

3. Such notes may be useful not only during transport, but also when transferring care at the ED.

Possible Complications

Using incorrect, deceptive, or unclear terminology, or failing to distinguish the paediatric report from the more frequent adult-oriented report, may delay preparation by the receiving ED.

Think Point

Do not give long pre-alerts when there is a distressed child in the ambulance.

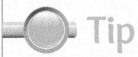

Tip

Report the patient's assessment using the PAT.

Procedure 1-1

Pre-alerting

① State the child's age, sex, and estimated body weight. Always give the body weight in kilograms or length-based resuscitation tape colour. This will allow the ED to prepare for the paediatric patient in advance. Using the patient's name is generally not pertinent to treatment, triage, or transport, so do not use names in the pre-alert. Emergency medical channels are easily monitored, and omitting the patient's name protects his or her identity and medical confidentiality.

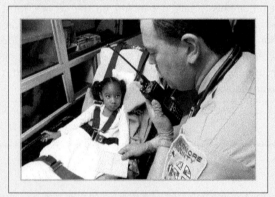

② Give the child's presenting complaint.

③ Provide in one sentence the mechanism of injury or history of illness, and state pertinent past medical history (usually none or brief).

④ Summarise the assessment and establish the level of severity and urgency for treatment using the Pae-

diatric Assessment Triangle (PAT). Address all three elements of the PAT, using appropriate descriptive words and terms, as listed in **Table P1-1.**

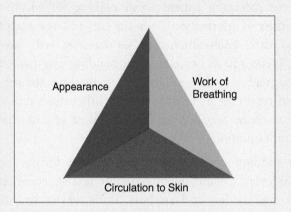

⑤ Report any abnormalities in the ABCDEs including any abnormal observations.

⑥ State treatment and response, using the PAT.

⑦ Estimate time of arrival.

⑧ **Table P1-2** is a sample paediatric pre-alert template.

Table P1-1 Examples of Paediatric-Specific Terminology for PAT

Appearance (use TICLS mnemonic to recall individual features)	Work of Breathing	Circulation to Skin
Tone Active, vigorous, good muscle tone Limp, listless, motionless, will not sit or walk	Apnoeic	Pink, good colour
Interactiveness Alert, interactive, attentive, playful Restless, agitated, screaming	Abnormal positioning (sniffing position, tripoding)	Mottled, dusky
Consolability Consolable or distractible by caregiver, comfortable Cannot be consoled	Abnormal airway sounds (snoring, stridor, wheezing, grunting)	Pale
Look/Gaze Fixes gaze, maintains good eye contact Will not engage or make eye contact	Retractions (supraclavicular, intercostal, subxiphoid)	Cyanotic
Speech/Cry Strong cry, normal speech Weak cry, cannot speak	Nasal flaring	

Table P1-2 Sample Paediatric Pre-alert Template (ASHICE)

Age	The patient's age in years or months.
Sex	The sex of the patient.
History	A short sentence describing what happened.
Injuries / **I**llness	Presenting complaint.
Condition	PAT triangle findings: • Appearance: Describe the patient's appearance using descriptive terms.* • Work of breathing: Describe the work of breathing using descriptive terms. • Circulation to skin: Describe the circulation to skin using descriptive terms. Summarise key findings from the ABCDEs and any abnormal observations. Summarise key interventions and patient's response to the interventions
ETA	Our ETA to [state receiving ED] is _____ minutes. Do you have any advice or questions?

*See Table P1-1 for examples of paediatric-specific descriptive terminology.

Procedure 2: Oxygen Delivery

Introduction

Hypoxia in the infant or child causes cardiopulmonary distress and may lead to organ failure. Careful assessment of the child's cardiopulmonary status includes standard physical assessment techniques and pulse oximetry. A normal room air pulse oximetry reading is 95% or greater. A pulse oximetry value of less than 95% on room air is an indication for supplemental oxygen. A value less than 90% with the child on 100% oxygen is usually also an indication for ventilatory support. Acute hypoxia is usually easy to treat. Rapid intervention may slow or reverse cardiopulmonary distress or failure and avoid the need for ventilatory support. Although respiratory disease is usually the cause of hypoxia in children, other conditions, such as hypovolaemic shock, severe poisonings, or seizures, may also result in hypoxia.

There are different procedures for giving oxygen to children that vary the amount of actual oxygen supplementation. Use an oxygen delivery technique that matches the child's clinical condition, age, and need for oxygen. For example, give oxygen by nasal cannula or simple mask to the child in no or mild distress who has an open airway. Give oxygen by a non-rebreathing mask or bag-valve-mask device to the child with moderate to severe respiratory distress. Rarely, a critical child requires endotracheal intubation for positive pressure ventilation and oxygen administration. When supplemental oxygen does not improve the child's condition, consider other possibilities, such as a cardiac disorder (e.g., cyanotic congenital heart disease); a circulatory disorder (e.g., hypovolaemic shock); or, rarely, a toxicological disorder (e.g., methaemoglobinemia).

Be creative in delivering oxygen to young children. Under some circumstances, giving blow-by oxygen may avoid agitating the child and increasing his or her distress. In the newly born be careful about oxygen delivery, because it is unnecessary if the newborn has a normal pulse oximetry and supplemental oxygen may be harmful to the immature brain.

Indications

Respiratory distress

Pulse oximetry less than 95% on room air

Respiratory failure

Partial upper airway obstruction

Partial lower airway obstruction

Worsening of chronic lung disease

Status epilepticus

Overdose

Shock from any cause

Multiple trauma

Any condition possibly causing decreased oxygen delivery to tissues

Smoke inhalation

Carbon monoxide poisoning

Contraindications

There are few absolute contraindications to oxygen delivery to a child who may be hypoxic. There are, however, rare relative contraindications to certain oxygen delivery techniques that do not match the child's clinical condition. For example, shunted cyanotic cardiac patients whose saturation goals are 75%–85% should not receive oxygen to increase saturation greater than 85%. Oxygen has proper doses and routes of administration for maximum benefit, minimum toxicity, optimal feasibility, and reasonable cost.

Rationale

A child's immature anatomy and physiology make respiratory distress and failure common paediatric emergencies. When apnoea or hypoventilation occurs, hypoxia develops quickly. Therefore, give oxygen to any child with clinical signs of cardiopulmonary distress or failure, or with a history suggesting possible abnormalities in gas exchange. *Children seldom have a condition where excess oxygen turns off their respiratory drive, so it is better to over-treat with oxygen than to under-treat.*

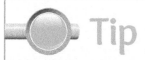

The appropriate oxygen delivery technique is based on the child's condition, age, and need for oxygen.

Preparation

Match the correct oxygen delivery device with the patient assessment (child's condition, age, and need for oxygen; **Table P2-1**) and connect to the delivery system.

Equipment

Subject to local availability:

Infant and paediatric nasal cannula

Paediatric mask sizes

Paediatric non-rebreathing mask

Oxygen connecting tubing

Oxygen source

Possible Complications

Injury, if the pressurised tank is punctured or a valve breaks off

Potential for fire, because oxygen supports combustion

Respiratory arrest if high concentrations of oxygen are given to the child with chronic lung disease (rare)

Agitation and worsening of hypoxia if delivery technique is overly aggressive

Hypothermia in an infant younger than 6 months of age with an endotracheal tube in place, who receives cool, unhumidified oxygen for more than 30 minutes

In newborns with normal pulse, brain injury may occur because of unnecessary supplemental oxygen

Table P2-1 Oxygen Delivery Technique and Patient Assessment

Device	Flow Rate	Concentration Delivered	Considerations
Nasal cannula	1–6 l/min	Up to 44%	• Low-flow system • Least restrictive • Slowly start flow of oxygen after cannula is secured to avoid frightening child • May help to tape cannula to child's cheeks • Use in infants who are obligatory nose breathers or if there is difficulty in obtaining a correctly sized mask
Simple mask	6–10 l/min	35–60%	• Low-flow system • Infant, paediatric, and adult sized masks are available • Use minimum flow rate to flush the mask
Non-rebreathing	12–15 l/min	60–90%	• High-flow system mask • Consists of face mask and reservoir bag with a valve on the exhalation mask port to prevent drawing in room air during inhalation and a valve between the reservoir bag and mask to prevent exhalation of air into the reservoir bag • Use in spontaneously breathing patients who require highest concentration of oxygen available (children with respiratory distress and shock) • Make sure the flow rate keeps the reservoir bag inflated • With a snug fit, delivers highest oxygen concentration available by mask • Paediatric and adult masks are available • Partial rebreather masks are indicated in neonates and infants who cannot overcome valve resistance
Blow-by	6–10 l/min	Depends on flow rate and proximity to face	• Indicated for infant or young child requiring oxygen who will not tolerate mask on the face • Start oxygen flow through simple mask, corrugated tubing, or oxygen tubing threaded through the bottom of a cup • Hold the delivery device as close to the child's nose and mouth as tolerated

Source: Emergency Nurses Association. Respiratory distress and failure. *Emergency Nursing Pediatric Course, Provider Manual.* Park Ridge, IL; 1999.

Think Point

Do not give oxygen to a newborn who is not hypoxic. It may cause injury in immature patients.

Tip

Add humidification to nasal cannula flow greater than 5 l/min to avoid nasal irritation and bleeding.

Tip

An oxygen mask may frighten a child. Consider involving parent or caregiver to reduce the fear.

Tip

For nasal cannula: percent oxygen delivered is affected by respiratory rate, tidal volume, and extent of mouth breathing. An infant may receive higher FiO_2 concentration than older patients (e.g., 30%–35% with 1 l/min oxygen, 26%–32% with 0.5 l/min oxygen).

Think Point

Do not force the child to lie down because it may increase the child's anxiety and agitation. Consider using positioning with parent or caregiver.

Procedure 2-1

Oxygen Delivery

1 Explain to the child and family why oxygen is needed and how the device works. Use developmentally appropriate language. **Table P2-2** suggests methods to ease anxiety in the child who does not want to cooperate with oxygen delivery. For blow-by oxygen using a paper cup, punch a hole in the bottom of the cup and insert the tubing through the hole. Placing stickers on the cup or drawing smiley faces may decrease the child's anxiety.

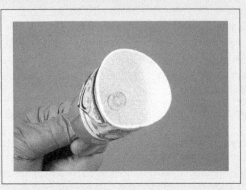

2 Allow the child to remain in a position of comfort, which may be sitting on the caregiver's lap. In the ambulance, the child must be safely restrained.

3a To apply a mask, select the correct size. The mask should extend from the bridge of the nose to the cleft of the chin. Avoid placing pressure on the eyes.

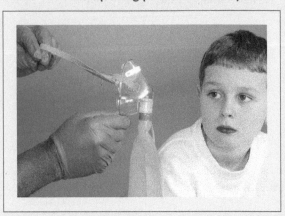

Procedure 2-1 (continued)

3b Place the mask over the child's head, starting from the nose downward. Squeeze the nose clip and adjust the head strap.

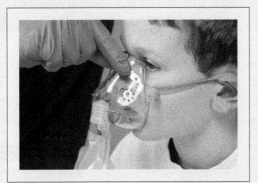

4 To apply a nasal cannula, curve the plastic prongs back into the nostrils. Loop the tubing around the ears.

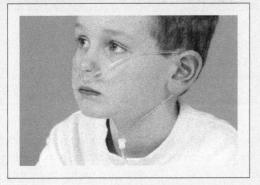

5 For blow-by oxygen, instruct the caregiver to hold the tubing or paper cup close to the child's face to maximise oxygen delivery.

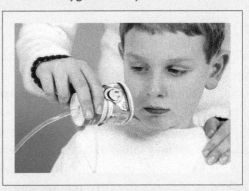

Table P2-2 Methods to Gain Child's Cooperation for Oxygen Delivery

Allow the child to hold the mask before placing it on his or her face.
Allow the child to feel the flow of oxygen before placing the mask on his or her face.
Consider involving parent or caregiver to support oxygen delivery as required.
If the child struggles, consider using the blow-by technique to avoid agitation and increasing the oxygen demands. Placing stickers or drawing smiley faces on the cup may decrease the child's anxiety.

Controversy

The amount of oxygen to give routinely to children with chronic lung disease is unknown and probably differs for each individual. Administration of oxygen to patients with chronic lung disease who retain carbon dioxide at baseline can result in hypoventilation, but rarely does so in actual practice in paediatrics. If the child has a history and assessment suggesting acute hypoxia and increased work of breathing, give oxygen but be ready to assist ventilation with a bag-valve-mask device.

Procedure 3: Suctioning

Introduction

Children of all ages are prone to airway obstruction from secretions, vomitus, pus, blood, oedema, and foreign bodies. In newborns, airway obstruction from amniotic fluid, meconium and blood is a common and potentially critical problem that is usually treatable with suction alone. In infancy and childhood, conditions, such as closed head injury or status epilepticus, may cause the loss of airway protective reflexes and put the child at risk for loss of airway patency from aspiration or airway obstruction. Children needing endotracheal intubation often have diseases or trauma associated with fluid in the endotracheal tube, airways, or air sacs; this fluid must be removed to ensure adequate oxygenation and ventilation. Children with tracheostomy tubes may get fluids or foreign bodies in the tubes, which must be evacuated.

Indications

All newborns

Infants or children with fluids or foreign bodies in the nasopharynx or oropharynx

Intubated patients with fluids or secretions in the endotracheal tubes

Patients with tracheostomy tubes with fluids or mucus in the tubes

Contraindications

Children with severe airway obstruction and suspected airway foreign body, prior to seeing the airway with laryngoscopy

Minimise suctioning in intubated children with increased intracranial pressure and herniation

Equipment

Endotracheal tube suction catheters, sizes 8 to 14 French

Feeding tubes, size 5 or 7 for small infants

Large-bore rigid suction catheter

Rationale

Suctioning is a basic technique to maintain an open airway. Children have tiny airways that are easily obstructed. The type of suction device and suctioning procedure to use depends on the child's age and clinical problem (**Table P3-1**). When suctioning newborns, avoid suctioning vigorously or deeply. Deep suctioning can cause vagal stimulation, bradycardia, and laryngospasm in the newborn, particularly in the first hours during initial transition to extrauterine life. Brief, gentle suctioning (mouth, then nose) is usually adequate to remove secretions. Suction catheters remove thin secretions from the mouth, nose, or throat, and are useful in all age groups. Suction catheters are also necessary for endotracheal tube suctioning. Large-bore rigid suction catheters are useful in infants and children (not newly borns) to remove thick secretions, vomitus, pus, blood, or particulate matter from the mouth.

Preparation

1. Select an appropriate suction device based on clinical condition or type of obstruction and age. This could be a vacuum outlet, battery-powered or electric portable suction, or hand-powered portable suction.

2. Make sure the suction device is operational.

3. Determine correct catheter size with the paediatric length-based resuscitation tape. The suction catheter should be smaller than the nostril.

4. Open catheter package.

5. Connect suction tubing or rigid suction catheter to connecting tubing and suction source.

6. Set suction force (maximum, 120 mm Hg), being careful to avoid injuring sensitive tissues.

7. Maintain sterile technique. Consider changing catheters between insertions to reduce infection risk.

Table P3-1 Suction Technique Based on Age and Type of Obstructing Material

Newborns	Suction catheter
Infants and children with thin secretions	Suction catheter
Newborns, infants, and children with endotracheal tube	Suction catheter
Infants and children with thick secretions or particulate matter	Large-bore suction catheter

Possible Complications

Injury to the mouth, nose, airway, or lung

Gagging, vomiting

Aspiration of stomach contents

Hypoxia from prolonged suctioning

Pushing foreign body into trachea with suction device

Increased intracranial pressure

Procedure 3-1

Oropharyngeal/Nasopharyngeal Suctioning With Suction Catheter

1 Suction the mouth, then the nose. Open the mouth and advance until the tip touches secretions.

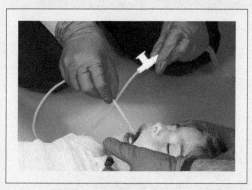

2 Block the side port and begin suctioning. Do not do deep suctioning beyond what is in direct vision. Remove catheter with twisting motion.

3 Insert the catheter into the nostril.

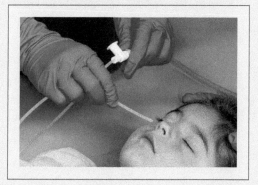

4 Block the side port to begin suctioning when the tip touches secretions. Remove the catheter with a twisting motion. Never suction longer than 5 seconds.

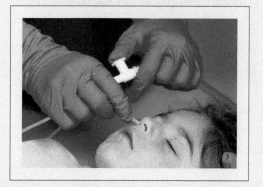

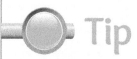

Tip

In suspected foreign body aspiration, look at the airway prior to suctioning.

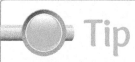

Tip

Suction for less than 5 seconds, but use enough time to remove secretions.

Procedure 3-2

Tracheal Tube Suctioning With Suction Catheter

1 Ask partner to pre-oxygenate the patient five to six times with a bag-valve-mask device using 100% oxygen.

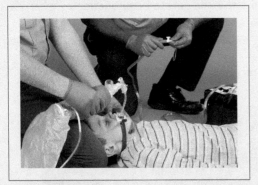

2 Reduce suction by not obstructing side port or kink the catheter, insert suction catheter through endotracheal tube and down the trachea until resistance is met.

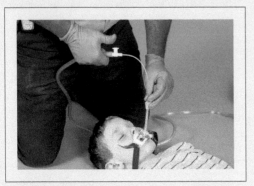

3 Apply suction off and on by placing thumb over the side port while withdrawing and twisting catheter (maximum, 5 seconds).

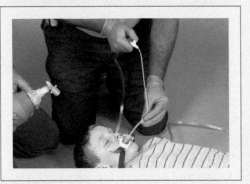

4 Irrigate catheter with normal saline poured into separate vessel to avoid contamination of container.

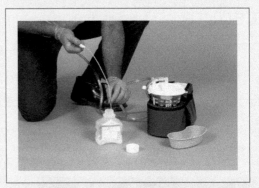

5 Ask partner to oxygenate five to six times. Repeat, as necessary. Consider using new sterile catheter to reduce infection risk.

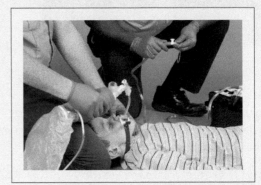

Procedure 3-3

Oropharyngeal Suctioning With Large-Bore Rigid Suction Catheter

1 Open the mouth and advance catheter until it touches secretions.

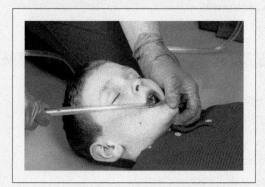

2 Close the side port or turn on suction to begin suctioning. Remove the catheter with a twisting motion. Do not suction more than 5 seconds.

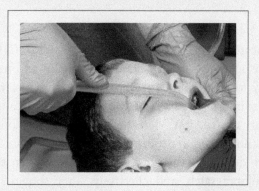

References

American Academy of Pediatrics, American Heart Association. *Textbook of Neonatal Resuscitation*. 7th ed. Elk Grove, IL: AAP; 2016.

Great Ormond Street Hospital for Children NHS Foundation Trust, 2018, *Suction*. Available at: www.gosh.nhs.uk/health-professionals/clinical-guidelines/suction. Accessed June 8, 2018.

Procedure 4: Airway Adjuncts

Introduction

An oropharyngeal (OP) or nasopharyngeal (NP) airway adjunct is often helpful to maintain an open airway for optimal ventilation. Sizing is important, because improperly sized OP or NP airways may cause further obstruction. The prehospital professional must know when to use an OP or NP airway adjunct, how to determine the proper size, and how to insert the adjunct safely and effectively. They should be mindful to manage the patient's airway with as little intervention as possible.

Indications

Respiratory insufficiency

NP or OP airway obstruction

Seizures, including postictal state (NP airway)

Contraindications

OP airway

    Intact gag reflex

    Ingestion of a caustic or petroleum product

NP airway

    Complete nasal obstruction

    Possible basilar skull fracture (Caution)

    Major maxillofacial trauma

Equipment

NP airways

OP airways

Rationale

Opening the airway of a small infant or child by positioning alone, with the head-tilt/chin-lift manoeuvres or jaw thrust, may not keep the tongue from obstructing the airway. Adequate ventilation often requires placement of airway adjuncts. They are easy to insert and may markedly improve airway patency. Adjuncts may immediately improve the efficacy of the child's spontaneous ventilation. In addition, they may allow more effective bag-valve-mask ventilation, reduce gastric inflation, and avert the need for endotracheal intubation.

Preparation

1. Position patient's airway:

   Medical patient

   - Perform the head-tilt/chin-lift manoeuvre to open the airway. Avoid hyperextension of the neck because it may cause airway obstruction.

   - Use padding under the shoulders of an infant or small child to get neutral airway position.

   Trauma patient

   - Use the modified jaw thrust manoeuvre with in-line spinal stabilisation to open the airway.

2. Select the properly sized adjunct:

   OP airway

   - Measure the device on the patient:

     ○ Place OP airway next to face with the flange at the level of the central incisors, and the bite block segment parallel to the hard palate.

     ○ The tip of the appropriate-sized OP airway should reach the angle of the jaw.

   NP airway

   - Measure the device on the patient:

     ○ The outside diameter of the NP airway should be less than the diameter of the nostril.

- Place the NP airway next to the face and measure from the tip of the nose to the tragus of the ear.
- Adjust movable flange (if present) up or down to get appropriate length.

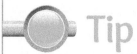

Tip

An NP airway is useful in maintaining an open airway during an active seizure.

Procedure 4-1

OP Airway Insertion

❶ Depress tongue with a tongue depressor (if available). Then insert oral airway with the tip down to avoid injury to the palate until the flange rests against lips.

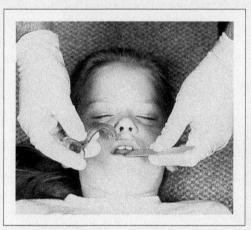

❷ If a tongue depressor is not available, and if trained, an appropriately sized laryngoscope blade could be used.

❸ Insert OP airway until the flange is resting against the lips.

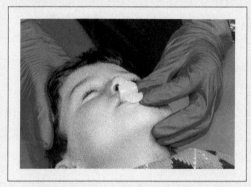

Procedure 4-2

NP Airway Insertion

1 Lubricate NP airway.

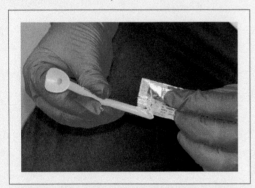

2 Insert with bevel toward septum (centre of nose).

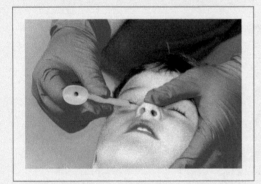

3 Gently advance tip along floor of nasal cavity.

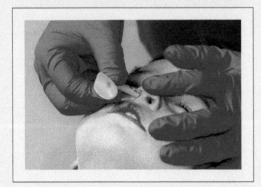

4 If using the right nostril, advance until flange is seated against outside of nostril. The tip should be in the nasopharynx.

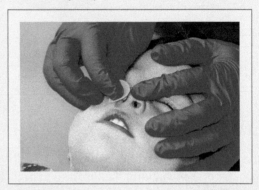

5 If using the left nostril, begin inserting the airway with the curvature upward until resistance is felt (about 2 cm), and then rotate the device 180 degrees and advance until flange is against outside of nostril.

6 Consider using both nostrils to insert two NP airways.

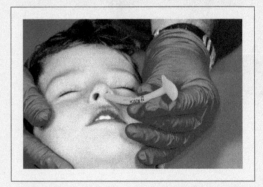

Possible Complications
OP Airway

If OP airway is too small, the tongue may get pushed back into the pharynx, obstructing the airway

If OP airway is too large, it may obstruct the larynx

Pharyngeal bleeding

Laryngospasm

Vomiting

NP Airway

Adenoidal tissue laceration

Pharyngeal bleeding

Obstruction of tube with fluids or soft tissues, causing airway obstruction

If an NP airway is too long, vagal stimulation or oesophageal entry with gastric distention may occur

Laryngospasm

Vomiting

Controversy

The use of airway adjuncts in facial trauma is sometimes questioned. If the child has an open fracture of the craniofacial bones, the device could penetrate into the brain and cause further brain injury or haemorrhage. However, the likelihood of that occurring is slight.

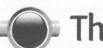

Think Point

Never attempt to insert an OP airway in a conscious child.

Think Point

Do not insert an OP airway that is too small, or it will push the tongue back and obstruct the airway.

Reference

Roberts K, Whalley H, Bleetman A. *The nasopharyngeal airway: dispelling myths and establishing the facts. Emergency Medical Journal.* 2005;22:394–396.

Procedure 5: Foreign Body Obstruction

Introduction

Foreign body obstruction of the airway is an uncommon cause of hypoxic brain injury and death in toddlers and pre-school-aged children, who place objects in their mouths as part of the exploratory behaviour normal for patients in these age groups. Liquids are the most common cause of choking in infants, whereas balloons, small objects, and food (e.g., round sweets, nuts, and grapes) are the most common causes of foreign body airway obstruction (FBAO) in children. The infant or child with a completely obstructed airway poses the ultimate medical challenge because a moment's delay can result in permanent disability or be fatal. When treating a patient with foreign body obstruction, it is important to begin with basic manoeuvres to clear the airway, but sometimes more advanced techniques are necessary.

Indications
Severe airway obstruction

Severe partial airway obstruction and respiratory failure

Contraindication
Partial airway obstruction with maintenance of the airway

Equipment
Laryngoscope and straight blades

Paediatric Magill forceps

Bag-valve-mask devices (infant and paediatric)

Rationale

In the setting of severe airway obstruction, prehospital professionals can make the difference between life and death. Immediate removal of an airway foreign body can often be achieved using basic life support (BLS) procedures, yet every year many children suffer grave injury and death because of failure to use basic clearance manoeuvres. Sometimes, the foreign body is deeper in the airway or embedded in tissue, so that basic manoeuvres are unsuccessful. In such cases, using Magill forceps and direct laryngoscopy may be the best option for removal.

Preparation

1. Attempt BLS manoeuvres first (see Procedure 5-1).
2. Move to advanced life support (ALS) manoeuvres if BLS manoeuvres fail.
3. Attach appropriately sized straight blade to laryngoscope handle.
4. Ensure light is working on laryngoscope blade.

Possible Complications

Hypoxia

Foreign body is pushed farther into airway

Laryngeal and tracheal injury

Teeth and mouth injury

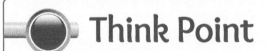 **Think Point**

Do not perform blind finger sweeps, which may push the foreign body further into the airway.

Procedure 5-1

BLS Manoeuvres

1 If FBAO is mild, do not interfere. Allow the victim to clear the airway by coughing while you observe for signs of severe FBAO.

2 If the FBAO is severe (i.e., the victim is unable to make a sound), you must act to relieve the obstruction.

3 For a child, perform subdiaphragmatic abdominal thrusts (Heimlich manoeuvre) until the object is expelled or the victim becomes unresponsive.

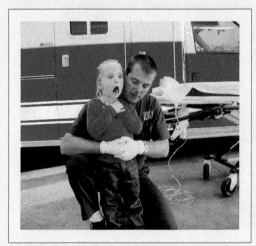

4 For an infant, deliver repeated cycles of five back blows (slaps) followed by five chest compressions until the object is expelled or the victim becomes unresponsive. Abdominal thrusts are not recommended for infants because they may damage the infant's relatively large and unprotected liver.

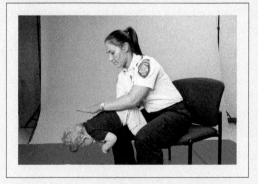

5 If the victim becomes unresponsive, start CPR with chest compressions (do not perform a pulse check).

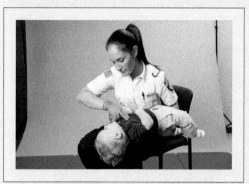

6 After 30 chest compressions, open the airway. If you see a foreign body, remove it but do not perform blind finger sweeps, because they may push the obstructed object farther into the pharynx and may damage the oropharynx. Attempt to give two breaths and continue with cycles of chest compressions and ventilations until the object is expelled.

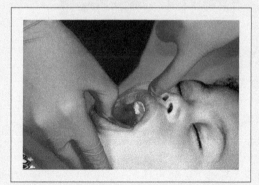

Procedure 5-2

Laryngoscopy and Magill Forceps

① Grasp laryngoscope handle in the left hand. Use trigger-finger technique.

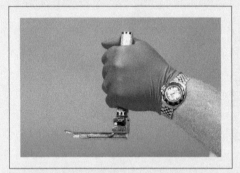

② Open mouth by using thumb pressure on chin. Insert paediatric straight laryngoscope blade into mouth.

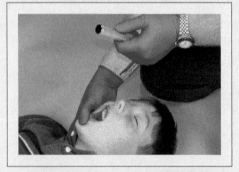

③ Lift tongue with blade. Exert gentle traction upward along the axis of the laryngoscope handle at a 45-degree angle. Do not use teeth or gums for leverage. Advance blade. Watch the tip until foreign body is visible. Do not go past vocal cords. Use suction to improve visibility and maintain airway.

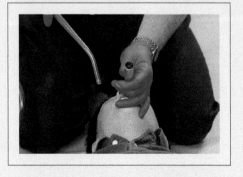

④ Grasp closed Magill forceps in right hand, palm down. Insert Magill forceps into mouth, tips closed. Open forceps and move tips around foreign body. Grasp foreign body and remove while looking directly at it. Look at the airway and make sure it is clear of foreign bodies or debris. Remove laryngoscope blade. After removal of foreign body, reassess respiratory status. Use suction if needed. Attempt to ventilate if the child does not breathe spontaneously. Return to BLS manoeuvres if no foreign body is seen by direct laryngoscopy.

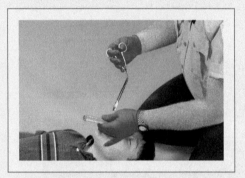
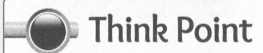

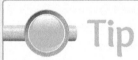 **Think Point**

Suctioning may push the foreign body farther into the airway, so look at the airway before suctioning.

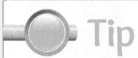 Tip

Repeat BLS procedures if no foreign body is seen by direct laryngoscopy.

Tip

Attempt BLS manoeuvres before using Magill forceps.

Reference

American Heart Association. 2015 American Heart Association Guidelines Update for CPR and ECC. *Circulation.* 2015; 132:18(suppl 2):S1–S293.

Procedure 6: Bronchodilator Therapy

Introduction

Wheezing from bronchospasm is one of the most common out-of-hospital paediatric problems. Children who are wheezing are usually in acute respiratory distress and may be anxious, agitated, and uncooperative. The prehospital professional must use a developmentally appropriate approach with the child and the caregiver when giving general non-invasive respiratory care and using a bronchodilator with or without anticholinergic medication. The caregiver can help by holding, soothing, and supporting a scared child. Although not specifically studied in the out-of-hospital setting, the metered dose inhaler (MDI) with use of a spacer should be the first line treatment for a child who is wheezing. Where required, or if an MDI and spacer is not available, bronchodilators can be given via an oxygen-powered nebuliser.

Indications

Salbutamol:

- Acute asthma attack.

- Expiratory wheezing associated with allergy, anaphylaxis, smoke inhalation or other lower airway cause.
- Exacerbation of chronic obstructive pulmonary disease.

Ipratropium Bromide:

- Acute, severe or life-threatening asthma
- Acute asthma unresponsive to salbutamol
- Exacerbation of chronic obstructive pulmonary disease, unresponsive to salbutamol.

Contraindication

Salbutamol:

None in the emergency situation.

Equipment and Medicines

Metered dose inhaler (MDI) and spacer

- Salbutamol (100 mcg/dose)

Appropriate bronchodilator for nebulisation

- Salbutamol (2.5 mg in 2.5 ml or 5 mg in 2.5 ml)
- Ipratropium bromide (250 mcg in 1 ml or 500 mcg in 2 ml)

Nebuliser mask and acorn

Oxygen source

Rationale

For asthma, early bronchodilator therapy, on the scene and on the way to the emergency department (ED), helps immediately open airways, relieve respiratory distress, and improve oxygen delivery. Early bronchodilator therapy may reduce the need for more aggressive hospital therapy, shorten ED and hospital times, and decrease the chances of complications or death. The addition of anticholinergic medication may also be beneficial. *Continuous inhalation treatment with a nebulised beta agonist is the best initial approach with* **severe** *wheezing and respiratory distress.*

Preparation
Inhalation Therapy

1. Have the caregiver hold the child on his or her lap. An older child can sit alone.

2. Have the child in an upright position of comfort.

3. Explain what is happening. Most children need only inhalation bronchodilator therapy with an MDI and spacer or by oxygen-powered nebuliser or with an MDI and spacer.

Possible Complications of Salbutamol and/or Ipratropium Bromide

Anxiety

Chest pain

Cough

Dizziness

Dry mouth

Dysrhythmias

Headache

Hypertension

Nausea

Nasal stuffiness

Palpitations

Restlessness

Tachycardia

Tremors

Vomiting

Procedure 6-1

Inhalation Therapy

1 If the child can cooperate, deliver nebulised bronchodilator, with or without anticholinergic medication, through a mouthpiece or mask. The caregiver can hold the mask to the child's face, if necessary.

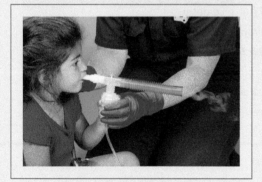

2 If an MDI is used, attach spacer and mask when the child is too young or unable to trigger aerosol effectively.

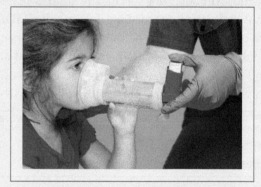

3 Monitor respiratory rate, heart rate, and pulse oximetry during therapy.

Specific pre-hospital treatment of asthma includes inhaled bronchodilators and hydrocortisone or intramuscular (IM) adrenaline, depending on the severity of the attack. Please see Figure 3-14 for further details on assessing and managing asthma in children.

Procedure 7: Bag-Valve-Mask Ventilation

Introduction

Bag-valve-mask ventilation is a highly effective way to deliver assisted ventilation to a child in respiratory failure. Oxygen at 60%–95% concentration can be given safely by choosing a well-fitted mask, connecting the oxygen reservoir to a supplemental oxygen source at 15 l/min, and ventilating at an age-appropriate rate.

Indication

Apnoea or respiratory arrest

Respiratory failure

Cyanosis despite supplemental oxygen*

Consider when oxygen saturation (SaO_2) less than 90% despite administration of 100% oxygen by non-rebreathing mask

Equipment

Transparent masks with soft rim, sizes neonate through adult

Self-inflating bag, at least 450 ml volume

*N.B. children with certain types of uncorrected cyanotic heart disease may have low oxygen saturations at baseline.

Rationale

Assisted ventilation is a way to oxygenate and ventilate a child who is unable to breathe adequately on his or her own. Although the technique does not provide the definitive airway control that endotracheal intubation does, in many cases bag-valve-mask ventilation will be the only technique available for assisting ventilation during resuscitation and transport. Effective bag-valve-mask ventilation is one of the prehospital professional's most useful skills in paediatric out-of-hospital care.

Preparation

1. Measure the mask on the patient. The mask should extend from the bridge of the nose to the cleft of the chin, avoiding compression of the eyes. The right-sized mask will have a small volume to minimize dead space and to prevent rebreathing of expired carbon dioxide. Transparency allows the clinician to observe the child for cyanosis of the lips and for any vomiting.

2. Select an appropriate resuscitator bag. Although a small child can be safely and effectively ventilated using a big bag, a small bag will not work for a large child. Paediatric tidal volume is approximately 8 ml/kg. The bag should have a volume of 450–750 ml. An adult bag is acceptable for larger children or adolescents.

3. Connect one end of oxygen tubing to the resuscitator bag and the other end to the flow meter, set to 15 l/min.

Possible Complications

Hypoxia

Barotrauma

Gastric distention

Vomiting and aspiration

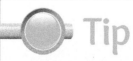 Tip

In children with pending respiratory failure due to an obstructive process (i.e., status asthmaticus), listening for the end of expiration may minimise risk of barotrauma.

Procedure 7-1

Bag-Valve-Mask Ventilation

1 Open airway. *Medical patient:* Use head-tilt/chin-lift manoeuvre. *Trauma patient:* Use jaw thrust with manual in-line stabilisation.

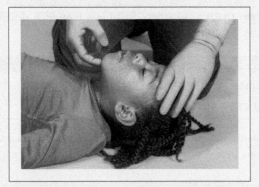

2 Ensure neutral positioning (sniffing position). Because infants and toddlers have large heads, place a small roll under the shoulders to achieve the sniffing position. Avoid hyperextension of the neck because this may cause airway obstruction or spinal injury.

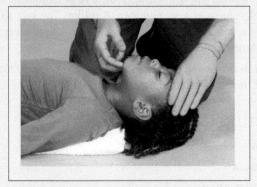

3 Insert appropriate airway adjunct if airway patency cannot be maintained with the head-tilt/chin-lift or jaw thrust manoeuvres (see **Procedure 4, Airway Adjuncts**). Use an oropharyngeal (OP) airway if the patient does not have a gag reflex, or use a nasopharyngeal (NP) airway if the patient has an active gag reflex.

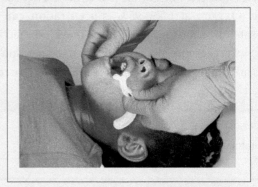

4 Begin ventilation.

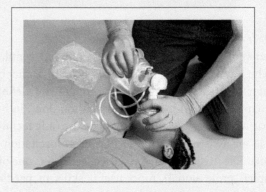

 Think Point

Avoid hyperextension of the neck, which may cause airway obstruction or spinal injury.

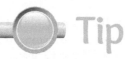 **Tip**

Use an OP or NP airway with the bag-valve-mask device if airway patency cannot be maintained with the head-tilt/chin-lift or jaw thrust manoeuvres.

Procedure 7-2

Bag-Valve-Mask Ventilation Using One-Clinician Technique

1 Apply the mask to the face and get an airtight seal by placing the thumb and index finger on the mask, and place the third, fourth, and fifth fingers on the bony portion of the jaw (mandible). This is called the E-C clamp technique.

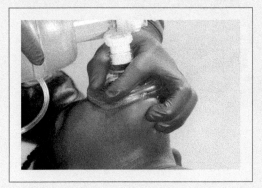

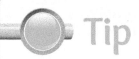 **Tip**

Pull the jaw into the mask, instead of pushing the mask into the face.

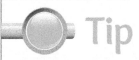 **Tip**

Seeing the chest rise is the best indicator of adequate tidal volume.

2 Pull the child's jaw into the mask, instead of pushing the mask into the face, to establish a seal. Failure to provide a tight seal may result in delivery of lower oxygen concentrations or an inadequate volume of air. Avoid placing pressure on soft tissues under the chin because this may compress the airway. Squeeze the bag with the dominant hand, watching for chest rise. Squeeze the bag only until the chest rise is visible, then release. Say, "Squeeze, release, release" during ventilation to achieve the correct inspiratory volume and to allow for expiration. Child and infant: 12–20 squeezes/minute. Adult: 12–16 squeezes/minute.

3 Assess effectiveness of ventilation. Look for adequate bilateral rise and fall of chest. Auscultate for lung sounds at the mid-axillary line bilaterally. Monitor oxygen saturation.

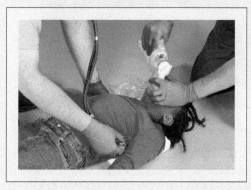

Procedure 7-3

Bag-Valve-Mask Ventilation Using Two-Rescuer Technique

The two-rescuer technique is preferable in trauma patients or if the one-rescuer technique does not create an effective seal.

1 Rescuer applies the mask to the face and maintains a seal. *Medical patient*: Hold the mask to the face with the thumb and index fingers of both hands; use the other fingers to perform a chin lift (bilateral E-C clamp technique). *Trauma patient*: Perform a jaw thrust manoeuvre, lifting the jaw into the mask with both hands, while maintaining manual in-line stabilisation.

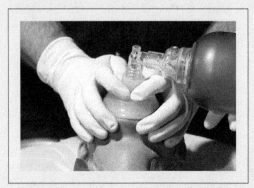

2 Pull the child's jaw into the mask, instead of pushing the mask into the face, to establish a seal. Avoid placing pressure on soft tissues under the chin because this may compress the airway.

3 Second rescuer ventilates. Avoid gastric distention. Watch the abdomen for signs of enlargement during ventilation. If this happens, reposition the airway and observe the chest rise carefully, squeezing the bag only until the chest starts to rise.

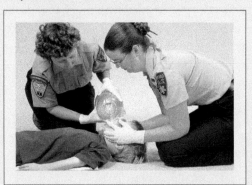

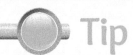
Tip

The two-rescuer technique is preferable in a trauma patient or if the one-rescuer technique does not get a good seal.

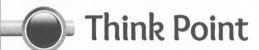
Think Point

A bag less than 450 ml will not generate enough inspiratory pressure to ventilate a large child.

Procedure 8: Pulse Oximetry

Introduction

Pulse oximetry, which measures oxygenation and pulse rate, can be a useful adjunct in the management of the ill or injured child. Use of the pulse oximeter does not replace clinical assessment of the child. Monitoring changes in pulse oximetry readings may help the prehospital professional to determine the patient's response to interventions and guide additional interventions.

However, there are caveats. If the child is in shock, inadequate circulating red blood cells may have such low flow states that the pulse oximeter probe will be unable to sense flow, resulting in an inability to obtain a reading or waveform. Where there is suspected carbon monoxide (CO) poisoning, do not rely on pulse oximetry. The probe detects gaseous saturation of the haemoglobin molecule and does not discriminate between oxygen and CO. A child with CO poisoning may have a pulse oximetry reading of 100% and be hypoxic.

Indications

Hypoxia

Need for oxygen therapy

Respiratory distress

Major trauma or other clinical conditions with the potential for hypoxia

Equipment

Pulse oximeter probes in sizes for newborns, infants, and children

Monitoring cable and pulse oximetry monitoring device

 Tip

In the newborn the Spo$_2$ probe needs to be located on the baby's right hand/wrist. This is to ensure a pre-ductal reading.

Preparation

1. Prepare the child for application of the pulse oximeter probe. This may be explained as being similar to putting on a plaster.

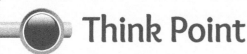 **Think Point**

Do not rely on pulse oximetry in carbon monoxide poisoning.

Possible Complications

Using incorrect probe placement or size

Poor perfusion with poor tracing or waveform

Inability to obtain a Spo$_2$ reading

Causes of Inability to Obtain a Reading or Waveform

- Using incorrect probe placement or size
- Poor perfusion with poor tracing or waveform

Procedure 8-1

Pulse Oximetry

1 Obtain equipment in the appropriate size. Place probe on a fingertip, toe, earlobe, or wrist as indicated on the manufacturer's instructions.

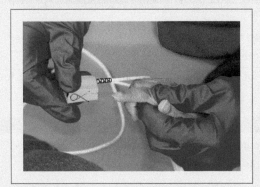

2 Connect the probe to the monitoring cable. Some portable monitoring devices have a reusable probe that has a spring-loaded clip for use only on a finger-tip or toe. Note oxygen saturation (SpO_2) and document. If the monitoring device being used shows a waveform, observe for correlation with heart rate.

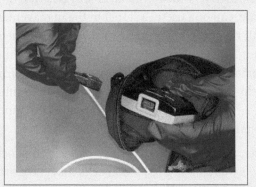

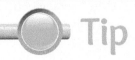 **Tip**

Use pulse oximetry in the primary assessment of every acutely ill or injured child.

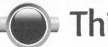 **Think Point**

Even when the pulse oximetry is normal, if there is increased work of breathing or significantly increased respiratory rate, the child may need additional therapy.

Procedure 9: Endotracheal Intubation

Introduction

Endotracheal intubation is the definitive advanced airway manoeuvre that can be a life-saving procedure for some critical patients. However, this procedure has important modifications and pitfalls in children. There are several anatomical considerations that make the paediatric airway different from the adult airway:

- The child's vocal cords are more anterior and superior.
- The tongue is proportionally larger.
- The mandible and oral cavity are smaller.
- The diameter and length of the trachea are less.
- The soft tissues are more fragile.
- The narrowest area of the airway for children 5 years of age and younger is the cricoid cartilage.

Performing the procedure confidently and competently in the field can be tricky. Inappropriate or unsuccessful intubation attempts may result in hypoxia or injury to the child's airway.

Indications

Respiratory or cardiopulmonary arrest

Respiratory failure

Inability to maintain patent airway

Loss of protective airway reflex

Need for controlled ventilation as in traumatic brain injury

Need for endotracheal administration of resuscitative medications

Severe shock (to decrease myocardial oxygen demand)

Contraindications

Permanent tracheostomy (relative)

Good response to bag-valve-mask ventilation and short transport time (relative)

Anatomical abnormalities that would probably prevent successful intubation (large tongue haematoma, massive facial injuries) (relative)

Equipment

Uncuffed ETTs in paediatric sizes (2.0–5.0), in addition to cuffed tubes (2.5–7.0)

Paediatric laryngoscope with fresh batteries

Paediatric laryngoscope blades, curved (sizes 2–4) and straight (sizes 0–4)

Laryngoscope bulb

Large-bore rigid suction catheter

Suction catheters, sizes 5–12 French

Paediatric stylets

Paediatric bougie

Water-soluble lubricant

Oropharyngeal airways

Paediatric bag-valve-mask device, at least 450 ml volume

Paediatric face masks

Adhesive tape

Commercial ETT securing devices/tape

Skin adhesive

Pulse oximeter

Oxygen source

Device for confirmation of ETT placement (e.g., capnography, end-tidal CO_2 device)

Rationale

Successful endotracheal tube (ETT) placement allows optimal oxygenation and ventilation and decreases the risk of aspiration and loss of airway control. A properly placed and secured ETT is a good tool for managing critical patients, but the procedure must be undertaken safely and by a clinician who is competent to carry out this skill.

Preparation

1. Make sure oxygen delivery equipment is connected to an oxygen source.

2. Select an appropriately sized ETT (**Tables P9-1** and **P9-2**) for oral endotracheal intubation.

3. For a properly selected uncuffed ETT:

   - Allow a minimal air leak. The absence of an air leak may indicate excessive pressure at the cricoid cartilage.

4. For a properly selected cuffed ETT: Check cuff for leaks, maintaining aseptic technique, as follows:

   - Inflate cuff with appropriate volume of air

   - Remove syringe

   - Feel cuff for integrity

   - Deflate cuff before insertion

5. Attach blade to laryngoscope handle, and make sure the bulb is secure and works.

6. Test the large-bore rigid suction catheter.

7. Insert stylet into the ETT (if not using a bougie), stopping the stylet at least 1 cm from the end of the ETT.

8. Bend the ETT into a gentle upward curve. In some cases, bend the tube into the shape of a hockey stick.

9. Lubricate tube with a water-soluble lubricant (optional).

10. Prepare device for confirmation of ETT placement.

11. To predict correct ETT tube position at gum line, either:

    - Calculate ETT position with formula: gum line position (in cm) = ~3 × tube size

12. Have partner prepare for:

    - Ongoing patient assessment

    - Providing time counts for ventilation rates

    - Watching monitors (heart rate, pulse oximetry)

    - Handling suction devices

    - Handling ETT

    - Applying gentle cricoid pressure

    - Stabilising neck, if child has possible spinal trauma

13. Position patient (avoid hyperextension or hyperflexion of neck).

    - Medical patient: Place the child in the "sniffing" position.

    - If spinal trauma is a possibility, place the child in neutral position with manual in-line stabilisation.

Table P9-1 Suggested Uncuffed Endotracheal Tube and Suction Catheter Sizes

Age	ETT Size (mm)	Suction Catheter Size (French)
Premature newborn	2.0–2.5	5
Newborn	3.0–3.5	6–8
6 months	3.5	8
12–18 months	4.0	8
3 years	4.5	8
5 years	5.0	10
6 years	5.5	10
8 years	6.0	10
12 years	6.5	12
16 years	7.0–8.0	14

Table P9-2 Selecting Endotracheal Tube Size

Uncuffed	Cuffed
Remembering numbers 　Newborns and infants 　　Preterm infants: 2.0- or 2.5-mm tube 　　Term newborns or small infants: 3.0- or 3.5-mm tube 　Infants 6–12 months: 3.5-mm tube 　Infants 12–18 months: 4.0-mm tube OR Use the resuscitation tape or resuscitation software. OR The diameter of the tracheal tube is approximately the same size as the child's fingernail on the fifth finger. Size = $\dfrac{\text{(age in years)}}{4} + 4$ (formula for child older than 2 years of age)	For a child younger than 2 years old $\dfrac{\text{(age in years)}}{4} + 3$ It is appropriate to approximate: 　3.0 or 3.5 ETT for a child younger than 1 year old 　3.5 or 4.0 ETT for a child 1–2 years old For a child 2–10 years old $\dfrac{\text{(age in years)}}{4} + 3.5$

Procedure 9-1

Insert Endotracheal Tube

1 Oxygenate and ventilate patient five to six times with bag-valve-mask device and 100% oxygen, at a rate of one ventilation every 3 seconds. Say "squeeze, release, release" to reinforce proper rate.

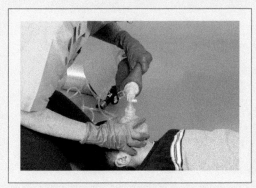

2 Grasp laryngoscope in left hand. Stop ventilating and begin timing, giving 20- to 30-second counts.

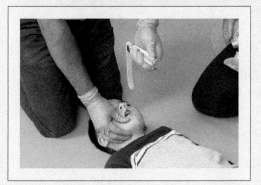

3 Open mouth by applying thumb pressure on chin; check mouth for foreign bodies or loose teeth; remove oropharyngeal airway if present.

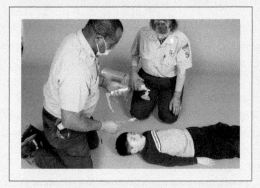

4 Hold laryngoscope in trigger finger position.

5 Insert paediatric straight laryngoscope blade into mouth.

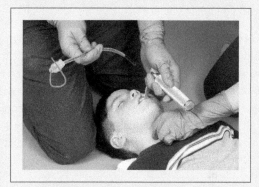

6 Lift tongue with blade.

7 Exert gentle traction upward along the axis of laryngoscope handle at a 45-degree angle. Do not use teeth or gums to gain leverage.

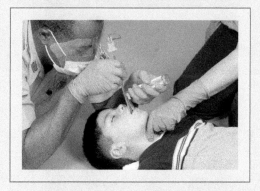

(continues)

Procedure 9-1 (continued)

8 Advance blade straight along tongue. Continue looking at blade tip, until tip is just beyond epiglottis. Do not take your eyes off of the vocal cords once visualised. Your partner should be handing the bougie and ETT to you while you are maintaining visualisation.

9 You may instruct the airway assistant to perform Backward-Upwards-Rightwards-Pressure (BURP) if required. If there is difficulty seeing the vocal cords, you have four options: (1) advance or retract laryngoscope blade; (2) modify amount of BURP; (3) remove vomitus, blood, other fluids, or particulate matter with rigid, large-bore suction device; or (4) repositioning of the head or degree of extension.

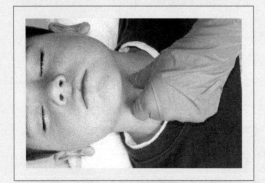

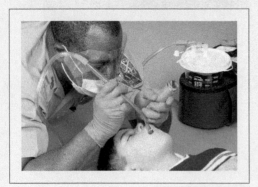

10 If gastric reflux occurs, stop laryngoscopy attempt and begin methods to clear the airway.

11 Continue to look at vocal cords and suction.

12 Remove large solid matter with paediatric Magill forceps.

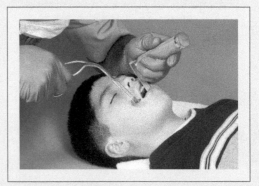

13 Insert bougie and once through the cords, ask for the ETT. Insert ETT. Hold tube in dart-like fashion with right hand and insert tip of tube from right corner of mouth down between vocal cords. Do not insert tube in channel of laryngoscope blade because this blocks the view of the vocal cords. Watch the ETT go through the vocal cords. Advance tube until vocal cord marker on ETT is situated beyond the vocal cords with an uncuffed tube. Advance a cuffed tube until the balloon passes through the vocal cords. Look for centimetre marking on ETT in relation to the gum line. Remove bougie.

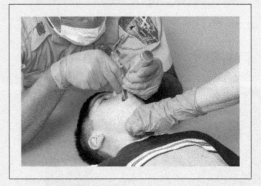

14 Remove laryngoscope blade, holding ETT in place.

Procedure 9-1 (continued)

15 Remove stylet from ETT (if bougie was not used).

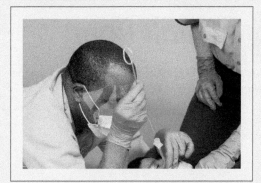

16 If using an ETT with a cuffed end, inflate cuff with pilot balloon. Maintain tube position by holding ETT against upper lip. If large amount of fluid is evident in ETT, use a suction catheter to clear the airway. Have partner maintain ETT position and ventilate patient with bag-valve-mask device.

17 Confirm ETT correct placement using an end-tidal CO_2 device or quantitative capnography as explained in **Procedure 10, Confirmation of Endotracheal Tube Placement**.

18 Assess correct position in trachea. Do general patient evaluation (appearance, heart rate, pulse oximetry). Look for bilateral chest rise. Make sure there are no bubbling, gurgling sounds in epigastric area indicating air-water interface (check for two breaths). Auscultate for bilateral lung sounds at the mid-axillary line, third intercostal space (check for two breaths on right and then two breaths on left). Use device to confirm-endotracheal positioning. If breath sounds are heard only on one side (usually the right), pull back ETT slightly until breath sounds are heard on both sides.

19 Record tube position on patient care record. Use centimetre mark at teeth or gum line or mark on ETT with indelible pen.

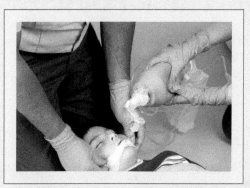

20 Secure tube with tape or commercially available ETT securing device, tape or tube tie. Reassess proper location of tube and make sure the patient is stable.

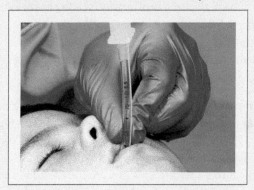

Indications for Tube Removal
Immediate Tube Removal

- No chest rise with ventilation.

- Presence of epigastric gurgling sounds.
- Failure to confirm endotracheal placement with detection device(s).

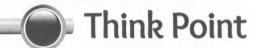

Think Point

Beware of inadequate spinal stabilisation during intubation attempts in trauma patients.

Think Point

Never assume the ETT is in the trachea unless you see the tube passing through the vocal cords.

Procedure 9-2

Secure Endotracheal Tube

1. Insert correctly sized oral airway (see **Procedure 4, Airway Adjuncts**) and make sure ETT is not compressed. Do not use a bite block in paediatric patients. Carefully hold the ETT in place while the second rescuer secures.

2. If a commercial device is available, it can be used; otherwise, in medical patients, one method of securing the ETT is by wrapping the tape around the back of the patient's neck. In trauma patients, cut two pieces of tape into a Y: secure one end around the tube and the other on the face. Do the same with the other piece of tape from the other side of the face.

3. Bring tape up to opposite side of face and wrap around the tube twice, crimping end of tape so it can be easily removed.

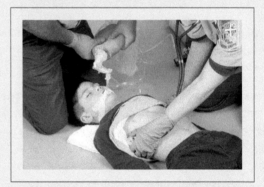

Procedure 9-3

Reconfirm Endotracheal Tube Placement

1 Recheck to make sure there is no bubbling, gurgling noise in epigastric area (air-water interface) for two breaths.

2 Reassess breath sounds bilaterally at the mid-axillary line, third intercostal space (two breaths on right and then two breaths on left). Take extra care handling an ETT in a paediatric patient because it can be easily dislodged. Reassess after patient is in ambulance (and after change of position or change in patient status). Report and record findings.

Possible Complications

Aspiration of stomach contents

Dislodgment of ETT from trachea

Oesophageal intubation

Hypoxia

Increased intracranial pressure

Laryngeal, tracheal, pharyngeal, or oesophageal injury

Teeth and mouth injury

Vocal cord injury

Procedure 9-4

Extubation

1 Postresuscitation extubation is rarely indicated in the field. All three situations must be present: (1) spontaneous breathing with adequate rate and tidal volume; (2) conscious patient; and (3) coughing and gagging causing inability to maintain oxygenation and ventilation. Ensure rigid large-bore suction device is functioning.

2 Suction oropharynx.

3 Turn patient on left side.

4 Deflate cuff completely (if cuff is inflated).

5 Remove ETT quickly at end-inspiratory phase, while suctioning.

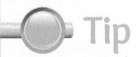

Tip

Make sure proper equipment is available and functioning before intubation attempt. Equipment should be laid out ("dumped") and checked by the airway assistant. Checklists can be useful here.

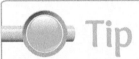

Tip

Chest rise is the best indication of correct endotracheal placement of the ETT. Qualitative end-tidal CO_2/capnography is also useful.

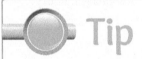

Tip

Always reassess tube location after patient movement or when there is a change in patient status.

Controversy

The value of performing endotracheal intubation in children in the out-of-hospital setting is controversial. More studies are necessary to define which groups of children benefit from this procedure, especially in light of the well-known risks of hypoxia, oesophageal intubation, tube dislodgment, airway injury, and transport delay.

Procedure 10: Confirmation of Endotracheal Tube Placement

Introduction

Performing paediatric endotracheal intubation in the out-of-hospital setting may be difficult or impossible even for experienced prehospital professionals. Confirming position of the endotracheal tube (ETT) in the trachea is a major challenge because oesophageal intubation is a common and dangerous complication of endotracheal intubation. Intubation is often **not** necessary in the field if there is effective bag-valve-mask ventilation with appropriate chest rise. Furthermore, portable quantitative capnography does not require intubation and may be used in line with bag-valve-mask ventilation as long as there is a good mask seal on the patient's face. Currently there are four methods to confirm placement of the ETT:

1. Clinical assessment

2. Use of exhaled carbon dioxide detection device

3. Use of digital capnometry (quantitative end-tidal CO_2)

4. Use of oesophageal aspiration bulb or syringe

Indications

Endotracheal intubation

Contraindications

An adult carbon dioxide detector device cannot be left in place in a child weighing less than 15 kg

Equipment

Stethoscope

Oesophageal detector bulb or syringe OR

Colorimetric end-tidal carbon dioxide detector device OR

Quantitative end-tidal CO_2 device, if available

Rationale

A properly positioned ETT makes it possible to effectively oxygenate and ventilate children with critical illnesses or injuries. Oesophageal placement of ETT, however, is usually harmful or fatal. Moreover, if the child is moved, a correctly placed ETT may easily dislodge from the trachea to the oropharynx or oesophagus. Delayed detection may result in hypoxia. Clinical assessment of placement of the ETT can be inaccurate, especially in infants and small children. Often, there is a lot of noise in the surrounding area (family members or traffic) that may make it hard to hear breath sounds. Also, breath sounds may be transmitted from the oesophagus or stomach throughout the chest of a child and mislead the listener. Fortunately, several mechanical adjuncts are available to supplement clinical assessment and help confirm correct ETT placement in the trachea.

Preparation

1. Intubate the infant or child with a correctly sized ETT (see **Procedure 9, Endotracheal Intubation**).
2. Determine the weight of the patient.
3. Suction any fluid from the ETT.

Oesophageal Detector (Aspiration) Bulb or Syringe

1. Remove oesophageal detector bulb or syringe from packaging.
   - Use only in children who weigh ≥20 kg.

Colorimetric Exhaled Carbon Dioxide Detector

1. Determine correct size of the carbon dioxide detector.
   - Use a paediatric device if the child weighs less than 15 kg.

- Use an adult device if the child weighs 15 kg or more.
- If an adult device is used on a small child, remove after six breaths (initial confirmation of placement).

2. Check the expiration date on the carbon dioxide detector package.

3. Remove the carbon dioxide detector from its packaging.

4. Inspect the carbon dioxide detector before use for bright purple colour and dryness.

Digital Capnometry

1. Place sensor as indicated by manufacturer.

2. Attach sensor probe to monitoring cable.

3. Observe for square waveform that indicates correct ETT placement.

4. Absence of square waveform indicates improperly placed ETT or low exhaled CO_2.

Procedure 10-1

Clinical Assessment

1 Look for bilateral rise and fall of the chest. Remove ETT if there is no chest rise with assisted ventilation. Listen for breath sounds over the stomach. If gurgling is present (like a straw in milk), the ETT is in the oesophagus. If breath sounds only are present in the stomach, continue assessment and do not remove the tube unless there is desaturations or bradycardia, as they may be transmitted from the lungs.

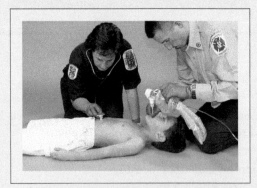

2 Listen for breath sounds in the right mid-axillary line, then in the left mid-axillary line. If breath sounds are equal, secure the tube. If breath sounds are greater on the right side than on the left side, then the tube may be in the right mainstem bronchus. Slowly pull back the ETT until breath sounds are equal.

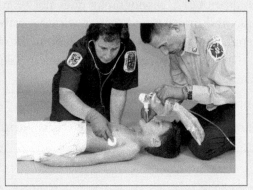

 # Think Point

Do not remove the ETT just because breath sounds are heard in the stomach. They may be transmitted sounds from the lungs. If the patient has continued desaturations or bradycardia, perform a direct laryngoscopy to ensure the ETT is through the vocal cords. If it is not, or you are unsure, and the patient has continued desaturations despite giving effective breaths with positive end expiratory pressure (PEEP), then removing the ETT is appropriate to deliver oxygen with bag-valve-mask ventilation.

Procedure 10-2

Oesophageal Detector Bulb or Syringe

1 Attach the device to the end of the ETT right after intubation and before breaths are given.

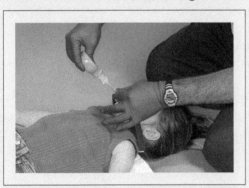

2 Aspirate slowly over 3–5 seconds. If resistance is felt, then the ETT is in the oesophagus. Remove it. If air is aspirated, the ETT is in the trachea. Secure it.

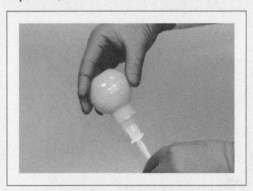

Possible Complications

A faulty device or misinterpretation of results of a carbon dioxide detector or oesophageal detector device may result in incorrect ETT placement or incorrectly removing an ETT that was correctly placed.

Rebreathing carbon dioxide may cause hypercarbia in an infant weighing less than 15 kg if an adult-sized detector is left in line. If the child weighs less than 15 kg, use a paediatric device. If the child weighs 15 kg or more, use an adult device.

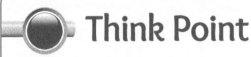 **Think Point**

Do not use an oesophageal detector bulb or syringe if the child weighs less than 20 kg.

Procedure 10-3

Colorimetric Carbon Dioxide Detector Device

1 Attach the device to the end of the ETT and attach the other end to the bag-valve-mask device.

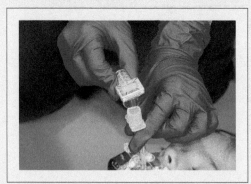

2 Begin ventilation.

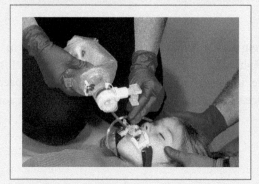

3 Observe the carbon dioxide detector for colour change during exhalation. Read only after a total of six breaths. Check the colour and act accordingly (**Table P10-1**). Regardless of whether the ETT is in the trachea, the carbon dioxide detector will change to a purple colour when 100% oxygen is squeezed through the bag-valve-mask device and ETT into the lungs. The colour on exhalation is the one to pay attention to because the colour in the expiratory phase of breathing reflects carbon dioxide production. However, do not leave an adult carbon dioxide detector in place after initial confirmation of tube position on a patient weighing less than 15 kg because the adult device has too much dead space and an infant can rebreathe carbon dioxide if it is left in line. Document observations and interventions.

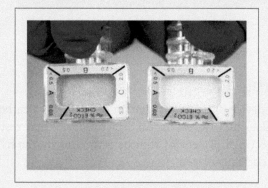

Table P10-1 Use of Colorimetric Exhaled Carbon Dioxide Detector in ETT Placement

Colour	Patient With Pulse	Patient Without Pulse
Yellow	Yes—tube correctly placed Leave tube in place and secure it	Yes—tube correctly placed Leave tube in place and secure it
Tan	Think about it Ventilate six more times (while reassessing tube placement) Reassess detector for colour change. If still tan, leave tube in place and secure it Attempt to correct any possible cause of low perfusion or low carbon dioxide	Think about it Ventilate six more times (while reassessing tube placement) Reassess detector for colour change. If still tan, leave tube in place and secure it Attempt to correct cause of low perfusion or low carbon dioxide
Purple	Problem—tube incorrectly placed or the child is in cardiac arrest or dead and is not producing measurable amounts of carbon dioxide or delivering it to the lungs. Extubate Ventilate with bag-valve-mask device Reintubate	Problem—tube may be incorrectly placed, or the child is dead and not producing measurable amounts of carbon dioxide Look at vocal cords with laryngoscope If tube is incorrectly placed: Extubate Ventilate with bag-valve-mask device Reintubate If tube is between vocal cords, and vocal cord marker is below vocal cords: Leave tube in place Check adequacy of CPR Proceed with ALS protocol

Tip

Remove the carbon dioxide detector from the ETT if endotracheal drugs are given, because a wet detector may not show a correct colour change from purple to yellow.

Tip

If the child is in cardiac arrest and not receiving chest compressions, no colour change will occur, even if placement is correct, because there is no carbon dioxide being delivered to the lungs.

Controversy

An important controversy is whether a carbon dioxide detector or oesophageal detector (aspiration) bulb or syringe is better. There is not enough data on efficacy, safety, and feasibility to clearly support one technique alone.

Tip

If the child weighs less than 15 kg, use a paediatric colorimetric exhaled carbon dioxide detector. If the child weighs 15 kg or more, use an adult device.

Procedure 10-4

Quantitative End-Tidal CO_2 ($ETCO_2$)

1 If quantitative $ETCO_2$ is used, a number should register quickly. Accuracy of the $ETCO_2$ number relies on a good mask seal if the patient is not intubated OR minimal leak if an ETT is in correct airway position.

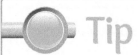

Tip

If there is a lot of pulmonary oedema or pulmonary haemorrhage, an $ETCO_2$ value may not register.

2 Remember that the number will be low in cardiac arrest and will hopefully improve with high-quality CPR and return of spontaneous circulation (ROSC).

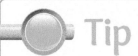

Tip

Pulse oximetry requires a pulse and will not register with a cardiac arrest and may be difficult to pick up with delayed capillary refill as may be seen with shock.

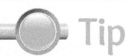

Tip

If the child is pulseless and no chest compressions are being performed, there will be a very low (or zero) number on quantitative assessment. Assess quality of CPR (depth, rate, recoil). Patients that have been pulseless for a period of time may not be revivable even with high-quality CPR.

3 Use waveform capnography tracing for quantitative assessment.

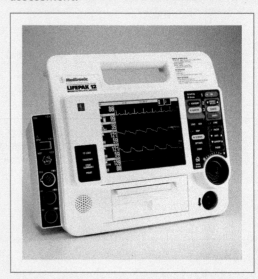

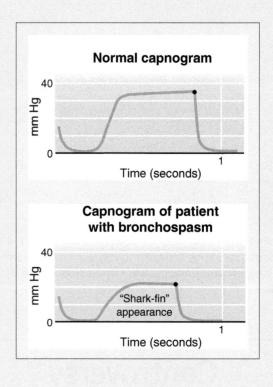

Procedure 11: Advanced Airway Techniques

Introduction

Rarely, standard bag-valve-mask ventilation fails and endotracheal intubation (ETI) is difficult or impossible. Examples of such patients are children with massive head trauma and airway oedema or haematomas of the mouth or upper airway, children with multisystem injuries and long transport times, or infants with significant congenital or acquired airway abnormalities that cannot be ventilated. In such dire circumstances, some ambulance services allow prehospital professionals to perform advanced airway techniques. These include use of a supraglottic airway device (SAD) and the gum-elastic bougie. Needle cricothyrotomy is another option and is explained in detail in this procedure. None of these techniques have been well evaluated in children in the out-of-hospital setting, and each procedure has important benefits, limitations, and contraindications.

Characteristics of children that are red flags for possible problems managing the airway include the following history or physical findings:

History:

1. Past history of difficult intubation or problems with ventilation.

2. Children with congenital anomalies affecting facial bones and oropharyngeal structures including the tongue.

3. History of recurrent stridor or upper airway obstruction.

Physical Findings:

1. Unable to open the mouth widely.

2. Difficulty in fully extending the neck.

3. Presence of a large tongue or dysmorphic facial features.

4. Inability to visualise the entire uvula when depressing the tongue with a tongue blade.

5. Trauma to the face, mouth, tongue, or neck.

Supraglottic Airway Device (SAD) i-gel®

The i-gel is a device used frequently by EMS services as an advanced airway device in adults. i-gel has a soft, gel-like, non-inflatable cuff, designed to provide an anatomical impression fit over the laryngeal inlet. A bag-valve-mask device can then be connected to the tube to provide rescue breathing.

The safety and efficacy of this procedure in children in the out-of-hospital setting is largely unreported. However, the procedure is simple and fast, the success rates in adults are excellent, and the risks are small. EMS practitioners must still maintain the skill of laryngoscopy to ensure the airway is clear of foreign bodies or obstruction before insertion of the i-gel.

A child who requires ventilation

Failed bag-valve-mask ventilation

Failed ETI attempt

Contraindications

Severe upper airway obstruction

An awake patient with intact airway reflexes

Patients requiring high pressures to ventilate (asthma, bronchiolitis)

Equipment

i-gel have seven sizes: 1, 1.5, 2, 2.5, 3, 4, and 5

Water-soluble lubricant

Oxygen source

Suction

Ventilation bag

Monitors (pulse oximeter, capnography)

Preparation

Select the i-gel size for the patient (see **Table P11-1** for sizing).

1. Select an appropriate resuscitator bag: although a small child can be safely and effectively ventilated using an adult bag, a paediatric bag will not work for a large child. Paediatric tidal volume is approximately 8 ml/kg. The bag should have a volume of 450–750 ml. Avoid using adult bags due to the risk of over inflation.

2. Connect the oxygen tubing.

3. Once inserted, connect the bag device to the end of the LMA.

Table P11-1 i-gel Size by Weight

i-gel Size	Weight of Patient
1	2–5 kg
1.5	5–12 kg
2	10–25 kg
2.5	25–35 kg
3	30–60 kg
4	50–90 kg
5	90+ kg

Tip

The i-gel is a fast and simple device and is widely used for adults and children in the prehospital setting.

Procedure 11-1

i-gel Insertion Method

1 Open the i-gel package and transfer the i-gel into the lid of the cage.

2 Place a small amount of lubricant (such as K-Y jelly) onto the middle of the smooth surface of the cage.

3 Lubricate the back, sides, and front of the cuff with a thin layer of lubricant.

4 Position the device so that the cuff outlet is facing towards the chin of the patient. The chin should be gently pressed down to open the mouth.

5 Introduce the leading tip of the i-gel into the mouth and in a direction towards the hard palate.

6 Glide the device into the mouth and along the hard palate with a continuous but gentle push, until a definitive resistance is felt.

7 The tip of the airway should be located into the upper oesophageal opening, and the cuff should be located against the laryngeal framework. The incisors should be resting on the bite block.

8 I-gel should be taped down from maxilla to maxilla or with tube tie.

9 If there is any resistance during insertion, a jaw thrust or insertion with rotation is recommended.

iGum-Elastic Bougie

Sometimes it is difficult to visualise the vocal cords for ETI. There are many reasons for failure to see the anatomy, especially if the child has muscle tone. The gum-elastic bougie or endotracheal tube (ETT) introducer is a long flexible stylet that facilitates insertion of an ETT. There are several versions of this device that are available and may prove useful in facilitating intubation. The cartilaginous rings structure of the trachea allows the operator to feel the gum-elastic bougie in the correct location. The semi-rigid tube or rod can be angled to pass into the trachea and as the device brushes against the tracheal rings, the rod can be palpated to be in position. Once in place, the device serves as a guide for placement of the ETT. Airway injury also is a risk.

Indication
An adjunct for the difficult airway when direct visualisation of the vocal cords is impossible because of secretions or blood obstructing the view

Contraindications
Major facial trauma
Laryngeal fracture
Severe upper airway obstruction

Equipment
Gum-elastic bougie device in paediatric and adult sizes
All equipment described under ETI

Preparation

1. Prepare the child for ETI (see **Procedure 9, Endotracheal Intubation**).
2. Ensure the gum-elastic bougie points upward in a J-shape configuration.

Procedure 11-2

Gum-Elastic Bougie Device

1. Place the lubricated ETT over the straight end of the gum-elastic bougie.

2. Visualise the cords with laryngoscopy.

3. Insert the J-shaped end of the gum-elastic bougie through the cords, advancing the device until clicks are palpated indicating the presence of tracheal rings.

4. Slide the ETT over the gum-elastic bougie into the trachea.

5. Remove the laryngoscope, then the gum-elastic bougie.

6. Ensure the ETT is in the trachea by end-tidal CO_2 detection or an oesophageal detector device, and that the tube has a correct position at the lips.

7. Secure the ETT.

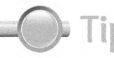 Tip

A gum-elastic bougie is particularly helpful when a very anteriorly placed larynx makes visualisation of the vocal cords difficult.

Needle Cricothyroidotomy

Indication
Can't ventilate and can't oxygenate situation
Obstructed or disrupted larynx

Contraindications
Presence of a secure airway
Traumatic destruction of the cricothyroid membrane
Surgical cricothyroidotomy is relatively contraindicated in children under the age of 5 years. In this group, perform needle cricothyroidotomy.

Equipment
Oxygen source
Oxygen cylinder
Transtracheal jet insufflation device (3-way tap, connected to oxygen tubing)
14-gauge cannula
10-ml syringe

Preparation

1. Declare an emergency and brief the team.

2. Ensure all equipment is available.

3. Place something under the shoulders to prevent hyperflexion of the neck and to improve visualisation of the anterior neck anatomy.

Procedure 11-3

Needle Cricothyroidotomy

1 Ensure equipment is readily available and where possible use an airway assistant.

2 Palpate the hyoid bone high in the neck and move caudally to identify the thyroid and cricoid cartilages.

3 Stabilise the cartilage using the thumb and index finger of the non-dominant hand.

4 With a 10-ml syringe attached to the 14-gauge cannula, insert just superior to the cricoid cartilage. Angle the cannula caudally at approximately a 45° angle to the skin.

5 As you insert the cannula, withdraw on the syringe and you should feel a rush of air enter the syringe once you pass into the trachea. Alternatively, you can place some saline in the syringe and you should notice air bubbles indicating entry to the trachea.

6 Advance the catheter into the trachea and remove the needle and syringe. Do not let go of the catheter until it is secured.

7 Attach the pre-prepared jet insufflation device (3-way tap and oxygen tubing) and begin to oxygenate the patient.

8 Administer 100% oxygen (15 l/min) via the insufflation device. Occlude the port to deliver oxygen for 1 second (inspiration), then release for 5 seconds (expiration).

9 Secure the ETT.

Complications

Bleeding can occur, but it is rare with this needle cricothyroidotomy technique.

Inappropriate placement of the needle can cause injury to the larynx, vocal cords, great vessels of the neck, nerves, or oesophagus.

High-pressure oxygen may cause barotrauma, surgical emphysema, or pneumothorax.

This is a temporary measure that may provide oxygenation for about 30 minutes and therefore, once performed, you should expedite transport to an emergency department capable of delivering advanced airway management.

Procedure 12: Intramuscular Injections

Introduction

The intramuscular (IM) route is acceptable for giving several important medications to children. These medications include adrenaline and morphine sulphate. The IM route has limitations, but when inhalation, intravenous (IV), or intraosseous (IO) delivery of medication is not possible, IM administration may be life-saving.

Indication

Administration of medications when vascular access is not possible or practical, or when IM is the required delivery route.

Contraindications

Poor perfusion

Availability of alternative effective routes: oral, inhalation, IV, IN, or IO

Equipment

Syringe

22- or 25-gauge needle (2.5 cm)

Rationale

IM administration allows the medication to absorb slowly but steadily. The advantages of the IM technique is easy delivery and high safety. The disadvantages are poor patient acceptance and delayed effect. Avoid IM medications in patients with low perfusion because absorption is unpredictable. Sometimes, in situations involving a child with low venous pressures, such as in anaphylaxis, IM is an excellent first choice for delivery while vascular access is attempted.

The IM route may result in nerve damage, particularly if the injection is in the buttocks of an infant or small child.

Preparation

1. Explain the procedure using developmentally appropriate terminology. Be honest and tell the child it will hurt but be over as quickly as possible. Describe the needle stick as a pinch or a bee sting.

2. Select the medication. Confirm that the child is not allergic to any medications.

3. Select the appropriate syringe and needle. Keep needles out of the child's sight.

Needle Length for IM Injection

- For the ventrogluteal or dorsogluteal sites, use a needle slightly longer than one half of the distance between the thumb and finger when the skin at the injection site is grasped.

- For the deltoid and vastus lateralis sites, use a 2.5 cm needle if the skin is grasped.

4. Cleanse the top of the medication vial with an alcohol wipe or open the ampule.

5. Withdraw the appropriate volume of medication, based on the child's milligram per kilogram dose. Calculate the dose using the page for age JRCALC guidelines.

- The maximum volume IM is:

    o 2 ml in older children

    o 1 ml in small children and older infants

    o 0.5 ml in small infants

6. Select the appropriate injection site (**Table P12-1**). Consider the following factors:

- The volume of medication

- The condition of the muscle

- The type of medication

- The child's ability to be properly positioned

7. Position and secure the child. Consider letting the caregiver hold the child in one of the following ways:

    - Have the child sit on the caregiver's lap, facing to the side. Put one of the child's arms around the caregiver's waist and have the caregiver hold the child close to his or her chest. The caregiver can hold the child's arms or legs.

    - Position the child straddling the caregiver's lap, sitting chest to chest. Tell the caregiver to hug the child. The caregiver can help to hold an arm or leg.

Possible Complications

Abscess

Cellulitis

Damage to blood vessel, nerve, or tendon

Redness or swelling at the site

Adverse reaction to the medication

Pain at site

Table P12-1 Appropriate Sites for IM Injections

Site	Indications	Landmarks	Considerations	Disadvantages
Vastus lateralis muscle: Largest muscle group in children under 3 years of age	Use in infants and small children Preferred site for all ages	Palpate the greater trochanter and the knee joint; divide the distance into thirds Use middle third for injection site	Can be used for IM injections in young children	Possible thrombosis of the femoral artery More painful than deltoid or gluteal sites.
Ventrogluteal muscle: Large muscle with few nerves and blood vessels	Use in children over 3 years of age	Have the child lie on his side and bend the upper leg forward in front of the lower leg Palpate greater trochanter and anterior and posterior iliac crests Place palm over greater trochanter with fingers open in a V shape pointing towards iliac crests Inject into centre of the V shape	Well-defined landmarks to identify the site	None
Dorsogluteal site	Use in children over 3 years of age	Have the child lie on his stomach and rotate his legs and toes inward Palpate greater trochanter and posterior iliac spine; draw an imaginary line between these two points Inject lateral and above the imaginary line	In an older child, larger volumes of medication (2 ml) can be injected because the muscle mass is larger.	Contraindicated in children under 3 years of age and those who have not been walking for at least 1 year Medication may inadvertently be given into fat in older child with a large fat mass May damage the sciatic nerve, which tracks out from the lower lumbar spine and goes underneath the gluteal muscles
Deltoid	Use for small volumes of medication Used in children 18 months of age and older	Palpate the shoulder and go two fingerbreadths below Give the injection in the upper third of the muscle	Faster absorption rate than gluteal site Fewer side effects from the injection and less painful site	May damage the radial nerve in young children Because of the limited muscle mass, only small volumes of medication can be injected

Procedure 12-1

IM Injection

1. The vastus lateralis site is preferable. Use the ventrogluteal or dorsogluteal sites if the thigh muscle is not accessible in children older than 3 years.

2. Grasp the body of the muscle between the thumb and forefingers.

3. Insert the needle at a 90-degree angle.

4. Release the skin and pull back on the plunger to aspirate for blood.

5. If no blood appears, inject the medication. If blood appears, remove the syringe and start the procedure again.

6. Apply gentle pressure to the site with a gauze pad. Do not massage the site.

 Tip

Select the injection site based on age, anatomical considerations, and volume of medication to be given.

 Think Point

Avoid injecting close to a major nerve because it may cause nerve damage.

Procedure 12-2

After the Injection

1. Praise the child. Apply an adhesive bandage to the site.

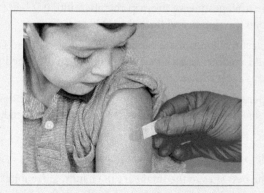

2. Dispose of the syringe in a sharps container.

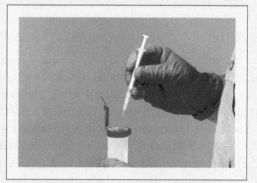

3. Write down the name of the medication, dosage, route, time, and any effects.

 Controversy

Some experts believe that the dorsogluteal site should not be used until the child has been walking for at least 1 year.

Procedure 13: Intravenous Access

Introduction

Establishing intravenous (IV) access is a long-established method of fluid and drug administration. However, unlike the situation with an adult, securing IV access in a paediatric patient is often difficult or impossible in the out-of-hospital setting. Fortunately, the majority of paediatric patients do not require IV access before emergency department (ED) arrival, and many out-of-hospital medications do not require an IV route for administration.

Indications

Cardiopulmonary arrest

Shock

Cardiac dysrhythmia

Illness or injury possibly requiring immediate IV drug or fluid administration

Contraindications

Availability of another reliable administration route

Equipment

IV cannula, 14- to 24-gauge

IV tubing (giving set)

IV fluid

Tourniquet

Occlusive dressing or adhesive tape

Gauze pad

IV flush

Skin cleansing solution

Rationale

IV access makes it easier to give medications and provides a route for fluid therapy in illness or injuries where there is possible blood or fluid loss. IV delivery is an excellent route for giving medications because it permits predictable delivery and more rapid onset of action for most important drugs. The indications for IV access must be carefully weighed against common complications and risks associated with the procedure. These include diversion from airway and breathing management, possible delays to ED care, and pain to the child. Also, there is a risk to the prehospital professional from exposure to blood-borne pathogens. However, in certain children, such as the critically ill child with shock, IV therapy in the field can be life-saving.

Preparation

1. Assemble the equipment. Select the appropriate IV fluid and giving set.

    - Inspect the solution for cloudiness, expiration date, leakage, or contamination.

    - Spike the fluid bag with the IV giving set, clamp the tubing, squeeze the drip chamber until it is half full, open the clamp, and flush the tubing.

    - Select the appropriate cannula, depending on need for fluid volume. Use a smaller cannula when only medications are indicated.

2. Prepare the child and family for the procedure. Use developmentally appropriate language to explain the procedure.

3. Select the site.

    - The scalp is a potential site in newborns.

    - The best sites in the infant are the hands, antecubital fossa, and saphenous vein at the ankle or feet. The dorsum (back) of the hand is a good site in chubby infants. To access that site, grasp the child's hand with the fingers closed and flex the wrist downward.

    - In toddlers and older children, potential sites are the hands and antecubital areas. Use the child's non-dominant extremity if possible.

    - Ideally, avoid inserting the cannula over a joint.

- Consider the antecubital fossa when fluid boluses are required because veins that are more distal in the forearm or hand are usually smaller.
- Hand veins are often mobile under the skin and may move with contact with the cannula.

4. Position the patient supine, or in the caregiver's lap if the child is under school age. Secure the child's legs to avoid kicking. The caregiver can help hold the child and immobilise the insertion site.

5. Apply the tourniquet proximal to the entry site. Do not make it too tight. The tourniquet should not block arterial flow. If it is necessary to make the vein more visible, do the following:
   - Place the extremity in a dependent position.
   - Tap or massage the site.
   - Ask the older child to clench and unclench their fist.

6. Cleanse the site with antiseptic solution.

Troubleshooting

1. If the fluid is not infusing properly, assess the following:
   - Make sure the tourniquet has been released.
   - Make sure the child's arm is not bent.
   - Make sure the tape is not too tight.
   - Make sure the tubing is not kinked.
   - Make sure the clamp is open.
   - Lower the fluid bag below the extremity and assess for a backflow of blood into the tubing.
   - Raise the fluid bag higher if possible.

2. If none of the above measures are effective, discontinue the IV and restart in another site.

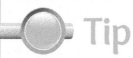

Reward and comfort the child after the procedure.

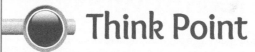

Never delay transport in any critically injured infant or child; consider IV attempts on the way to the hospital.

Procedure 13-1

Intravenous Access

1 Insert the needle. Stabilise the vein by pulling the skin taut distally from the insertion site. Insert the cannula through the skin with the bevel up, at a 30-degree angle. Insert the cannula slowly; blood return may be delayed for a few seconds. When there is a flashback of blood, advance the needle and cannula into the vein and then remove the needle. Never pull the cannula back over the needle because this may cause shearing of the catheter tip. Dispose of the needle in a suitable sharps bin. Release the tourniquet. Compress the vein proximal to the site to prevent blood loss through the cannula while connecting the tubing. It is also helpful to position a gauze pad under the cannula at this time. Connect the giving set or male Luer lock to the cannula. If a saline lock (male Luer lock with injection port) is used, a 2- to 5-ml saline flush should be used to maintain patency.

2 Stabilise the cannula with an occlusive dressing or tape. Avoid placing an excess amount of tape or gauze over the site because it obstructs the view of the site. Use an occlusive dressing that is purpose-made for fixing cannulas because these are clear to allow visualisation of the site.

3 Be careful to ensure the child is not going to pull out the cannula or block it by moving their limb too much.

4 Monitor the solution drip rate to avoid giving too much or too little fluid.

Possible Complications

Pain

Infiltration (look for pain or oedema at the site, inability to infuse fluids, or lack of blood return; discontinue IV and insert at another site)

Hypothermia from giving too much room-temperature fluid to an infant

Skin infection

Thrombophlebitis

Inadvertent fluid overload

Cannula shear

Inadvertent arterial puncture

Think Point

Do not use words like "stick" or "needle" when describing the procedure to the child. Instead, consider an explanation such as, "I will be putting a soft tube into your arm to give your veins a drink".

Controversy

Few children require IV access in the field or on the way to the ED. Injured children must always be transported before attempting IV access. For ill children, especially if there is a short transport time, it is controversial which ones need IV access.

Tip

Position the child and secure the site before beginning the procedure.

Procedure 14: Intraosseous Needle Insertion

Introduction

Establishing vascular access is often difficult or impossible during life-threatening emergencies in infants and young children. The intraosseous (IO), intramedullary, or marrow route for the delivery of resuscitation fluids and medications has been used for more than 50 years in children and adults. Many studies have confirmed that the IO space is an excellent route for medications and fluids. The primary technical problem is successfully piercing the bony cortex (outer layer of the bone) in older children. The bones of neonates and infants are usually soft and the IO space is relatively large, so needle insertion is easier in children of these younger age groups. Good equipment, preparation, and effective technique are especially important for success.

Indication

Severe illness or injury requiring immediate drugs or fluids, when intravenous (IV) access is impossible or unlikely to be successful

Contraindications

Available secure IV line

Fracture or prior failed IO attempt

Equipment

IO needles

Skin cleansing solution

Normal saline and IV tubing

10-ml syringe

Extension connector and 3-way tap (optional)

Rationale

Using an IO needle to give drugs or fluids is an excellent alternative to cannulating peripheral veins in critically ill or injured children. The IO space is highly vascular and functions as a non-collapsible vein. Needle insertion into this space is a rapid, safe, effective, and acceptable route. In the setting of cardiac arrest, time should not be wasted attempting intravenous access. There are several possible sites, but the easiest location is the proximal tibia. The IO space is suitable for infusion of all parenteral medications, crystalloid fluids, or blood products—which quickly traverse the small veins of the bone and eventually enter into the central circulation. Complications are usually minor and infrequent.

Possible Complications

Compartment syndrome

Failed infusion

Growth plate injury

Bone infection

Skin infection

Bone fracture

Landmarking

Proximal Tibia Site

1. Use the flat surface of the proximal medial tibia, just below and medial to the tibial tuberosity on the flat side of the bone.

2. Introduce the IO needle in the skin at 90 degrees, ensure that the needle is placed away from the growth plate.

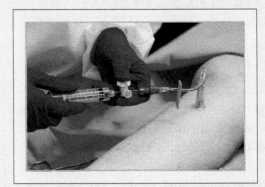

Landmarking

Distal Tibia Site

1. Use the flat surface of the medial distal tibia above the medial malleolus.

2. Introduce the IO needle in the skin at 90 degrees, ensure that the needle is placed away from the growth plate.

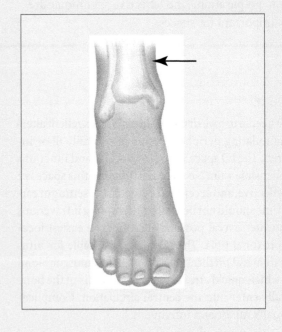

Landmarking

Distal Femur Site

1. Use the distal third of the femur, estimate distance through soft tissue to reach the bony surface of femur, and ensure that an IO needle has been chosen to a length that allows bony penetration.

2. Introduce the IO needle in the skin, at 90 degrees to the femur, making sure to avoid the growth plate.

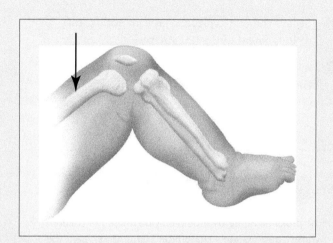

 Think Point

Although IO access is easy, quick, and safe, it is painful in a conscious child and therefore is only practical in a critically ill or injured child.

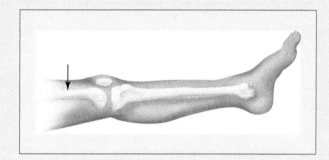

Landmarking

Proximal Humerus Site

1. With the child's hand resting on the abdomen and elbow held close to the body, palpate up the length of the humerus until a "notch" or "groove" followed by a protrusion is felt. This groove represents the surgical neck of the humerus.

2. The insertion point for the IO needle is located approximately 1 cm above the surgical neck.

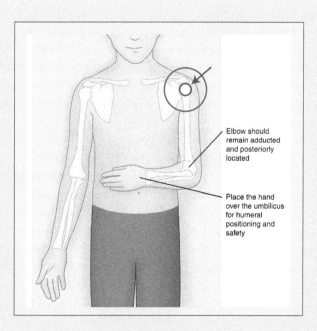

Elbow should remain adducted and posteriorly located

Place the hand over the umbilicus for humeral positioning and safety

(continues)

Landmarking *(continued)*

3 Secure the arm in place to prevent accidental dislodgement of the IO catheter.

4 A larger size IO needle will be required to access the site.

 Think Point

The proximal humerus should only be utilised in children whose appropriate anatomical landmarks can be identified.

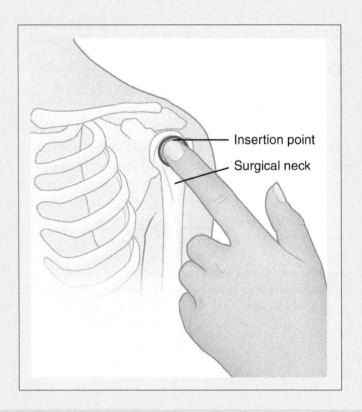

Insertion point
Surgical neck

Insertion technique

Traditional IO Insertion

1 Pierce the bony cortex with a firm, twisting motion. Use a back-and-forth twisting motion to enter the marrow space. Do not push hard on the needle. A "pop" may be felt as the needle passes through the bony cortex and into the marrow cavity.

2 Remove the stylet. Any bone marrow aspirated may be used for a glucose check or other testing. However, sometimes marrow cannot be aspirated. Confirm correct placement by infusing 10 ml of normal saline without resistance or swelling around the site due to leakage of fluid.

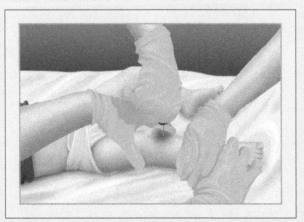

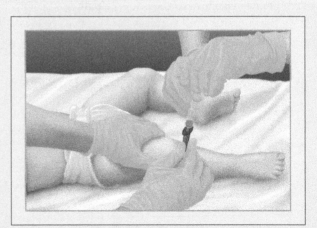

Insertion technique (continued)

3   Attach IV line to the hub, or to an extension-connector and 3-way tap, and infuse fluids or drugs directly into IO space.

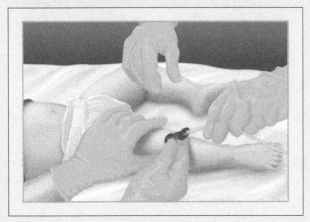

4   Secure the needle in situ with an appropriate dressing or with tape. Monitor the surrounding tissue to ensure that there is no swelling to indicate leakage of fluid.

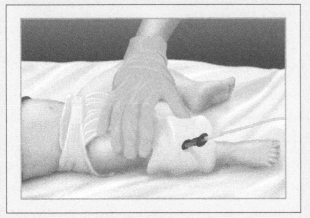

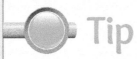 **Tip**

When placing a traditional IO needle, use firm pressure and a twisting motion.

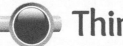 **Think Point**

Insert the IO needle gently. Too much force may push the needle all the way through the bone and into the soft tissues.

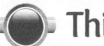 **Think Point**

Avoid placing your hand behind the insertions site while placing the IO to prevent possible injury from through-and-through IO needle penetration.

Insertion technique

EZ-IO Insertion

An alternate to the traditional manual IO is the EZ-IO (**Figure P14-1**).

1 Select the appropriate needle for the patient's age. The adult set (for patients ≥40 kg) is 25 mm in length and red. The paediatric set (for children 3–39 kg) is 15 mm in length and blue. There is also a larger adult needle (for those ≥40 kg with excessive tissue at the insertion site), which is 45 mm in length and yellow. Weight guidelines are rough estimates. Make sure at least 1 black line can still be seen on the needle when inserted through the skin, but prior to drilling through the cortex of the bone.

2 Attach the needle to the EZ-IO drill.

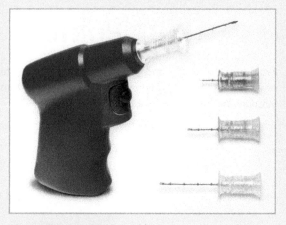

Figure P14-1 EZ-IO tool.

3 Position the needle and EZ-IO drill at 90 degrees to the bone. Press the trigger on the drill handle and apply moderate pressure, while letting the drill do the work for you. When you feel the "pop", you're in. (The pain from the EZ-IO insertion is generally similar to that of peripheral IV insertion.) As with traditional IO insertion, refrain from placing your other hand behind the insertion site to prevent possible palm penetration from excessive force.

4 Disconnect the EZ-IO drill while leaving the needle in place.

5 Withdraw the needle stylet and confirm placement by aspiration of blood with the syringe; however, the inability to aspirate blood does not necessarily indicate improper placement. Confirm correct placement by infusing 10 ml of normal saline without resistance or swelling around the site due to leakage of fluid.

Procedure 15: Cardiopulmonary Resuscitation

Introduction

Cardiopulmonary arrest (CPA) occurs when a patient's heart and lungs stop functioning. In children, CPA usually begins as a primary respiratory arrest. This is in contrast to adults, in whom CPA or "sudden death" is almost always a primary cardiac event that occurs with onset of ventricular fibrillation (VF) and an abrupt change in the heart's electrical activity. Because cessation of effective breathing is often the precipitating factor in paediatric CPA, airway management and ventilation are to children in CPA what defibrillation is to adults. Cardiopulmonary resuscitation (CPR) refers to basic airway management, artificial ventilation, and chest compressions to provide oxygen and circulation to core organs: the heart, brain, and lungs. In children, CPR has been shown to improve survival from drowning, and it may also benefit patients in CPA from other causes. Asphyxial cardiac arrest is more common than VF cardiac arrest in infants and children, and ventilations are extremely important in paediatric resuscitation.

Indications

Newborn, neonate, infant, or child of any age who is apnoeic and pulseless

Newborn with a heart rate less than 60 beats/min and not improving after standard newborn care

Neonate, infants, and children with a heart rate less than 60 beats/min and poor perfusion

Contraindication

Newborn, infant, or child with effective perfusion (palpable central or peripheral pulse)

Equipment

Mouth-to-mask device

Bag-valve-mask device, infant, or child

Airway adjuncts

Appropriate mask sizes

Rationale

CPR encompasses the basic procedures for sustaining critical oxygenation, ventilation, and perfusion recommended by the European Resuscitation Council (ERC). The paediatric techniques are slightly modified from the adult techniques to reflect the known differences in CPA between age groups. Furthermore, there are specific differences between infants and children, including number of rescuers, placement of hands and fingers, rates of ventilation, and rates and depth of chest compressions.

Preparation

1. Position a child on a hard surface. It is NOT appropriate to position any child on the forearm of the rescuer with the hand supporting the head.

Paediatric Assessment

1. Carry out a primary survey using the <C>ABCDE approach.

2. If no pulse detected in 10 seconds, start chest compressions (see ratios in **Table P15-1**).

3. If definite pulse greater than 60 per minute, then administer one breath every 3 to 5 seconds.

   - Infant BLS guidelines apply to infants less than 1 year of age.

   - Child BLS guidelines apply to children 1 year of age until puberty. For teaching purposes, puberty is defined as breast development in girls and the presence of axillary hair in boys.

   - Adult BLS guidelines apply at and beyond puberty.

High-Quality CPR

High-quality CPR is defined by:

1. Chest compressions of appropriate rate and depth.

2. Push fast: push at a rate of 100–120 compressions per minute.

3. Push hard: push with sufficient force to depress at least one-third the anteroposterior (AP) diameter of the chest or approximately 4 cm in infants and 5 cm in children.

4. Allow complete chest recoil after each compression to allow the heart to refill with blood. Incomplete recoil during CPR is associated with higher intrathoracic pressures and significantly decreased venous return, coronary perfusion, blood flow, and cerebral perfusion.

5. Minimise interruptions of chest compressions.

6. Avoid excessive ventilation.

7. See ratios in Table P15-1 for ratio of chest compressions to ventilation.

8. Rescuers should rotate the compressor role every 2 minutes to avoid fatigue.

9. Ratios do not apply if patient is intubated. Deliver breaths at a rate of 8–10 per minute and continuous chest compressions (one breath approximately every 6 seconds)

10. If the patient has return of spontaneous circulation (ROSC) with a perfusing rhythm and pulse, then breaths can be delivered at a rate of approximately 20 per minute (one breath every 3 seconds).

Table P15-1 Chest Compressions to Ventilation Ratios

Age	Compressions (min)/Ratios	Depth (inches)	Hand Placement
Newborn	3:1 ratio of compressions to ventilations (90 compressions to 30 breaths every minute); consider 15:2 if cardiac in origin	Compress approximately one-third of AP chest diameter	Two thumbs encircling the chest and supporting back (may prefer higher coronary perfusion pressure than two-finger technique)
Infant	100–120/min; 15:2 ratio of compressions	Compress at least one-third the depth of the chest or about 4 cm	Lone rescuers (whether lay rescuers or health care providers) should compress the sternum with two fingers placed just below the intermammary line; do not compress over the xiphoid or ribs
Child	100–120/min; 15:2 ratio of compressions	Compress at least one-third of the AP dimension of the chest or approximately 5 cm	Lone rescuers (whether lay rescuers or health care providers) should compress the lower half of sternum with heel of one or two hands
Adolescent	100–120/min; 30:2 ratio of compressions to breaths	Compress at least one-third of the AP dimension of the chest or approximately 5 cm	Place the heel of one hand on the centre of the chest (lower half of the sternum). Place the heel of your other hand over the first hand.

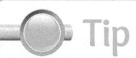

Tip

Manipulation of the head to keep the airway in a neutral position is essential for effective ventilation. A towel roll under the shoulders of the infant or small child may help maintain neutral head position.

Procedure 15-1

Performing CPR on an Infant

1 Position the infant on a firm surface. Place two fingers in the middle of the sternum just below a line between the nipples. Use two fingers to compress the chest at least one-third the AP diameter of the chest or about 4 cm at a rate of 100–120 per minute. Allow the sternum to return to its normal position between compressions.

2 Co-ordinate compressions with ventilations in a 15:2 ratio, pausing for two ventilations at the end of each cycle. Perform mouth-to-mask ventilation with 100% oxygen. Give two breaths of 1 second each. Continue cycles of compressions and ventilations until an automated external defibrillator (AED) becomes available or the infant shows signs of spontaneous breathing.

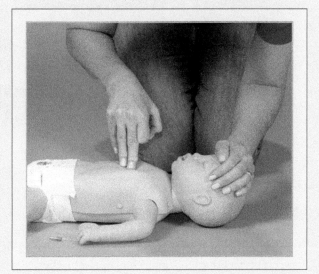

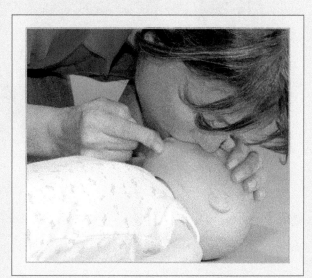

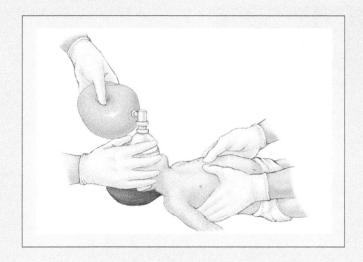

Procedure 15-2

Performing CPR on a Child

1 Place the child on a firm surface. Prepare to place the heel of one or both hands in the centre of the chest, in between the nipples, avoiding the xiphoid process.

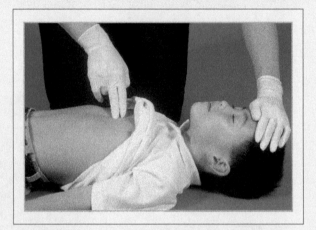

2 Compress the chest at least one-third the AP diameter of the chest or approximately 5 cm at a rate of 100–120 per minute.

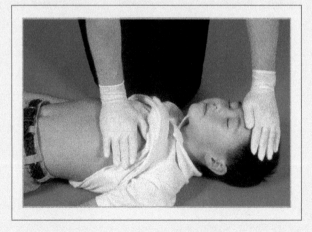

3 Co-ordinate compressions with ventilations in a 15:2 ratio. At the end of each cycle, pause for two ventilations. Perform mouth-to-mask ventilation with 100% oxygen. Give two breaths of 1 second each.

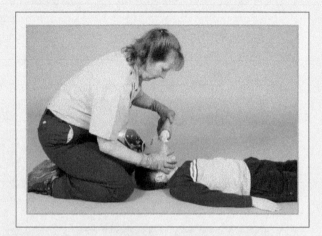

4 Continue cycles of compressions and ventilations until an AED becomes available or the patient shows signs of spontaneous breathing. If the child resumes effective breathing, place him or her in a position that allows for frequent reassessment of the airway and vital signs during transport.

Possible Complications

Coronary vessel injury

Diaphragm injury

Haemopericardium

Haemothorax

Interference with ventilation

Liver injury

Myocardial injury

Pneumothorax

Rib fractures

Spleen injury

Sternal fracture

Use of End-Tidal Carbon Dioxide (ETCO$_2$) for Quality of Compressions

1. Exhaled CO_2 is reflective of cardiac output during a cardiac arrest, because pulmonary blood flow must exist for ETCO$_2$ to register.

2. Quantitative ETCO$_2$ may be used to monitor quality of CPR. Normal ETCO$_2$ with a good mask seal or if the patient is intubated is approximately 35–45 mm Hg (or 4.5–6 kPa). During a cardiac arrest, the ETCO$_2$ value will be much lower and can theoretically reach 0 if the patient has no pulse and is not receiving chest compressions.

3. Potential goals for quantitative ETCO$_2$ during a pulseless arrest are greater than 15 mm Hg (or 1.9 kPa) .

4. If ROSC is achieved, the ETCO$_2$ will begin to rise, reflecting increasing blood flow for cardiac output.

5. After circulation (ROSC) is restored, monitor systemic oxygen saturation. It may be reasonable, when appropriate equipment is available, to titrate oxygen administration to maintain the oxyhaemoglobin saturation greater than or equal to 94%.

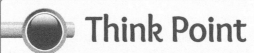 **Think Point**

Take the time to deliver meaningful interventions at the scene. While removal to hospital is nearly always indicated, this should not be at the loss of high quality basic and advanced life support at the scene.

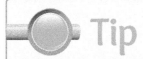 **Tip**

CO_2 may be lowered through prolonged O_2 administration above what is necessary due to lowering of systemic vascular resistance.

Procedure 16: AED and Defibrillation

Introduction

Synchronised cardioversion for tachydysrhythmias has long been part of adult emergency care. Ventricular dysrhythmias are rare in children, especially in infants, and paediatric supraventricular tachycardia (SVT) is usually treatable with medical therapy. However, all providers should be prepared to provide defibrillation in appropriate situations. Ventricular fibrillation (VF) is observed in 5%–15% of paediatric and adolescent arrest. When a child develops VF or pulseless ventricular tachycardia, early defibrillation may be life-saving. For those with the appropriate skill set, synchronised cardioversion may resuscitate a child in shock with SVT. Synchronised cardioversion provides a shock that is timed (synchronised) with the QRS complex, avoiding delivery during the refractory period of the cardiac cycle, when a shock could produce VF. Use the synchronised mode for selected cases of SVT or ventricular tachycardia with a pulse, and the asynchronised (defibrillation) mode for VF or ventricular tachycardia without a pulse.

Indications

Ventricular fibrillation

Pulseless ventricular tachycardia

Procedure for those who are trained to the relevant competency level

SVT with shock and no vascular access rapidly available (synchronised)

Ventricular tachycardia with shock and unresponsiveness with pulse

Contraindications

Conscious patient with good perfusion

Equipment

Automatic external defibrillator with pads appropriate for age

Standard defibrillator with paddles or pads appropriate for age

Rationale

When a child's heart rhythm deteriorates into ventricular tachycardia or fibrillation, there is usually a severe systemic insult, such as profound hypoxia, ischaemia, electrolyte abnormalities, electrocution, or myocarditis. Death may result if treatment is delayed. SVT, in contrast, is usually a more stable cardiac rhythm. When the child is pulseless and has VF or ventricular tachycardia, perform defibrillation as quickly as possible with the appropriate technique. If a child has SVT or ventricular tachycardia with a pulse and demonstrates the clinical signs of shock, synchronised cardioversion may be indicated. Do not attempt to perform synchronised cardioversion on a child with SVT who is well perfused.

Preparation

1. Open airway and ventilate with bag-valve-mask device with 100% oxygen if indicated, while assembling equipment for cardioversion or defibrillation.

2. If child is pulseless, begin cardiopulmonary resuscitation, until an automated external defibrillator (AED) or conventional defibrillator is available.

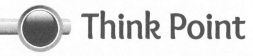 **Think Point**

Do not deliver synchronised cardioversion to a conscious child with SVT or ventricular tachycardia unless the child is in shock and has no intravenous (IV) or intraosseous (IO) access rapidly available for medical treatment.

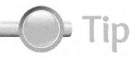 Tip

For a child with ventricular fibrillation or pulseless ventricular tachycardia, use the asynchronised (defibrillation) mode.

Procedure 16-1

Automated External Defibrillator (AED) Use

1 Apply the paddles or pads directly to the skin. Place one paddle or pad on the anterior chest wall on the right side of the sternum inferior to the clavicle and the other paddle or pad on the left mid-clavicular line at the level of the xiphoid process. As another option, use the anterior-posterior position.

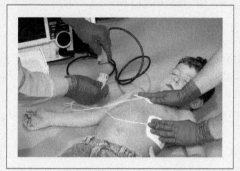

2 Clear the nearby area to avoid shocking someone. Check the top, middle, and bottom of the patient—confirm everyone is clear—prepare to deliver the shock (while looking at the patient).

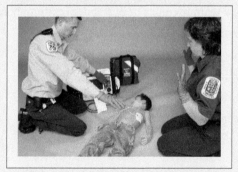

3 Deliver the shock and immediately resume CPR.

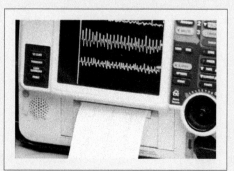

4 Continue CPR for 2 minutes. then check monitor for a change in rhythm, and check pulse.

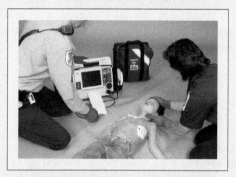

5 If the first electrical shock is unsuccessful, resume CPR, then re-analyse the rhythm after 2 minutes (five cycles) of CPR. Give specific dysrhythmia treatment with adrenaline or other drugs, as per service protocol.

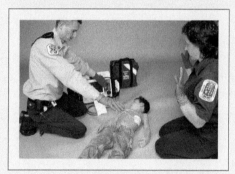

 ## Controversy

The preferred paddle location in children is controversial and no study in humans has compared the two techniques. Anterior chest wall placement has the advantage of a supine child and easier airway management. Anterior-posterior placement may allow larger paddles and more effective delivery of the charge.

Preparation
Conventional Defibrillator Use

1. Select the proper paddle or pad size.
2. Prepare paddles or skin electrodes with electrode jelly, paste, or saline-soaked gauze pads, or use self-adhesive defibrillator pads (now most commonly used). Do not let jelly or paste from one site touch the other and form an "electrical bridge" between sites, which could result in ineffective defibrillation or skin burns.

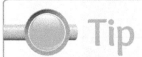 **Tip**

Maintain high-quality chest compressions until defibrillator is charged when you are analysing rhythm OR as long as possible when using AED mode. Immediately resume compressions once rhythm is analysed and does not suggest a shock OR immediately after a shock is delivered.

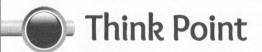 **Think Point**

Failure to firmly apply paddles to the chest wall decreases effective delivery of charge.

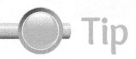 **Tip**

Consider giving a benzodiazepine before cardioversion if patient is awake.

Table P16-1 Appropriate Electrical Charge for Countershock

Dysrhythmia	Mode	Charge
Ventricular fibrillation Ventricular tachycardia without a pulse	Defibrillation (asynchronised)	4 J/kg Then 4 J/kg after CPR and each dose of medication.
IF TRAINED AND COMPETENT Ventricular tachycardia with pulse, SVT	Synchronised Cardioversion	0.5–1.0 J/kg. Repeat as needed.

3. Establish appropriate electrical charge: 4 joules/kg if using a manual defibrillator (**Table P16-1**). Automatically calculated if using an AED.
4. Charge the defibrillator while continuing high quality CPR

Possible Complications

Ineffective delivery of countershock because of failure to charge, improper positioning on the chest, incorrect paddle size, or improper conduction medium

Burns on the chest wall

Failure to "clear" before voltage discharge, leading to electrical shock of a team member or bystander (extremely rare)

Tachydysrhythmia

Bradycardia

Myocardial damage or necrosis

Cardiogenic shock

Embolic phenomena

Procedure 16-2

One Rescuer with an AED

For children younger than 8 years of age, use a child-pad cable system if available.

1 Verify unresponsiveness.

2 Look for no breathing or only gasping and check pulse.

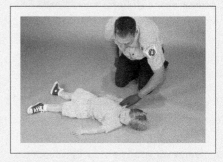

3 If not breathing but with a pulse, begin bag-valve-mask ventilations.

4 If no pulse, begin CPR with 15 compressions and 2 breaths.

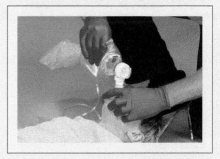

5 Apply AED as soon as it is available.

6 POWER ON the AED and follow voice prompts. Some devices will turn on when the AED lid or carrying case is opened.

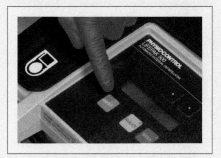

7 ATTACH the AED. Select the correct pads for victim's size and age (adult versus child). Peel the backing from the pads. Attach the adhesive pads to the victim as shown on the pads. (If only adult pads are available, and they overlap when placed on the chest, use an anterior (chest) and posterior (back) placement.) Attach the electrode cable to the AED (if not preconnected).

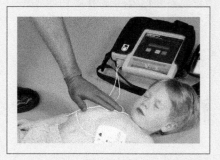

8 Allow the AED to ANALYSE the victim's rhythm ("clear" victim during analysis). Deliver a SHOCK if needed ("clear" victim before shock).

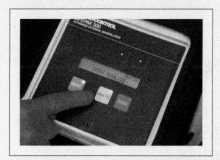

Reasonable variations in this sequence are acceptable.

9 Resume CPR.

Procedure 16-3

Two Rescuer AED Sequence of Action

1 Verify unresponsiveness. Have partner get AED.

2 Look for no breathing or only gasping and check pulse.

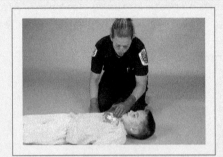

3 If no pulse, start CPR. If not breathing but with a pulse, begin bag-valve-mask ventilations.

4 Apply AED as soon as it is available.

5 Place the AED near the rescuer who will be operating it. The AED is usually placed on the side of the victim opposite the rescuer who is performing CPR. The rescuer begins performing CPR while the rescuer who was performing CPR prepares to operate the AED. (It is acceptable to reverse these roles.)

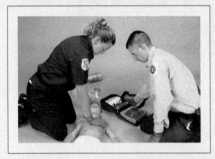

6 The AED operator takes the following actions. POWER ON the AED first (some devices will turn on automatically when the AED lid or carrying case is opened).

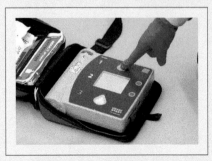

7 ATTACH the self-adhesive pads to the victim. Select correct pads for the victim's size and age. Peel the backing from the pads. Ask the rescuer performing CPR to stop chest compressions. Attach the adhesive pads to the victim as shown on the pads. (If only adult pads are available, and they overlap when placed on the chest, use an anterior (chest) and posterior (back) placement.) Attach the AED connecting cables to the AED (if not preconnected). Press the ANALYSE button to start rhythm analysis (some brands of AEDs do not require this step). ANALYSE rhythm. Clear the victim before and during analysis. Check that no one is touching the victim.

"Shock Indicated" message. Resume CPR until AED is charged and ready to deliver shock. Clear the victim once more before pushing the SHOCK button ("I'm clear, you're clear, everybody's clear"). Check that no one is touching the victim. Press the SHOCK button (victim may display muscle contractions).

"No Shock Indicated" message. Resume CPR immediately after the shock is given.

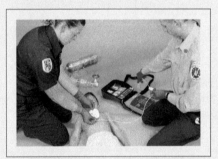

8 After about two minutes of CPR (or when prompted by the AED), analyse rhythm, then follow the "shock indicated" or "no shock indicated" steps as appropriate.

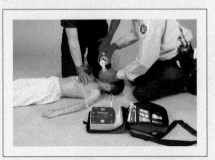

Procedure 17: Rectal Administration of Benzodiazepines

Introduction

Rectal drug administration is a well-known delivery technique in children and is useful for many medications, including antipyretics and anticonvulsants. The only rectal medication approved in most services is diazepam for paediatric status epilepticus. Status epilepticus is a major paediatric medical emergency that may benefit from quick treatment. Although the first priority is airway and breathing, additional therapy may include medication to terminate the seizure. Rectal diazepam is an effective route with few added complications when other routes of administration are not immediately available. It is important to ask if the parents have administered a rectal gel form of diazepam prior to arrival of the ambulance service.

Indication

Status epilepticus

Contraindications

Newborn age (a month or less) (relative)

Recent rectal surgery (e.g., for Hirschsprung disease, imperforate anus) (relative)

Equipment

Lubricant

Rectal tube diazepam

Rationale

Establishing IV or intraosseous (IO) access is often time consuming and may delay delivery of essential advanced life support (ALS) drugs, especially in infants and toddlers. The rectum is an effective alternative route for emergency drug administration. The rectum is highly vascularised, and certain drugs are quickly absorbed through the lining or mucosa. Diazepam is a lipid-soluble benzodiazepine that is reliably absorbed through the rectum and terminates most seizures without further treatment. It takes a few minutes longer to stop the seizure after rectal administration of diazepam as compared to IV diazepam.

Preparation

1. Use a paediatric resuscitation tape or JRCALC recommendations to determine the weight of the child, or establish the patient's weight from information provided by the caregiver.

2. Unwrap the rectal tube and lubricate the end noting the insertion marks on the neck of the tube. Remove any caps or covers.

Possible Complications

Respiratory depression

Failed administration

Rectal tearing

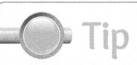

Tip

The most serious potential complication of rectal diazepam is respiratory depression, which is usually from the drug, but may be from the prolonged seizure or the underlying cause of the seizure.

Procedure 17-1

Rectal Administration of Benzodiazepines

1 Position the patient in the decubitus position, knee-chest position, or supine position with a second prehospital professional or the caregiver holding the legs apart.

2 Carefully introduce the rectal tube no more than 2.5 cm into the rectum. The tube neck has an insertion marker. Squeeze the solution into the rectum. Remove the tube remembering to keep the bulb squeezed. Hold buttocks closed for 10 seconds.

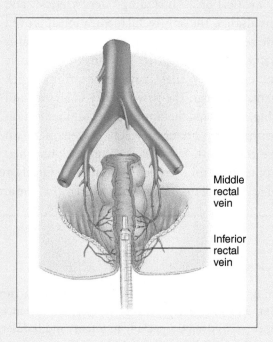

Middle rectal vein

Inferior rectal vein

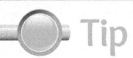

Tip

The rectal dose of diazepam is detailed in the JRCALC guidance. Onset of action for rectal diazepam is slower than IV dose.

Think Point

Administration of diazepam too high into the rectum may decrease its anticonvulsant effect, because the drug may be absorbed differently and broken down more quickly in the liver.

Procedure 18: Spinal Immobilisation

Introduction

Spinal injury may be subtle or difficult to recognise because of altered mental state, distracting injuries, or lack of obvious signs. Failure to recognise potential spinal injury can lead to death or permanent disability. Spinal immobilisation is therefore essential for every child who sustains a suspicious mechanism of injury (where the head, neck, or spine may be involved), who has pain or tenderness of the spine, or who has signs or symptoms of weakness or loss of sensation.

Rationale

The spinal column is made of 33 articulating bones, and its structure changes significantly during childhood growth. The age of the child and the physical state of spinal growth are important factors in the incidence and types of paediatric spinal injuries. Whenever the mechanism of injury, signs, or symptoms suggests possible spinal injury, the entire spine must be stabilised. Maintain the anatomical stability of the entire spinal column as carefully as possible, and use age-specific considerations in approaching the child to minimise spinal movement.

Preparation

1. If the child is unstable or the environment is unsafe, quickly remove the patient onto the stretcher or the long spine board using manual spinal stabilisation techniques.

2. Spinal boards or extrication devices can be used to move the child onto the stretcher.

3. Anatomical differences, specifically the large size of an infant or child's head, require modification of stabilisation procedures. For example, place a thin (2.55 cm) layer of padding beneath the child's body from the shoulder to the hips.

4. Prepare the child and caregiver for the procedure by explaining actions. Make a game of it for an alert, cooperative child.

Possible Complications

Airway obstruction

Impairment of ventilation

Obscuring haemorrhage or other injuries

Spinal injury from improper technique

Back pain

Procedure 18-1

Immobilising a Child

1 Use a towel under the shoulders of a small child to maintain the head in a neutral position.

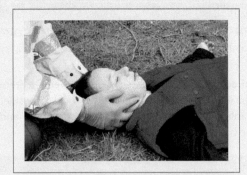

2 Apply an appropriately sized cervical collar.

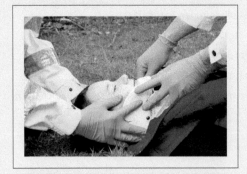

3 Log roll the child onto the immobilisation device.

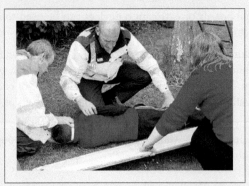

4 Secure the torso first.

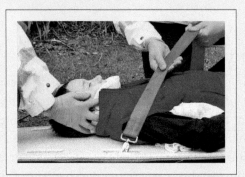

5 Secure the head last.

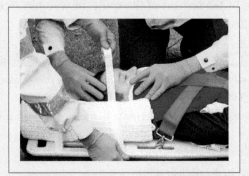

6 Ensure that the child is strapped in properly.

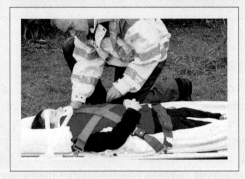

Based on American Academy of Orthopaedic Surgeons and College of Paramedics. Nancy Caroline's Emergency Care in the Streets, revised 7th Ed. Burlington: Jones & Bartlett, 2014.

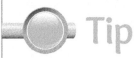 Tip

Reassure nervous children that the spinal stabilisation is only temporary, but it is necessary. Try distraction.

Procedure 18-2

Immobilising an Infant

① Stabilise the head in a neutral position.

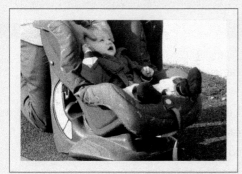

② Place an immobilisation device between the infant and the surface on which he or she is resting.

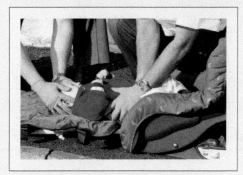

③ Slide the infant onto the board.

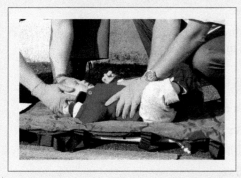

④ Ensure the neutral head position. Secure the torso first; pad any voids.

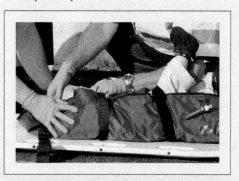

⑤ Secure the head.

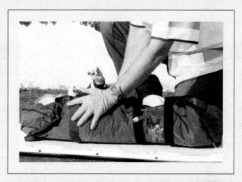

Based on American Academy of Orthopaedic Surgeons and College of Paramedics. Nancy Caroline's Emergency Care in the Streets, revised 7th Ed. Burlington: Jones & Bartlett, 2014.

Procedure 19: Removing and Replacing a Tracheostomy Tube

Introduction

Children with tracheostomy tubes are increasingly common in the out-of-hospital setting. Most of these children live at home and have trained caregivers. Rarely, a tracheostomy tube problem occurs with a technology-assisted child (TAC) and 999 is activated.

Indications

Decannulation

Obstruction

Contraindications

Inadequately sized tract or stoma for insertion of a new tracheostomy tube; in this case, insert an endotracheal tube

Lack of a replacement tracheostomy tube or appropriately sized endotracheal tube

New tract and breathing adequately

Equipment

Suction device

Sterile suction catheters

Oxygen

Bag-valve-mask device, standard paediatric and adult mask sizes

Tracheostomy cannulas, appropriately sized for patient

Endotracheal tubes, standard paediatric and adult sizes

Laryngoscope handle with blades

Tape or tracheostomy ties

Gauze pads

5- or 10-ml syringe

Water-soluble lubricant

Scissors

Sterile saline

Stethoscope

Rationale

Treatment of a tracheostomy tube problem usually requires simple techniques, such as suctioning or removal of the old tube and replacement with a new tube. Partial airway obstruction from clogging of the old tube may not be relieved by suctioning alone, or it may be impossible to ventilate a child through an existing tracheostomy tube because of decannulation or severe obstruction. Under these conditions, the prehospital professional may need to place a new tracheostomy tube to save the child's life.

Preparation

1. Ask the caregiver if there are any special problems with the child's trachea or special requirements involving the child's tracheostomy.

2. Ask the caregiver if a replacement tracheostomy tube is available.

3. Speak directly to the child about what to expect and attempt to enlist her cooperation.

Possible Complications

Creation of a false lumen

Subcutaneous air

Pneumomediastinum

Pneumothorax

Bleeding at insertion site

Bleeding through tube

Mainstem intubation with endotracheal tube (usually right mainstem)

Procedure 19-1

Removing an Old Tracheostomy Tube

1 Position the child with the head and neck hyperextended to expose the tracheostomy site.

2 Apply oxygen over the mouth and nose.

3 If the existing tube has a cuff, deflate it. Connect a 5- to 10-ml syringe to the valve on the pilot balloon. Draw air out until the balloon collapses. Cutting the balloon will not deflate the cuff.

4 Cut or untie the cloth ties that hold the tracheostomy tube in place.

5 Withdraw the tracheostomy tube using a slow, steady, outward and downward motion.

6 Assess airway for patency and adequate ventilation.

7 Provide oxygen and ventilation as needed (through the stoma if necessary).

Procedure 19-2

Replacing the Tracheostomy Tube

Insert a tracheostomy tube of the same size and model whenever possible. If this is not available, use a smaller tube or an endotracheal tube of the same inner diameter as the tracheostomy tube.

1 If the tube uses an insertion obturator, place this in the tube. If the tube has an inner and outer cannula, use the outer cannula and obturator for insertion.

2 Moisten or lubricate the tip of the tube (and obturator) with water, sterile saline, or a water-soluble lubricant.

3 Hold the device by the flange (wings) or hold the actual tube like a pencil.

4 Gently insert the tube with an arching motion (follow the curvature of the tube) posteriorly and then downward. Slight traction on the skin above or below the stoma may help.

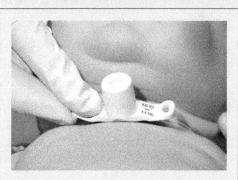

5 Once the tube is in place, remove the obturator, attach the bag-valve-mask device, and attempt to ventilate. If the tube uses an inner cannula, insert to allow mechanical ventilation with a bag-valve-mask device.

(continues)

Procedure 19-2 (continued)

6 Check for proper placement by watching for bilateral chest rise, listening for equal breath sounds, and observing the patient. Signs of improper placement include lack of chest rise, unusual resistance to assisted ventilation, air in the surrounding tissues, and lack of patient improvement.

7 If the tube cannot be inserted, withdraw the tube, administer oxygen, and ventilate as needed.

8 Use a smaller-size tracheostomy tube for the second attempt. If still unsuccessful with a smaller tracheostomy tube, insert an endotracheal tube through the stoma. Check the length of the original tracheostomy tube, note the markings on the endotracheal tube, and advance it to the same depth as the original tube. The inserted portion of the endotracheal tube will be approximately half the distance needed for oral insertion. Do not advance the tube too far, or it may go into a mainstem bronchus (usually the right).

9 If still unsuccessful, use a suction catheter as a guide. Insert a small, sterile suction catheter through the tracheostomy tube. Without applying suction, insert the suction catheter into the stoma. Slide the tracheostomy tube along the suction catheter and into the stoma, until it is in the proper position. Remove the suction catheter. Assess ventilation through the tracheostomy tube.

10 If still unsuccessful, consider orotracheal intubation or transport the patient with ventilation through the stoma using a stoma mask or newborn mask, or through bag-valve-mask device over the nose and mouth while covering the stoma with a sterile gauze.

11 After proper placement, cut the ends of the tracheostomy ties or tape diagonally (allows for easy insertion); pass through eyelets (openings) on the flanges; and tie around the patient's neck, so that only a little finger can pass between the ties and the neck.

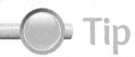

Tip

Talk to the caregiver about the size and type of tracheostomy tube and about known problems with the stoma or tube.

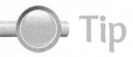

Tip

If unable to reinsert a tracheostomy tube, use a similarly sized or smaller endotracheal tube.

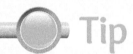

Tip

Keep the suction catheter close at hand.

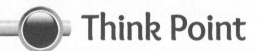

Think Point

Do not force a tracheostomy tube, especially through a new stoma site. Consider inserting a smaller-size tracheostomy or endotracheal tube.

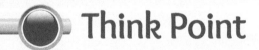

Think Point

Do not advance an endotracheal tube too far through the stoma.

Glossary

abdomen the anatomic portion of the anterior trunk below the ribs and above the pelvis; it contains the stomach, lower part of the oesophagus, small and large intestines, liver, gall bladder, spleen, pancreas, and bladder.

abdominal excursions the work of abdominal muscles in infants during the breathing cycle.

abrasion a portion of skin or of a mucous membrane scraped away as a result of injury.

absorb to take in or suck up.

acceleration deceleration event a type of injury caused when a moving body part, such as the head, stops its forward motion suddenly.

acid a corrosive substance with low pH.

acidosis excessive acidity of body fluids due to an accumulation of acids (as in diabetic acidosis or renal disease) or an excessive loss of bicarbonate (as in renal disease).

acrocyanosis cyanosis of the extremities; acrocyanosis of the hands and feet may be normal in the infant within the first hour after birth.

activation phase first of three phases in disaster response. This is the notification and initial response phase which includes establishment of the Incident Command System organisation and scene assessment.

acute characterised by sharpness or severity, or having a sudden onset, sharp rise, and short course.

adrenaline synonym for epinephrine. A hormone produced by the body that increases pulse rate and blood pressure; mediates the "fight-or-flight" response of the sympathetic nervous system when the body is under stress.

adsorb to take up and hold by adsorption.

afebrile seizures a seizure not accompanied by a fever.

airway adjunct an artificial device to maintain an open airway.

alert, verbal, painful, unresponsive (AVPU) scale the components of the AVPU scale are used to assess the level of consciousness: Alert, Voice, Painful, Unresponsive.

alkali a strong base with a high pH, usually corrosive to tissues.

alveoli the air sacs of the lungs in which the exchange of oxygen and carbon dioxide takes place.

amniotic fluid the liquid contained in the amnion, inside the uterus. This fluid is sterile, transparent, and almost colorless. The liquid surrounds and protects the fetus from injury and helps maintain an even temperature.

analgesia, analgesic a drug that relieves pain.

anaphylactic reaction an extreme, life-threatening systemic allergic reaction that may include shock and respiratory failure.

anaphylaxis a severe form of hypersensitivity reaction that produces dangerous physiologic changes, such as bronchospasm, shock, and airway oedema.

antecubital fossa the triangular area lying anterior to and below the elbow, bounded medially by the pronator teres muscle and laterally by the brachioradialis muscles.

anthrax a deadly bacteria (*Bacillus anthracis*) that lies dormant in a spore (protective shell); the germ is released from the spore when exposed to the optimal temperature and moisture. The route of entry is inhalation, cutaneous, or gastrointestinal (from consuming food that contains spores).

antibiotic any of a variety of natural or synthetic substances that inhibit growth of, or destroy, bacteria that are responsible for infectious diseases.

anticonvulsant agent that prevents or stops convulsions.

antigen protein recognised by the immune system which causes an allergic reaction.

antipyretic an agent that reduces fever.

antivenin a serum that counteracts the effect of venom from an animal or insect.

anxiolytic reduction of anxiety, agitation, or tension.

apnoea a temporary cessation of breathing.

apnoeic characterised by absence of breathing.

asphyxia a condition caused by insufficient oxygen.

assisted ventilation to provide ventilation mechanically.

asthma a disease caused by increased responsiveness of the tracheobronchial tree to various stimuli. The result is paroxysmal constriction of the bronchial airways. Clinically, there is severe dyspnea accompanied by wheezing.

asystole cardiac standstill; absence of contractions of the heart.

ataxia an abnormal gait.

atrioventricular heart block blockage of the electrical impulse from the atrium of the heart to the ventricle.

atrium one of two (right and left) upper chambers of the heart. The right atrium receives blood from the vena cava and delivers it to the right ventricle, which, in turn, pumps blood into the blood vessels of the lungs. The left atrium receives blood from pulmonary veins and delivers it to the left ventricle, which, in turn, pumps blood into the body.

auscultate to listen, as with a stethoscope.

auscultation the process of listening for sounds within the body with a stethoscope.

automatic implantable cardioverter-defibrillator (AICD) an implantable electronic device designed to monitor heart rhythm and determine if it is abnormal and needs to be corrected.

axial loading vertical pressure on the spine.

axillary temperature the temperature taken in the armpit.

axonal shearing a tearing of axons or nerve sheaths, caused by sudden movement, to produce severe brain injury.

baseline a known or initial value with which subsequent observations can be compared.

basilar skull fracture a fracture into the base of the skull, sometimes associated with brain haemorrhage or brain injury.

Battle sign bruising behind the ear; an indication of basilar skull fracture.

benzodiazepines a family of sedative-hypnotic drugs useful for treatment of seizures and agitation.

bilateral pertaining to, affecting, or relating to two sides.

biological agents organisms that cause disease, including viruses, bacteria, and toxins.

biological pathogens a microorganism that can cause disease in a host.

blister agents (vesicants) blister agents; the primary route of entry for vesicants is through the skin.

blood pressure the perfusing pressure of blood.

brachial pertaining to a main artery and vein of the arm.

bradycardia a slow heartbeat.

brain death cessation of brain function.

brain perfusion blood circulation in the brain.

brainstem the stemlike part of the brain that connects the cerebral hemispheres with the spinal cord.

brainstem functions bodily functions controlled by the brain stem that are necessary for life, such as breathing.

brainstem herniation bulging and compression of brain tissue; causes breathing to stop and death of the patient.

bronchiolitis inflammation of the bronchioles by a virus.

bronchoconstriction narrowing of the bronchial tubes.

bronchodilator a drug that helps open the airways to improve air movement and reduce wheezing.

bronchopulmonary dysplasia (BPD) iatrogenic chronic lung disease that develops in premature infants following a period of oxygen therapy.

bronchovesicular pertaining to the tree of pulmonary passages.

buckle fracture a minor fracture only partially through the bone, in which the top layer of bone on one side is compressed, forming a slight angle or "buckle" in the surface.

bulging fontanelle an elevation of the immature opening of bone in the front of the skull; this sign may suggest increased intracranial pressure.

calcium channel blockers a family of drugs that helps reduce the speed of conduction through the heart and the overall work of the heart.

cannulating to introduce a catheter through a vein or passageway.

capillary refill time (CRT) a test that evaluates distal circulatory system function performed by pushing on an area such as a nail bed and watching the speed of its return of pinkness after releasing the pressure.

capnometry the use of a capnometer, a device that measures the amount of expired carbon dioxide.

cardiac arrest the cessation of cardiac mechanical activity, determined by the inability to palpate a central pulse, unresponsiveness, and apnoea.

cardiac dysrhythmia an abnormal cardiac rhythm.

cardiac medication various medications used to treat for heart disease and cardiovascular conditions.

cardiogenic shock a reduced cardiac output secondary to abnormal cardiac function.

cardiomyopathy disease of the myocardium, especially due to primary disease of the heart muscle.

cartilage a specialised type of dense connective tissue, softer than bone, that is common in the skeletons of children.

cartilaginous growth plates the horizontal part of the bone which grows as the human body matures.

caustic corrosive and burning; destructive to living tissue.

central cyanosis slightly bluish, grayish, or dark purple discoloration of the skin (on the trunk and face) due to presence of hypoxia.

central nervous system (CNS) CNS consists of the brain and spinal cord; it controls vital body functions.

central venous catheter catheter inserted into the vena cava to permit intermittent or continuous monitoring of central venous pressure and to facilitate obtaining blood samples for analysis.

cerebral cortex the higher brain; the source of the senses, thinking, feeling, and voluntary movement.

cerebral oedema swelling of the brain.

cerebral spinal fluid (CSF) shunt tube that allows fluid manufactured in the ventricles of the brain from the subarachnoid space to drain in another part of the anatomy outside of the brain, such as the peritoneum. This can lower pressure in the brain.

cervical of, pertaining to, or in the region of the upper spine.

chest wall the musculoskeletal framework of the chest.

chicken pox (varicella) an acute viral disease with mild constitutional symptoms (headache, fever, malaise) followed by an eruption appearing in crops and characterised by macules, papules, and vesicles.

child maltreatment a general term applying to all forms of child abuse and neglect.

child neglect failure by those responsible for caring for a child to provide for the child's nutritional, emotional, and physical needs.

children with special health care needs (CSHCN) those who have or are at increased risk for a chronic, physical, developmental, behavioral, or emotional condition and who also require health and related services of a type or amount beyond that required by children generally.

cholinergic crisis a crisis involving cholinergic drugs, pesticides or "nerve gases" designed for chemical warfare. Cholinergic agents overstimulate normal body functions that are controlled by the parasympathetic nerves.

cholinergic impulses description of a neuron that secretes the neurotransmitter acetylcholine.

circadian rhythm the regular recurrence, in cycles of about 24 hours, of biological processes or activities, such as sensitivity to drugs and stimuli, hormone secretion, sleeping, feeding, etc. This rhythm seems to be set by a biological clock that seems to be set by recurring daylight and darkness.

clavicles the collarbone; a bone, curved like the letter f, that articulates with the sternum and scapula.

coin rubbing cultural ritual intended to treat an illness by rubbing hot coins, often on the back, which produces rounded and oblong red, patch, flat skin lesions.

colostomy the surgical establishment of an opening between the colon and the surface of the body for the purpose of providing drainage of the bowel.

commotio cordis sudden cardiac arrest from a blunt, nonpenetrating blow to the chest. The basis of the cardiac arrest is ventricular fibrillation (a chaotically abnormal heart rhythm) triggered by chest wall impact immediately over the anatomic position of the heart.

compensated shock a clinical state in which there are clinical signs of inadequate tissue perfusion, but the patient's blood pressure is in the normal range.

compensatory mechanisms physiologic responses, initiated to help return the body's vital functions to normal after a severe insult to breathing, perfusion, or metabolic function.

complex febrile seizure a self-limited seizure in a previously healthy child between the ages of 6 months and 6 years that is associated with an elevated fever, which lasts longer than15 minutes, and may have focal motor activity.

complex partial seizure characterised by alteration of consciousness with or without complex focal motor activity.

compression a squeezing together; state of being pressed together.

concussion a brain injury causing any type of altered state of consciousness.

congenital present at birth.

congenital anomalies an anatomic structure that is unusual or different at birth.

congenital diaphragmatic hernia a developmental defect of the diaphragm in which the abdominal organs herniate into the chest.

congenital heart disease heart disease that is present from birth.

congestive heart failure a disorder in which the heart loses part of its ability to effectively pump blood, usually as a result of damage to the heart muscle and usually resulting in a backup of fluid into the lungs.

consent permission to render care.

contact burn a thermal burn from direct contact with a hot object, fluid, or gas.

core perfusion blood circulation in the core of the human body.

cortical pertaining to or of the outer layer of the brain.

crackles rales; lung sounds that suggest fluid in alveoli.

cranium the area of the head above the ears and eyes; the skull. The cranium contains the brain.

crepitus the noise or feel of gas in soft tissues.

cupping the cultural practice of placing warm cups on the skin to pull out illness from the body. This results in red, flat, rounded skin lesions which are often more intensely red at the borders.

Cushing triad the combination of hypertension, bradycardia and irregular respirations that occurs with increased intracranial pressure.

cyanide a colorless gas that has an odor similar to almonds, and which is a chemical asphyxiant used in many industrial processes; exposure can occur from by-products of combustion at structure fires.

cyanosis slightly bluish, grayish, slatelike, or dark purple discoloration of the skin due to presence of hypoxia.

cyanotic heart disease a type of congenital heart disease with a right to left shunt resulting in partially oxygenated blood in the systemic circulation.

decerebrate a posture characterised by rigid extension of the arms and legs; indicates pressure on the brain stem at the level of the pons and may appear in patients with severe brain swelling.

decompensated shock a shock state characterised by low blood pressure, which will rapidly progress to cardiac arrest if not rapidly corrected.

decontamination the process of removing a poison.

decorticate a posture characterised by flexion of the arms and extension of the legs; indicates pressure on the cerebral cortex and subcortical white matter with preservation of brainstem function and may appear in patients with severe brain trauma.

demarcated a defined area in a boundary.

dendrite a projection from a neuron that makes connections with an adjacent cell.

dextrose a form of glucose (or sugar) found naturally in animal and plant tissue and derived synthetically from starch.

diabetes mellitus a metabolic disorder in which the ability to metabolise sugar is impaired, usually because of a lack of insulin.

diabetic ketoacidosis a form of acidosis in diabetes in which certain acids accumulate when insulin is not available.

diagnostic testing tests used to determine the cause of an illness or disorder.

diaphoretic a state of excessive perspiration because of high physiologic stress.

diaphragm the muscle separating the chest from the abdominal cavity, which allows breathing.

diaphysis the shaft of a long bone.

diastolic pressure the pressure that remains in the arteries during the relaxing phase of the heart's cycle (diastole) when the left ventricle is at rest.

diffuse axonal injury an injury to the brain, resulting in diffuse brain swelling

dirty bomb name given to a bomb that is used as a radiological dispersal device (RDD).

distal farthest from the center.

distal extremities structures that are farther from the trunk or nearer to the free end of the extremity.

distention inflation, enlargement.

distributive shock a clinical state characterised by maldistribution of blood volume and vascular tone.

diving reflex submersion of the face and nose in water to produce a vagal reaction; used to terminate an important dysrhythmia of childhood called supraventricular tachycardia.

Do Not Attempt Resuscitation (DNAR) written documentation giving permission to medical personnel not to attempt resuscitation in the event of cardiac arrest.

Down syndrome a congenital disorder in which a person is born with three copies of chromosome 21 (trisomy 21). Clinical features include mental retardation, slanting eyes, a broad short skull, broad hands and short fingers. Other congenital abnormalities include heart defects and oesophageal atresia.

dysphagia inability to swallow or difficulty in swallowing.

dysrhythmias abnormal, disordered rhythm.

effortless tachypnoea tachypnoea, without the signs of increased work of breathing; this represents the child's attempt to blow off extra carbon dioxide to correct the acidosis generated by poor perfusion.

electrocardiogram (ECG) a 12-lead electrocardiographic recording used to evaluate the heart and its rhythm.

emesis vomiting.

emotional abuse the intentional infliction of emotional harm to a child.

emotional neglect the intentional omission of emotional support to a child.

empathy the awareness of and insight into the feelings, emotions, and behavior of another person.

encephalitis inflammation of the brain.

enterovirus species of virus that causes gastrointestinal or respiratory disease in children.

envenomation the act of injecting venom, such as by a snake or insect.

epiglottis a leaf or omega-shaped structure located immediately posterior to the root of the tongue that prevents food and secretions from entering the trachea.

epiglottitis inflammation of the epiglottis.

epilepsy a condition of recurrent seizures.

epinephrine a substance produced by the body (commonly called adrenaline) and that has a vital role in the function of the sympathetic nervous system; also a drug produced by pharmaceutical companies that increases blood pressure and causes bronchodilation; the drug of choice for an anaphylactic reaction.

epiphysis the ends of the bone that are the secondary ossification centers.

evaporation change from liquid to vapor.

exhalation the process of breathing out.

extensor posturing see decerebrate.

extraocular movement of the eyes in various directions.

feeding tube a tube placed into the stomach through the mouth, nose, or skin.

fetus a human or mammal in an early form of intrauterine development.

flaccidity weak, lax, and soft.

flail chest an unstable condition of the chest wall due to two or more fractures of the ribs resulting in ineffective breathing.

flexion the act of bending.

flexural creases the creases behind the knees or inside the elbows.

focal limited to a part of the body.

fontanelle a soft spot of undeveloped bone lying between the cranial bones of the skull of a fetus or infant.

fulminant pneumonia sudden and intense inflammation of the lungs with infection.

gag reflex the protective reflex that keeps food, fluid, or secretions from getting into the trachea.

gastric feeding tube a tube that provides a channel directly into a patient's stomach, allowing removal of gas, blood, and toxins, or insertion medications and nutrition.

gastroenteritis inflammation of the stomach and intestinal tract.

gastrointestinal (GI) decontamination the removal of poison from the stomach.

gastrostomy tube (G-tube) a feeding tube placed directly through the wall of the abdomen.

generalised seizure characterised by movements (often tonic-clonic) that indicate involvement of both cerebral hemispheres.

gestation the length of time from conception to birth.

glial cells specialised cells that surround neurons, providing mechanical and physical support and electrical insulation between neurons.

glottis the sound-producing apparatus of the larynx, consisting of two vocal folds.

glucagon a hormone that has the property of increasing the concentration of sugar in the blood.

greenstick fracture a fracture involving only part of the outer layer or cortex of a bone.

grunting a short, low-pitched sound at the end of exhalation, present in children with moderate to severe hypoxia; it reflects poor gas exchange because of fluid in the lower airways and air sacs.

haematoma a swelling or mass of blood confined to a organ, tissue, or space and caused by a break in a blood vessel.

haemodialysis a form of dialysis in which the blood is removed from the patient through a catheter or fistula, and then returns to the body through another needle, removing various toxins, electrolytes, and fluid in the process.

haemopericardium accumulation of blood around the heart muscle in the pericardial sac.

haemophilia a congenital condition in which the patient lacks one or more of the blood's normal clotting factors.

haemostat instrument clamp; in its closed position it squeezes tissues or vessels and arrests the flow of blood.

hazardous materials (HazMat) any substance that is toxic, poisonous, radioactive, flammable, or explosive and causes injury or death with exposure.

head bobbing the head lifts and tilts back during inspiration, then moves forward during expiration; a sign of increased work of breathing.

hepatomegaly enlargement of the liver.

hives wheals; an itchy rash caused by contact with or ingestion of an allergic substance or food.

homeostasis the maintenance of a relatively stable internal physiologic environment.

hydrocarbon a basic organic compound made up only of hydrogen and carbon.

hydrocephalus the increased accumulation of cerebrospinal fluid within the ventricles of the brain.

hydrochloric acid a powerful and corrosive aqueous solution of hydrogen chloride (HCl).

hymenoptera insects such as bees, ants, and wasps.

hyperoxia increased oxygen in the blood.

hyperthermia unusually elevated body temperature.

hypertrophic cardiomyopathy (HCM) a condition in which the heart muscle is unusually thick, which means that the heart has to pump harder to get blood to leave.

hypnotic pertaining to sleep or sedation.

hypocarbia decreased carbon dioxide in the blood, usually from an excess rate of ventilation.

hypoglycaemia low blood sugar.

hypoperfusion inadequate circulation.

hypotension decrease of systolic and diastolic blood pressure below normal for age, representing decompensated shock.

hypotensive (decompensated) shock a shock state characterised by low blood pressure, which will rapidly progress to cardiac arrest if not rapidly corrected.

hypothermia having a body temperature below normal range.

hypotonia reduced muscular tension.

hypovolaemia diminished blood volume.

hypoxemia a decreased oxygen saturation in blood detected by pulse oximetry or direct measurement of oxygen saturation in an arterial blood gas sample.

hypoxia a pathological condition in which the body as a whole (generalised hypoxia) or region of the body (tissue hypoxia) is deprived of an adequate oxygen supply.

hypoxic stress a subnormal concentration of oxygen.

ileostomy the surgical establishment of an opening between the small bowel and the surface of the body for the purpose of providing drainage of the bowel.

impending brainstem herniation when brain tissue, cerebrospinal fluid, and blood vessels are moved or pressed away from their usual position inside the skull.

implementation phase second of the three phases in disaster response. Activities during this phase include: search and rescue, victim triage, initial stabilisation and transport, and definitive management of scene hazards and victims.

in utero within the uterus.

indwelling central venous catheter small, flexible plastic tube inserted into a large vein above the heart, usually the subclavian vein, through which access to the blood stream can be made. This catheter is left in place and allows drugs and blood products to be given and blood samples withdrawn painlessly.

informed consent permission for treatment given by a competent patient after the potential risks, benefits, and alternatives to treatment have been explained.

inspiratory the process of moving air into the lungs.

insulin a hormone produced by the islet of Langerhans (an exocrine gland in the pancreas) that enables sugar in the blood to enter the cells of the body; used in synthetic form to treat and control diabetes mellitus.

intercostal between the ribs.

intercurrent intervening.

intra-abdominal within the abdomen.

intracranial within the cranium or skull.

intracranial hypertension increased pressure of the cerebrospinal fluid that impairs brain function.

intramuscular medications injections into a muscle; a medication delivery route.

intravascular volume the water portion of the circulatory system surrounding the blood cells.

ischaemia deficiency of blood supply.

jaundice a condition characterised by yellowness of skin, whites of eyes, mucous membranes, and body fluids due to deposition of excess bilirubin in the blood (hyperbilirubinemia).

jugular venous distension a prominence of the jugular veins as they fill with blood; if patient is not supine, indication that the blood may be having difficulty flowing back into the right side of the heart. This can be caused by pericardial tamponade, tension pneumothorax, or right-sided heart failure.

lactic acidosis the metabolic acidotic state resulting from the accumulation of lactic acid secondary to anaerobic cellular metabolism.

laryngoscopy an examination of the interior of the larynx.

larynx the enlarged upper end of the trachea, below the root of the tongue, that contains the vocal cords.

lateral pertaining to the side.

lethargy listlessness; weakness.

leukaemia a cancerous condition in which certain cell lines begin to grow abnormally fast.

localises when a patient is able to respond to the site of a specific noxious or painful stimulus (e.g., when a patient reaches for and pushes away the hand that is pinching them during a neurologic exam).

long QT syndrome a condition characterised by a QT interval exceeding approximately 450 ms.

lordosis forward curve of the lumbar spine.

malaise discomfort, uneasiness, or generalised ill feeling, often indicative of infection.

malposition when something is in an incorrect or abnormal position.

mandible the horseshoe-shaped bone forming the lower jaw.

mass-casualty incident (MCI) an emergency situation involving more than one patient, and which can place such great demand on equipment or personnel that the system is stretched to its limit or beyond.

meconium the bowel contents of a fetus. The presence of meconium in amniotic fluid means the fetus may have suffered some type of stress, such as hypoxia, and may be depressed and need to be resuscitated.

mediastinum the space between the lungs, in the center of the chest, that contains the heart, trachea, mainstem bronchi, part of the oesophagus, and large blood vessels.

meninges a set of three tough membranes, the dura mater, arachnoid, and pia mater, that encloses the entire brain and spinal cord.

meningitis inflammation of the membranes of the spinal cord or brain.

meningococcal sepsis blood-borne infection with the bacteria *Neisseria meningitidis* leading to sepsis (fever or hypothermia, shock, and hypotension).

meningococcemia infection of the blood stream by the bacteria *Neisseria meningitidis*. This is usually a severe infection characterised by fever, shock and a characteristic purpuric rash (bruising of the skin) with or without meningitis.

metabolic acidosis a metabolic state of acidosis resulting from retention of hydrogen or other positively charged ions not related to respiratory compromise.

midaxillary (line) imaginary vertical line drawn through the middle of the axilla (armpit), parallel to the midline.

minute ventilation the volume of air exchanged per minute [minute ventilation =tidal volume × respiratory rate].

miosis abnormal contraction of pupils.

Mongolian spots blue-gray areas of discoloration of the skin caused by abnormal pigment, not by trauma or bruising.

motor activity muscle use.

mottling a condition of abnormal skin circulation, caused by vasoconstriction or inadequate circulation.

multisystem trauma injury involving more than one organ system, such as combined injury to the chest, abdomen, and brain.

myocardial depression when the heart muscle is not working adequately.

myocardial function a measure of how well the heart is working.

myocardial infarction the death of part of the heart muscle caused by partial or complete occlusion of one or more of the coronary arteries.

myocarditis inflammation of the myocardium.

nasal cannula an oxygen-delivery device in which oxygen flows through two small, tubelike prongs that fit into the patient's nostrils.

nasal flaring flaring out of the nostrils, indicating increased work of breathing and hypoxia.

nasopharyngeal airway (NPA) airway adjunct inserted into the nostril of a conscious patient who is not able to maintain a natural airway.

needle decompression the removal of air from a closed space, such as from the pleura.

neonatal seizures seizures that occur in neonates.

nerve agents a class of chemicals including organophosphates; they function by blocking an essential enzyme in the nervous system, which causes the body's organs to become overstimulated.

neurogenic shock shock caused by paralysis of the nerves that control the size of the blood vessels, leading to widespread dilation and pooling of blood in the peripheral vessels to the extent that adequate perfusion cannot be maintained; seen in patients with spinal cord injuries.

neurovascular concerning both the nervous and vascular systems.

nonpulsatile fontanelle when the fontanelle or "soft spot" on an infant's head is full, usually tense and does not seem to beat or pulse with each beat of the heart.

nuclear bomb a bomb which is extremely powerful due to its use of atomic energy as a source of its explosive nature. In addition to the actual explosive force of the bomb, injury is caused in a wider area by the radiation released by the explosion.

obstructive shock shock or inadequate tissue perfusion that is caused by a restriction to blood flow out from the heart (e.g., shock due to a critical coarctation or severe narrowing of the aorta, tension pneumothorax, or cardiac tamponade).

obturator an inner stabilising structure that gives stiffness to a hollow tube, to allow insertion or clearing of an obstruction.

occlusion the closure of a passage.

occlusive dressing a dressing that covers completely.

occult illness an illness that is not immediately obvious or is "hidden." An illness that does not have obvious symptoms.

oedema a local or generalised collection of tissue fluid.

oesophagus a muscular canal that carries food from the pharynx to the stomach.

opiates see narcotics.

oral glucose a simple sugar that is readily absorbed by the bloodstream; it is carried on the EMS unit.

organophosphate insecticide a type of poison with cholinergic properties, used as an insecticide.

oropharyngeal airway (OPA) an airway adjunct inserted into the mouth to keep the tongue from blocking the upper airway and to make suctioning the airway easier.

oropharynx the part of the pharynx lying between the soft palate and upper portion of the epiglottis.

ossification the formation of bone. An ossification center is an area where cartilage is transformed through calcification into a new area of bone.

osteogenesis imperfecta a genetic disorder in which the bones are brittle, and results in fractures.

ostomies a surgical opening made in the skin as a way for waste products to leave the body.

otorrhoea any flow or discharge from the ear.

Paediatric Assessment Triangle (PAT) assessment tool that allows rapid formation of a general impression of the type and level of illness or injury in an infant or child without touching him or her; consists of assessing appearance, work of breathing, and circulation to the skin.

pallor lack of color; paleness.

palpation physical touching for the purpose of obtaining information.

paradoxical irritability a marker for possible serious paediatric illness, consisting of a particular type of irritability where attempts to console further distress the child.

pathology the study and diagnosis of disease.

pathophysiology the study of how disease or injury affects the body.

pedal related to the foot or feet (e.g., pedal pulses are pulses found in the foot).

pelvic fractures breaks through one or more bones of the pelvis (the hip bones and the sacrum and coccyx or lower parts of the spine).

percutaneous endoscopic gastrostomy (PEG) a procedure that places a tube through the abdominal wall and into the stomach.

perfusion blood circulation.

pericardial tamponade compression of the heart due to a buildup of blood or other fluid in the pericardial sac.

periosteum the membrane, made up of a double layer of connective tissue, that covers all bones, except the articular surfaces.

peripheral cyanosis slightly bluish or dark purple discoloration of the skin (on the hands and feet only).

peripheral vasoconstriction when the blood vessels in the outer extremities (hands and feet especially) constrict (get smaller in size through the contraction of the smooth muscle in the blood vessel walls) and therefore lead to a decrease in blood flow to those areas. This may produce peripheral cyanosis (bluish discoloration of the hands and feet) and prolonged capillary refill time.

peritoneal dialysis a type of dialysis in which a special solution is instilled through a catheter into the patient's abdomen, and that draws toxins, electrolytes, and other fluids from the body through the peritoneal membrane.

peritoneum the membrane lining the abdominal cavity (parietal peritoneum) and covering the abdominal organs (visceral peritoneum).

petechiae small, purplish, nonblanching spots on the skin that appear in certain severe fevers and may be indicative of possible sepsis.

petechial related to petechiae, small purplish, nonblanching spots on the skin. Petechiae represent small areas of haemorrhage into the skin and may be seen with infections, especially sepsis.

petechial rash rash which contains petechiae, small areas of haemorrhage into the skin that do not blanch when they are pressed on.

pharynx passageway for air from nasal cavity to larynx and food from mouth to oesophagus.

phencyclidine (PCP, Angel Dust) a hallucinogen, referred to as PCP or angel dust. Moderate doses cause elevated blood pressure, rapid pulse, increased skeletal muscle tone, and, sometimes, myoclonic jerks.

physeal plate pertaining to growth or to the segment of bone that is concerned with growth.

physical abuse see child maltreatment.

physical neglect see child neglect.

physiologic concerning body function.

Pierre Robin syndrome a condition present at birth marked by a small lower jaw (micrognathia). The tongue tends to fall back and downward (glossoptosis), and there is a cleft soft palate.

placenta the tissue attached to the uterine wall that nourishes the fetus through the umbilical cord.

plague an illness caused by infection with the bacteria *Yersinia pestis*. The disease is characterised by fever and chills followed by a severe illness with pneumonia, headache, and delirium. It is transmitted to humans by the bites of fleas from infected rodents and has a high fatality rate. It is an agent that could possibly be used as a weapon of bioterrorism.

pleura the serous membrane that enfolds both lungs and is reflected upon the walls of the thorax and diaphragm.

pleural space the space between the parietal and visceral layers of the pleura.

pneumomediastinum air or gas in the mediastinal tissues.

pneumonia an inflammation of the lungs caused primarily by bacteria, viruses, and chemical irritants.

pneumothorax a collection of air in the pleural cavity, which if under pressure may cause severe physiologic changes with poor venous return and inadequate cardiac output.

polypharmacy an ingestion involving more than one drug.

positive-pressure ventilation assisted ventilation.

postictal state the confused state of a patient after having a seizure.

postpartum after childbirth.

posturing abnormal body positioning after a brain injury; it may be in response to painful stimuli.

pre-term labour labor beginning prior to the 37th week of gestation.

primary brain injury injury resulting from the direct biomechanical effects of the impact forces on the brain which result in direct impact or sudden movement causing shear stress of the brain.

proximal nearest the point of attachment, center of the body, or point of reference; opposite of distal.

pulmonary contusion a bruise of the lung.

pulmonary intoxicants toxins or poisons which may be absorbed through (e.g., by inhalation) or cause harm to the respiratory system.

pulmonary oedema a build-up of fluid in the lungs.

purpura a rash that looks like bruising of the skin that is usually seen in overwhelming infections (sepsis) or when a patient has an inflammation of the blood vessels (vasculitis).

purpuric pertaining to bruising of the skin.

pus the liquid product of inflammation, generally yellow in color.

QRS complex the electrical shape of a major portion of the heart rhythm on the cardiac monitor, representing ventricular electrical activity.

quadriplegia a condition that causes paralysis of all four extremities (both arms and both legs) usually due to an injury in the upper cervical portion of the spinal cord.

radial pertaining to the radius, the larger and more lateral of the two bones in the forearm.

reactivity the capacity for reacting to a stimulus.

reassessment the part of the assessment process in which problems are reevaluated and responses to treatment are assessed.

recovery phase final of three phases in disaster response. Activities include: scene withdrawal, return to normal operations, and debriefing.

recovery position a side-lying position used to maintain a clear airway in unconscious patients who are breathing adequately and do not have suspected injuries to the spine, hips, or pelvis.

renal dialysis a technique for filtering the blood of its toxic wastes, removing excess fluids, and restoring the normal balance of electrolytes.

respiratory arrest the absence of respirations (i.e., apnoea) with detectable cardiac activity.

respiratory depression a condition in which there is a slowing of the respiratory rate and decreased respiratory effort usually due to some effect on the respiratory center in the medulla of the brain. This may be caused by trauma, illness, or the effects of drugs (e.g., morphine or diazepam) or toxins (e.g., ethanol).

respiratory distress a clinical state characterised by increased respiratory rate, effort, and work of breathing.

respiratory failure a clinical state of inadequate oxygenation, ventilation, or both.

respiratory syncytial virus (RSV) a virus that commonly causes bronchiolitis.

retractions physical drawing in of the chest wall between the ribs that occurs with increased work of breathing.

rhinorrhoea thin watery discharge from the nose.

ricin neurotoxin derived from mash that is left from the castor bean. When introduced into the body, ricin causes pulmonary oedema and respiratory and circulatory failure, leading to death.

salivation the act of secreting saliva.

SALT sort, assess, livesaving interventions, and treatment/transport: a triage system.

saphenous veins two superficial veins, the great and small, passing up the leg.

scald a burn to skin or flesh caused by moist heat and hot vapors, as steam.

scaphoid the wrist bone that is found just beyond the most distal portion of the radius.

scoliosis a lateral curvature of the spine.

secondary assessment a step in the patient assessment process in which a systematic physical examination of the patient is performed. The examination may be a systematic full-body evaluation or an assessment that focuses on a certain area or region of the body, often determined through the presenting complaint.

secondary brain injury injury to the brain resulting from factors occurring after the initial biomechanical effects of the primary brain injury (such as hypoxia and hypotension).

secretion the process of producing liquid materials into the blood or body cavities.

sedative an agent that relaxes.

sepsis a pathological state, usually in a febrile patient, resulting from the presence of invading microorganisms or their poisonous products in the bloodstream.

septic shock shock from infection, involving hypotension and signs of inadequate organ perfusion.

serum glucose the level of blood sugar.

sexual abuse rape, sexual assault, or sexual molestation.

shock a clinical syndrome in which the blood flow and oxygen delivery are inadequate for normal organ function.

sickle cell disease a hereditary disease characterised by abnormal clumping together of deformed red blood cells. The patients have painful crises, anemia, infection-risks, strokes, and other serious complications.

simple febrile seizure a brief (less than 15 minutes), self-limited, generalised convulsion in a previously healthy child between the ages of 6 months and 6 years that is associated with an elevated fever. Children with simple febrile seizures have relatively short postictal periods after which they return to their baseline with a nonfocal neurologic examination.

simple partial seizures a focal (localised) seizure which involves a motor or sensory abnormality (e.g., twitching of one hand or a visual disturbance) in a patient who remains conscious. In children, partial seizures are usually motor seizures and frequently will progress to generalised seizures.

sinus arrhythmia a variation in the resting heart rate often seen in children and adolescents. As the child breathes in the heart rate increases slightly and as they exhale the heart rate decreases. This is a normal variation in children and not truly an arrhythmia. On ECG each QRS complex is preceded by a P wave and there are no missed or skipped beats.

sinus tachycardia rapid heart rate in a child with normal conduction.

smallpox a rare, highly contagious viral disease; it is most contagious when blisters begin to form.

sniffing position an upright position in which the patient's head and chin are thrust slightly forward to keep the airway open; the child appears to be sniffing.

soft-tissue injuries injuries to the skin, fat, muscles, ligaments, and tendons.

spasticity increased tone or contractions of muscles causing stiff and awkward movements.

spina bifida a congenital anomaly where the posterior elements of the vertebrae have failed to fuse together. The spinal cord and its associated coverings (meninges) may protrude through this defect in the vertebrae leading to a range of neurologic impairment in the lower extremities depending on the degree and level of the protrusion. When the defect is isolated to the bony structures without spinal cord or meningeal abnormality this is termed spina bifida occulta.

spine the vertebral column.

spleen the major abdominal organ involved in the production and destruction of red blood cells and immune cells. It is filled with blood and can haemorrhage after injury.

splinting fixation with a splint.

(START) Simple Triage and Rapid Treatment a triage system.

status epilepticus a state of continuous seizures or multiple seizures without an intervening return to consciousness.

sterile free from living microorganisms.

stress forces that disrupt equilibrium or produce strain.

stridor a harsh sound during inspiration, high-pitched due to partial upper airway obstruction.

subcostal beneath the ribs.

subdural haemorrhage bleeding beneath the dura mater.

subglottic beneath the glottis.

substernal situated beneath the sternum.

sucking chest wound an open or penetrating chest-wall wound through which air passes during inspiration and expiration.

sudden unexpected death in infancy (SUDI) is the death of a baby less than 1 year of age that occurs suddenly and unexpectedly and whose cause of death is not immediately obvious before investigation.

superior vena cava one of the two largest veins in the body that carries blood from the upper extremities, head, neck, and chest into the heart.

supraclavicular located above the clavicle.

supraglottic the area above the glottis or true vocal cords.

suprasternal above the sternum.

supraventricular tachycardia (SVT) an abnormal heart rhythm with a rapid rate and narrow QRS complex.

symmetry correspondence in shape, size, and relative position of parts on opposite sides of a body.

sympathomimetic agents adrenergic drugs; producing effects resembling those resulting from stimulation of the sympathetic nervous system, such as effects following the injection of epinephrine.

symptomatic ventricular dysrhythmias abnormal ventricular electrical impulses (e.g., ventricular tachycardia) that are associated with symptoms on the part of the patient.

synaptic connections connections between two or more nerves (i.e., synapses).

tachycardia rapid heart rate.

tachypnoea rapid respiration.

tamponade compression of tissues.

tension pneumothorax an accumulation of air or gas in the pleural cavity that progressively increases and causes serious haemodynamic changes.

terrorism a violent act dangerous to human life, in violation of the law, to intimidate or coerce a government, the civilian population, or any segment thereof, in furtherance of political or social objectives.

thermoregulation heat regulation.

thoracic excursions the movements of the chest wall (rib cage and muscles) associated with respirations.

thoracic pertaining to the chest or thorax.

thoracostomy opening of the chest wall to allow drainage of the chest cavity.

tidal volume the amount of air that is exchanged with each breath.

titratable the ability to adjust the desired effect of an agent by giving more or less of that agent as needed over time (e.g., using an intravenous catheter to slowly give more analgesic or sedative agents until a patient is just quiet enough to effectively complete a procedure).

tonic-clonic a seizure that features rhythmic back-and-forth motion of an extremity and body stiffness.

totally implanted devices (mediport) a catheter totally implanted and not visible to the eye (mediport).

trachea a cylindrical cartilaginous tube from the larynx to the bronchial tubes. It extends from the 6th cervical to the 5th thoracic vertebra, where it divides at a point called the carina into two bronchi, one leading to each lung.

tracheitis an inflammation of the trachea.

tracheostomy operation of incising the skin over the trachea and making a surgical wound in the trachea in order to permit an airway during tracheal obstruction.

tracheostomy tube a tube inserted into the trachea in children who cannot breathe or maintain a clear airway on their own.

transdermal through the skin.

transient not lasting; of brief duration.

transmucosal to pass across a mucous membrane (e.g., the absorption of a toxin or pharmaceutical agent across the mucous membranes of the mouth).

Trauma Incident Management (TrIM) a team that provides support and counselling for prehospital professionals who have been exposed to stressful incidents in the course of their work.

traumatic brain injury (TBI) the preferred term for head trauma.

tripoding an abnormal position to keep the airway open; it involves leaning forward onto two arms stretched forward.

tympanic temperature body temperature measurement made by the use of a device which measures the reflectance of infrared light from the tympanic membrane (ear drum).

umbilical cord the attachment connecting the fetus with the placenta.

urostomy a surgical procedure to create an opening (stoma) that connects the urinary system to the surface of the skin and allows urine to drain through the abdominal wall.

vagal pertaining to the vagus nerve.

vagal nerve stimulator (VNS) a small device implanted under the skin near the collarbone as a treatment for epilepsy.

vaginal introitus the vaginal opening.

vagus nerve the cranial nerve (X) that provides motor functions to the soft palate, pharynx, and larynx and carries taste bud fibers from the posterior tongue, sensory fibers from the inferior pharynx, larynx, thoracic, and abdominal organs, and parasympathetic fibers to thoracic and abdominal organs.

vascular tone the amount of constriction in a blood vessel or more generally, the overall amount of constriction in the blood vessels of the body. This is a reflection of the acute cardiovascular health of the patient. Patients in shock often have marked vasoconstriction in an attempt to increase their vascular tone and blood pressure to maximise perfusion to vital organs. When there is a loss of vascular tone (e.g., in sepsis or spinal shock) there is often generalised vasodilatation and severe hypotension.

vasculitis inflammation of the blood vessels which usually is associated with pain, swelling, and often leakage of fluid and blood from the vessels into other organs. When this occurs in the skin a purpuric rash often develops.

vasoconstriction decrease in the calibre of blood vessels.

vasodilatation dilatation of blood vessels.

vasomotor pertaining to the nerves having muscular control of the blood vessel walls.

vasopressor agent a drug that increases vascular tone and increases blood pressure.

ventilation-perfusion mismatch a pathologic state where the oxygen going into the lungs is not mixing appropriately with the blood circulating through the lungs.

ventilator a mechanical device for artificial ventilation of the lungs.

ventricle one of two (right and left) lower chambers of the heart. The left ventricle receives blood from the left atrium (upper chamber) and delivers blood to the aorta. The right ventricle receives blood from the right atrium and pumps it into the pulmonary artery.

vertebral bodies the 33 bones that make up the spinal column.

viral myocarditis a viral infection of the heart which frequently leads to dysrhythmias, especially ventricular dysrhythmias and poor muscle function which produces congestive heart failure.

visual analogue scores (VAS) scales generated by asking a patient or subject to quantify the amount of a sensation they are feeling (usually pain) by pointing to where on a line their sensation is. By measuring how far along the line the patient points one can use this as a measure of that sensation. A frequently used technique for the measurement of pain in research studies.

vocal cords two small folds of tissue in the larynx which vibrate as air moves across them to produce sound.

volume resuscitation replenishing the blood volume.

wheezing production of whistling sounds during expiration such as occurs in asthma and bronchiolitis.

work of breathing an indicator of oxygenation and ventilation. Work of breathing reflects the child's attempt to compensate for hypoxia.

Index